Equine-Assisted Mental Health Interventions

Written by internationally renowned equine-assisted mental health professionals, this edited collection teaches counselors how to design and implement equine-assisted mental health interventions for different populations and various challenges. Supported by ethical considerations and theoretical frameworks, chapters cover common issues including depression, anxiety, grief, ADHD, autism, eating disorders, substance abuse, self-esteem, social skills and communication, couples and family work, and professional development. Each chapter provides practical tips for implementing treatment strategies, case studies with transcript analyses, and sample session notes. This book will appeal to both the expert equine-assisted mental health counselor and the seasoned counselor who is open to partnering with an equine practitioner to help their clients in new and innovative ways.

Kay Sudekum Trotter, PhD, LPC-S, RPT-S, NCC, CEIP-MH, is a licensed professional counselor supervisor, author, speaker, and consultant, as well as the founder of Kaleidoscope Behavioral Health in Flower Mound, Texas, where she has developed and taught animal-assisted therapy workshops. Dr. Trotter's groundbreaking research led to one of the first published studies on the effectiveness of equine-assisted mental health. She is the author of *Harnessing the Power of Equine Assisted Counseling: Adding Animal Assisted Therapy to Your Practice.*

Jennifer N. Baggerly, PhD, LPC-S, RPT-S, is a professor of counseling at University of North Texas at Dallas, a licensed professional counselor supervisor, and a registered play therapist supervisor who also provides counseling at Kaleidoscope Behavioral Health. She is a former chair of the board for the Association for Play Therapy. Dr. Baggerly has taught and provided counseling for children for more than 20 years. She is the coauthor of *Counseling Families: Play-Based Treatment*, *Group Play Therapy: A Dynamic Approach* and *Child-Centered Play Therapy Research: The Evidence Base for Effective Practice.*

Equine-Assisted Mental Health Interventions

Harnessing Solutions to Common Problems

Edited by Kay Sudekum Trotter and Jennifer N. Baggerly

Routledge
Taylor & Francis Group
NEW YORK AND LONDON

First published 2019
by Routledge
711 Third Avenue, New York, NY 10017

and by Routledge
2 Park Square, Milton Park, Abingdon, Oxon, OX14 4RN

Routledge is an imprint of the Taylor & Francis Group, an informa business

Library of Congress Cataloging-in-Publication Data
Names: Trotter, Kay Sudekum, editor. | Baggerly, Jennifer, editor.
Title: Equine-assisted mental health interventions: harnessing solutions to
common problems / edited by Kay Sudekum Trotter and Jennifer N. Baggerly.
Description: New York: Routledge, 2019. | Includes bibliographical references.
Identifiers: LCCN 2018015548 | ISBN 9781138037281 (hardcover : alk. paper) |
ISBN 9781138037298 (pbk. : alk. paper) | ISBN 9781315164144 (e-book)
Subjects: | MESH: Equine-Assisted Therapy | Mental Disorders–therapy
Classification: LCC RC1220.H67 | NLM WM 450.5.A6 | DDC 616.89/16581—dc23
LC record available at https://lccn.loc.gov/2018015548

ISBN: 978-1-138-03728-1 (hbk)
ISBN: 978-1-138-03729-8 (pbk)
ISBN: 978-1-315-16414-4 (ebk)

Typeset in Garamond MT & Futura BT
by codeMantra

To Kay's daughter, Kelly Widener, and Jennifer's daughter, Katelyn Jean Baggerly. They are both strong, free-spirited, and beautiful, like the healing horses described in this book.

To the children, adolescents, adults, and families we serve at Kaleidoscope Behavioral Health in Flower Mound, Texas.

Contents

PREFACE

Equines including horses, donkeys, and mules have aided humans for approximately 6,000 years. In the past, humans used equines for physical labor to move workers and their burdens. Currently, mental health counselors join with equines in emotional labor to move clients and their burdens. This joining with equines, which facilitates the magical movement of clients' burdens and souls, is what this book is about. You have heard "don't look a gift horse in the mouth." In this book, we will look at the gift of the horse to do what the mouth of the counselor cannot—reach an emotional depth in an experiential, equine relationship that exceeds cognitive reason.

Equine-assisted mental health is a relatively new mental health discipline. Kay Trotter explained this to me (Jennifer Baggerly) while at a networking banquet. In 2006, Kay completed her doctoral research dissertation on the efficacy of equine-assisted group counseling with at-risk children and adolescents. Since literature in the field was lacking, Kay made an important contribution in her 2012 edited book entitled *Harnessing the Power of Equine Assisted Counseling: Adding Animal Assisted Therapy to Your Practice.* Yet, just like the early years of life in a child, growth in equine-assisted mental health was rapid—becoming more and more sophisticated over the past six years. Since Kay was so excited by this rapid development, I encouraged her to make another contribution to the field by editing a book with the most prominent equine-assisted mental health professionals in the world. She did not look happy by my suggestion until I offered to lend my experience at editing mental health, primarily play therapy, books.

A perfect partnership was born. Kay is an equine expert. I serve as an editing expert. Kay knows how to join with horses to move clients' burdens and souls. I know virtually nothing about horses except for the few trail rides I have been on, but I am a counselor who is willing to be creative in helping my clients. We wanted to edit a book that appeals to both the expert equine-assisted mental health counselor and the seasoned counselor who is open to partnering with an equine practitioner to help their clients in new and innovative ways.

The process used to accomplish this balance for equine expert and novice was to lasso Kay's network of worldwide experts. Although the equine-assisted mental health community roams wide, we corralled chapter authors from the USA, England, Netherlands, Germany, and New Zealand. The chapter authors cover common problems that counselors treat including depression, anxiety, grief, ADHD, autism, oppositional defiant disorder, eating disorders, substance abuse, self-esteem, social skills and communication, couples and family, and professional development. Originally, we had included the topic of trauma but we had so many chapters that it exceeded our page limit. Therefore, we will have a separate book on *Equine-Assisted Mental Health for Healing Trauma.*

This book on common problems begins with an ethical and theoretical framework. Ethically, each chapter author clearly respects the value and dignity of horses and clients. The ethical guidelines of various professional equine interaction associations are followed to ensure the safety of both horses and clients. Theoretical counseling approaches are explained in each chapter and vary from psychodynamic to behavioral to Gestalt to Rogerian, depending on the author. This theoretical underpinning increases the quality and mental health professionalism in a way that seems to be missing from other books. Practical descriptions of how to implement treatment strategies are also provided in each chapter. Most chapters offer a case example with sample transcripts to provide a clearer understanding of treatment strategies.

Language and terms vary in this book because we wanted to honor each author's contribution. Some chapter authors use the term "equine-assisted therapy" while others use the term "equine-facilitated psychotherapy." However, in order to provide distinction between different types of therapy (e.g., physical therapy, occupational therapy), we recommend the term "equine-assisted mental health treatment" in an attempt to promote the mental health counseling field.

The treatment strategies described are not intended to be implemented by an equine professional without a mental health professional. Rather, these treatment strategies are intended to be implemented by a licensed mental health professional (e.g., licensed professional counselor, licensed psychologist, licensed social worker, or licensed marriage and family therapists) in cooperation with an equine professional. The treatment strategies described in this book are to be part of a comprehensive mental health treatment plan including assessment, diagnosis, goals, objectives, therapeutic relationship, theoretical grounding in a specific counseling theory, theoretical conceptualization of the client, and several treatment strategies to obtain the client's goals.

It is our hope that this book will help you grow as a mental health professional by developing equine-assisted mental health treatment knowledge and skills. As you respect the equine and respect the client while implementing these strategies, you will witness the magical movement of clients' burdens and souls that only equines can give.

Ride On,
Jennifer N. Baggerly

About the Editors

DR. KAY SUDEKUM TROTTER

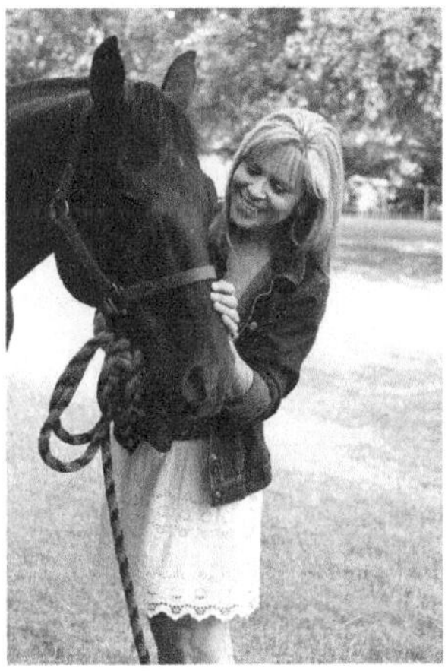

Dr. Kay Trotter is the founder of Kaleidoscope Behavioral Health, a group practice providing services to the whole family: children, teens, and adults. She has taught and spoken professionally on child development, such as treating anxiety in children, play therapy, parenting and equine-assisted mental health. Dr. Trotter has worked with children and their families over the past 20 years. She is a Licensed Professional Counselor Supervisor, Registered Play Therapist Supervisor, National Certified Counselor and Certified Equine Interaction Professional—Mental Health. Dr. Trotter currently serves on the Medical City Lewisville Board of Trustees and is the Past-President of the North Texas Chapter of Play Therapy. Dr. Trotter earned her master degree and PhD from the University of North Texas, with an emphasis on Play Therapy and Animal Assisted Therapy—Equine. Her PhD dissertation became groundbreaking research, and is one of the first published studies on the effectiveness of equine-assisted mental health. Contact Dr. Trotter: Kay@KayTrotter.com

DR. JENNIFER N. BAGGERLY

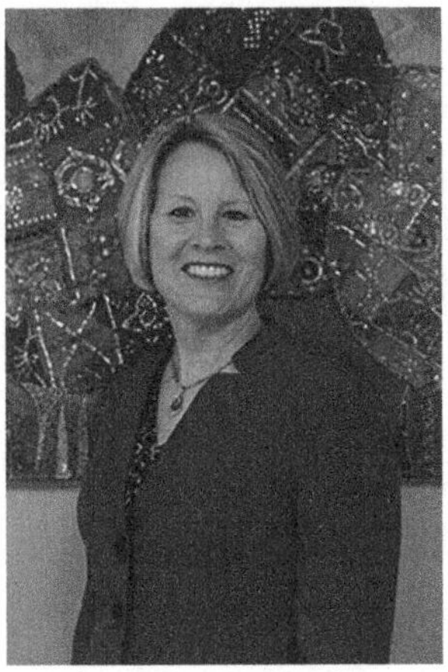

Dr. Jennifer N. Baggerly is a professor of Counseling at the University of North Texas at Dallas. Dr. Baggerly is a Licensed Professional Counselor Supervisor and a Registered Play Therapist Supervisor who also provides counseling at Kaleidoscope Behavioral Health. She served as Chair of the Board of Directors for the Association for Play Therapy from 2013 to 2014 and was a member of the board from 2009 to 2015. Dr. Baggerly has taught and counseled children for more than 20 years. Her published books include *Counseling Families: Play-Based Treatment*, *Group Play Therapy: A Dynamic Approach*, and *Child-Centered Play Therapy Research: The Evidence Base for Effective Practice*. Dr. Baggerly's multiple research projects and over 60 publications have led to her being recognized as a prominent expert in children's counseling. Contact Dr. Baggerly: Jennifer.Baggerly@untdallas.edu.

About the Contributors

Elizabeth Bailey is a registered nurse, board certified in psychiatric-mental health care. She worked at the Resnick Neuropsychiatric Hospital at UCLA for 11 years. She recently completed a Master's program in clinical psychology and is in the process of becoming licensed as an MFT in California. She occasionally works with the Transitioning Families program in the capacity of psychiatric RN, and is currently working on a second book with her sister, Dr. Rebecca Bailey. Contact Elizabeth Bailey: Ebaileyla@yahoo.com.

Dr. Rebecca F. Bailey, PhD, developed Transitioning Families, a family-based program for therapeutic reunification and reintegration. She is a nationally recognized expert in non-familial and familial abduction. Dr. Bailey is a consultant to the National Center for Missing and Exploited Children and is an active member of the Association of Family and Conciliation Courts as well as the International Association of the Chiefs of Police. Contact Dr. Bailey: DrBailey@TransitioningFamilies.com.

Dr. Alita Buzel, PhD, licensed Clinical Psychologist, holds a doctoral degree from the New School of Social Research. Her private practice in New York City includes individual, group, and couples psychotherapy. In addition, Dr. Buzel offers equine psychotherapy workshops at the GALLOPNYC facility in Forest Hills and in Bridgehampton, New York. She is the author of the book *Beyond Words: The Healing Power of Horses* and runs workshops teaching her therapeutic methods. Contact Dr. Buzel: Buzel12@aol.com.

Joanne Byrnes is Co-director at Peakgrove Solutions. Joanne is Registered Clinical Psychotherapist and has a BSc (Psych) and Master of Gestalt Therapy. She has operated as a Gestalt therapist for ten years and has been operating as equine assisted therapist since 2012 at Peakgrove, certified under the OK Corral Series. Byrnes provides and teaches Family and Systemic Constellations, specializing in in equine-assisted constellations. Contact Joanne Byrnes: Joanne.Byrnes@gmail.com.

Dr. Vallarie E. Coleman, PhD, PsyD is a psychologist and psychoanalyst who founded Stand InBalance, Equine Assisted Growth, Learning & Psychotherapy. Located in Westlake Village, CA, Dr. Coleman and her team integrate expertise in psychology, group dynamics, and systems to help people and organizations maximize their potential. An accomplished presenter, Coleman's TEDx talk on Finding your Authentic Self with the Help of Horses reflects her passion about relationships, authenticity, and how equines can help us become better humans. Contact Dr. Coleman: DrVal@ StandInBalance.com.

Corey L. DeMala-Moran, MA, LMHC, is a Licensed Mental Health Counselor and Co-Founder/President of the Amity Foundation for Healing with Horses, Inc., a non-profit organization providing equine-assisted psychotherapy for those suffering from trauma. Corey is a certified EMDR therapist and provides counseling for individuals, couples, and groups at Amity Counseling Center, her private practice in Warwick, NY. Contact Corey DeMala-Moran: CoreyDeMala@gmail.com.

Molly DePrekel, MA, LP, is in private practice at the Midwest Center for Trauma and Hold Your Horses. Molly received her MA in counseling and psychological services from St. Mary's University and BS in Animal Husbandry from Michigan State University. She holds a certificate in EMDR, Yoga Calm, and Sensorimotor

Psychotherapy. She is past President of the Equine Facilitated Mental Health Association, is a contributing author to the book *Harnessing the Power of Equine Assisted Counseling*, and has co-authored six manuals on animal-assisted interventions. Contact Molly DePrekel: Molly@mwtraumacenter.com.

Dr. Saan Ecker, PhD, is Co-director at Peakgrove Solutions. Dr. Ecker is a Certified Professional Counselor and a provisional registered psychologist with qualifications in Buddhist psychotherapy, psychology, and social science. Dr. Ecker has been providing equine-assisted psychotherapy at Peakgrove since 2011 and is certified under the OK Corral Series. She is undertaking research into the evidence base of EAP. Contact Dr. Ecker: SaanE@westnet.com.au.

Dr. Phyllis Erdman, PhD, is a professor in the counseling psychology program and Executive Associate Dean for Academic Affairs, in the College of Education, Washington State University, Pullman, WA. She is a licensed mental health counselor and Clinical Member of the American Association for Marriage and Family Therapy. Contact Dr. Erdman: Perdman@wsu.edu.

Tracie Faa-Thompson, MA, AASW, PGdipNDPT, is a specialist social worker in adoption and a British Association of Play Therapists registered nondirective play therapist. Faa-Thompson teaches social work and conducts workshops on attachment theory, life story work, and Filial Therapy. Her AAPT program, Turn About Pegasus, serves at-risk youth and families and operates year-round in rural north Northumberland in the UK. She is a cofounder of the International Institute for Animal Assisted Play Therapy™. She has written on AAPT and Filial Therapy. Contact Tracie Faa-Thompson: Tracie.j.faa@gmail.com.

Dr. Natasha Filippides, PhD, is an Eagala-certified Equine Assisted Psychotherapist at Stand InBalance, LLC. Through her passion for horses and Depth Psychology, Dr. Filippides has formed a Depth Psychological approach to equine-assisted psychotherapy. Her particular areas of interest include working with individuals to develop a greater capacity for self-awareness, relationship satisfaction, and career success. She specializes in working with depression, anxiety, trauma, addiction, and dual diagnosis. Contact Dr. Filippides: Natasha@StandInBalance.com.

Dr. Karen Frederick, PhD, is an Assistant Professor at Houston Baptist University's College of Education and Behavioral Sciences. She is the program coordinator for HBU's Master of Education in School Counseling program. She is also a Licensed Professional Counselor. Her passion is working with at-risk youth. She has been actively involved in the Equine-Assisted Growth and Learning Association (Eagala) since 2006. Contact Dr. Frederick: Kef@hopeunbridled.org.

Dr. Shelley Green, PhD, LMFT, is Professor of Family Therapy at Nova Southeastern University (NSU); she is also Co-Founder and also serves as Clinical Director of Stable Place. A Clinical Fellow and Approved Supervisor with the American Association for Marriage and Family Therapy (AAMFT), she is in private practice in Ft. Lauderdale. Dr. Green has published widely and presents at state, national, and international conferences on sexuality, clinical training and supervision, and equine-assisted therapies. Contact Dr. Green: Shelley@nova.edu.

Dr. Maya Gupta, PhD, earned her MS and PhD from the University of Georgia focusing on animal cruelty and its connections to interpersonal violence. Dr. Gupta has been director, researcher, and consultant for human–animal interaction and animal welfare organizations; teaches for the Anthrozoology program at Canisius College and the Veterinary Forensic Sciences Program at the University of Florida; and holds governance/advisory roles with the National Link Coalition, the Association of Prosecuting Attorneys, and APA's **Section** on Human–Animal Interaction. Contact Dr. Gupta at MayaCarless@gmail.com.

Sue Jacobson is the director of Palouse Area Therapeutic Horsemanship (PATH) at Washington State University's College of Veterinary Medicine. She is a PATH Intl. certified Therapeutic Riding Instructor and Equine Specialist in Mental Health and Learning. She co-founded the PATH to Success equine-facilitated learning program with Phyllis Erdman. Sue is a lifelong horsewoman and has been involved in equine assisted activities and therapies for 11 years. Contact Sue Jacobson: Sjacobson@vetmed.wsu.edu.

Tim Jobe, BS, has spent the past 50 years learning from the horse how to build a connected relationship that seamlessly transfers to human relationships. For the past 30 years he has partnered horses and people while developing a model of therapy that is healing for both. He and his wife, Bettina Shultz-Jobe, developed the Natural Lifemanship model of TF-EAP in which they continue to train and certify individuals across the globe. Contact Tim Jobe: Tim@NaturalLifemanship.com.

Valerie Bruce Judd, M.A., is the Executive Director and Co-founder of Stable Place, a community-based non-profit agency providing equine-assisted clinical services in the South Florida community. Valerie attended the Juilliard School and Manhattan School of Music, earning both her Bachelors and Master's degrees in music performance. As a PATH-certified Equine Specialist, Valerie has worked in clinical settings with children, couples, groups, and individuals since 2009. Contact Valerie Bruce Judd: Valbj@me.com.

Dr. Veronica Lac, PhD, LPC, is the Executive Director and Founder of the HERD Institute. Dr. Lac specializes in working with eating disorders, trauma, and attachment, and has developed equine- and canine-assisted programs for at-risk adolescents in collaboration with residential treatment centers and eating disorder clinics. She is also a PATH-registered therapeutic riding instructor. Veronica is passionate about training EFPL practitioners and research in the field of equine-facilitated psychotherapy. Contact Dr. Lac: Veronica@herdinstitute.com.

Katarina Felicia Lundgren, BA, lives in the south of Sweden. She is Eagala-certified, Human–Animal Consultant trained through the Learning Animals program in equine cognition and interspecies relationships, and a certified mindfulness instructor. In 2013, she and her team opened up MiMer, a research and education center that funds and supports research on horses and horse–human interactions. Much of her time is spent on researching and educating on horses' abilities and horse–human interactions. Contact Felicia Katarina: Felicia@horseandnature.se.

Dr. Leslie McCullough, PhD, LCSW, is assistant professor teaching social work at Washburn University, PATH Intl. certified Therapeutic Riding Instructor, Equine Specialist in Mental Health and Learning. Over the past 35+ years Dr. McCullough has taken her clinical talents for working with at-risk populations—including those having experienced interpersonal trauma and violent juvenile offenders—into children's psychiatric and residential facilities, group homes, halfway houses, and her outpatient equine-facilitated psychotherapy program. Contact Dr. McCullough: Leslie@legendsequestrian.com.

Dr. Laura McFarland, PhD, holds a doctorate in Multicultural Special Education from the University of Texas at Austin where she taught and facilitated culturally and linguistically responsive pedagogy among pre-service special educators. As Director of Education with Natural Lifemanship, she develops research-based educational content and programs, ensuring that those trained and certified in Natural Lifemanship acquire the competencies needed to effectively employ the model in their professional practices. Contact Dr. McFarland: Laura@NaturalLifemanship.com.

Ritva Mickelsson, MEd, SPHT®, PhD candidate, holds a Master of Education degree in Behavioral Science and Special Education from the University of Helsinki. She is a Registered Instructor of Equine Assisted Social Education (EASE). Mickelsson has completed a Professional Development Workshop on Equine-Assisted Interactions at the University of Denver, Graduate School of Social Work and Institute for Human–Animal Connection. Her research interest is to compare impact of three interventions, one of them being EASE, on special pupils' well-being. Contact Ritva at: Mickelssonritva@gmail.com

Cynthia Penalva, MS, is currently a doctoral student in the Marriage and Family Therapy program at Nova Southeastern University in Ft. Lauderdale, Florida, a registered Marriage and Family Therapy intern in the State of Florida, and a staff therapist at Stable Place, in Davie, Florida. During the past year, she completed her doctoral internship at Stable Place. Penalva obtained her Master's degree in Family Therapy at Nova Southeastern University. Contact Cynthia Penalva: Cp1149@mysnu.nova.edu.

Rob Pliskin, MSSA, LSW, CDCA, International NHS Clinician, Eagala (Duel Certified) Professional. In 1998, Pliskin began his exploration of equines and healing while gentling wild horses and burros in the American West. Pliskin co-founded the EAP program at Big Heart Ranch in Malibu, CA for adolescents in 2005. Since 2010 Pliskin has been an adjunct instructor at Lake Erie College, teaching Equine Assisted Therapy. He holds Advanced Certification as an Eagala Mental Health Professional and Equine Specialist. Contact Rob Pliskin: RobPliskin@icloud.com.

Michael Rolleston, MS, is currently a doctoral student in the Family Therapy program at Nova Southeastern University. He worked as an intake coordinator and therapist at the NSU Brief Therapy Institute's Family Therapy Clinic for four years. He has been intake coordinator and a staff therapist at Stable Place for the past three years. Contact Michael Rolleston: mr1755@mynsu.nova.edu.

Natalie Runge, MA, LPCC, holds a Master of Arts degree in Counseling Psychology from the University of St. Thomas. She is a Licensed Professional Clinical Counselor and provides individual, couples, family, and group counseling to children, adolescents, and adults. She also holds a certificate in Animal-Assisted Therapy, Learning, and Education through the Animals and Human Health program at the University of Denver, Graduate School of Social Work and Institute for Human–Animal Connection. Contact Natalie Runge: Natalie.Runge@icloud.com.

Vanessa M. Sanford, MD, LPC-S, RPT-S, NCC, CDWF, is a bilingual therapist and was awarded the 2007 Texas Mental Health Professional of the Year for Child Advocacy Centers of Texas. She has been included in educational films bringing awareness to child abuse, including *The Little Voice* made by Texas Young Lawyers Association. Sanford is a licensed Professional Counselor/Supervisor, Registered Play Therapist/Supervisor, National Certified Counselor, and Certified Daring Way Facilitator based on the research by Brené Brown. Contact Vanessa Sanford: Vanessa@SanfordSupportSystem.com.

Patti Schlough, LPC, is a Licensed Professional Counselor in Pennsylvania and Maryland providing counseling and therapy in her private practice and in Harford County Public Schools; Schlough has provided counseling and therapy to children, adolescents and families for the past 30 years; she is a member of the Eagala Ethics committee; she is an Eagala mentor. She is currently participating in a year-long certification program with Mindful Schools. Contact Patti Schlough: Patti@peacellc.org.

Monica Schroeder, MS, is currently earning her PhD in Family Therapy at Nova Southeastern University. She works at NSU's College of Arts, Humanities, and Social Sciences as a graduate assistant within the Department of Family Therapy and has been a staff therapist at Stable Place for three years. Monica completed her Master's externship at Stable Place. Contact Monica Schroeder: ms3299@mynsu.nova.edu.

Dr. Hallie Sheade, PhD, LPC, RPT, NCC, holds a Doctorate in Counseling from the University of North Texas. She's a Licensed Professional Counselor, Registered Play Therapist, and National Certified Counselor. She maintains a full-time equine assisted counseling practice, Equine Connection Counseling, that provides individual, couples, family, and group counseling to children, adolescents, and adults. Hallie developed the evidence-informed models Relational Equine-Partnered Counseling and Equine-Partnered Play Therapy. Contact Dr. Sheade: Hallie@EquineConnectionCounseling.com.

Bettina Shultz-Jobe, MA, LPC, holds a Master of Arts degree in Counseling and is a Licensed Professional Counselor. She is trained in a variety of experiential, body-based, equine, and trauma therapies, and has served a variety of clients for more than 15 years. She and her husband, Tim Jobe, developed the Natural Lifemanship model of TF-EAP in which they continue to train and certify individuals across the globe. Contact Bettina Shultz-Jobe: Bettina@NaturalLifemanship.com.

Dr. Carlene Taylor, EdD, LMHC, LPC, CPCS, holds an EdD in Counseling Psychology/Counselor Education & Supervision from Argosy and an MEd in Counseling from Auburn. She has more than 20 years of practice experience working with children, adolescents and adults specializing in AAT/EFP and yoga. She is a Visiting Professor at the Brooks College of Health at UNF in Jacksonville, FL and maintains an office practice in Fernandina Beach and EFP practice at LightHorse Healing, Inc. in Kingsland, GA. Contact Dr. Taylor: DrCarlene@drcarlenetaylor.com.

Sara B. Willerson, LCSW, and the Horses, Heart & Soul™, LLC program provide Equine Facilitated Psychotherapy services for children and adults in North Texas. She is a graduate of Smith College School for Social Work and an Eponaquest Advanced Approved Instructor. Together with her equine partners, Sara invites everyone to experience the transformational healing power of the horse outside of the traditional office environment. Contact Sara Willerson: Swillerson@aol.com.

Dr. Kirby Wycoff, PsyD, NCSP, is an Assistant Professor of School Psychology at Worcester State University in Central Massachusetts and a Nationally Certified School Psychologist. She is a former member of the Governing Board of the American Psychological Associations **Section** on Human–Animal Interactions. Dr. Wycoff teaches and supervises graduate students and her clinical work and research focuses on at-risk children, human–animal interactions and trauma impacted youth and families. Contact Dr. Wycoff: Kwycoff@worester.edu.

Section 1

Ethical Considerations and Theoretical Framework

1

Ethical Considerations in Equine-Assisted Interventions

Meeting the Needs of Both Human and Horse

Kirby Wycoff and Maya Gupta

INTRODUCTION

Across our country, on a daily basis, we are seeing more and more animals serving humans in need. From miniature horses providing trauma-based relief work at natural disasters and school shootings to prison programs working with off-the-track thoroughbreds, and mustang herds teaching executives about leadership, not a day goes by where we do not hear about the use of animals to alleviate human suffering or improve the human experience. Advocates of animals used in service of humans believe that serious attention must be given to the animal's physical ability and training for the work, as well as the handler's ability to advocate for his/her animal-assisted intervention (AAI) partner (Wycoff, 2014). Ethical consideration is needed for both the human who is being served and the animal who is doing the serving. Specifically, there are three key foundational ethical concerns of providing equine-assisted interventions. First, there are the goals of the interaction, then the appropriateness of the client for the specific modality, finally the suitability and preparation that the horse has for the work. As clinicians, it is our objective to honor and respect our human clients and our equine partners to deliver high-quality, ethical services.

The principle of also honoring and respecting the animal and those that care for the animal is often overlooked in animal-assisted interventions. As a human-centric society, we often put the needs of humans above those of animals. While there may be nothing inherently wrong with this perspective, as clinicians we have a responsibility to consider our animal partners if we are going to have them provide professional services. Those that have chosen to read this book are likely doing so because they have an interest in equine-assisted interventions. Note that the term equine-assisted interventions (EAI) will be used here to include a wide range of activities, therapies, and educational experiences. Maybe you are already doing EAI and want to improve your practice or perhaps you are just delving into the field for the first time. You may have a lifetime of experience with horses or perhaps have never set foot inside a barn. You chose your professional path into the helping field, to advance your knowledge by reading this book, and considered this line of work. You, like these authors, made a choice. However, our equine partners have no choice; they are drafted into the role. It is our responsibility, both ethically and morally, to give our animal partners choice in the work they do, for how long they do it, with whom they do it, and if they even do it at all (Wycoff, 2014).

ETHICAL CODES AND EQUINE-ASSISTED INTERVENTIONS

Ethics codes in the helping professions are put into place to protect the rights and needs of the humans that are being served. All major mental health organizations include an ethical code as part of their professional training guidelines and licensing practices. Ethical codes set professional standards and define appropriate and inappropriate behavior. Generally speaking, these codes put forth a set of guidelines that are intended to mitigate risk to the client above all else. The law indicates a minimum standard that will be tolerated and enforced, while ethics represent an ideal set of standards (Corey, Corey, & Callahan, 2014). Ethical codes typically express the professional values of a field as well. Most start by noting that the ethical code is intended to build trust in the public and honor the public trust in the professional services provided therein (American Association for Marriage and Family Therapy, 2017). Through the means of the ethics code, aspirational core values and an obligatory set of rules are put forth to those in the profession.

American Psychological Association

In its *Ethical Principles of Psychologists and Code of Conduct*, the APA noted that the goals of the document are to:

> provide a common set of principles and standards upon which psychologist's build their professional and scientific work... It has as its goal the welfare and protection of the individual and groups with whom psychologists work and the education of members, students and the public regarding ethical standards of the discipline.
>
> (American Psychological Association (APA), 2017, p. 3)

The ethical code is more than just a code of conduct, however; it is also intended to be a way of thinking, being and viewing oneself. As noted above, the APA's code focuses on the "welfare and protection" of clients. However, there are some statutes that are relevant to the provision of equine-assisted interventions and may also consider the welfare and protection of our equine partners (Allen & Colbert, 2016). Kirsten Allen and Lindsey Colbert, from the Graduate School of Professional Psychology at the University of Denver, considered the specific APA code statues specific relevance for those clinicians practicing in animal-assisted interventions. Competence and human relations from the APA code are highlighted below and can be found at: www.apa.org/ethics/code/index.aspx. Standard 2: Competence. Standard 2.01: Boundaries of Competence.

Standard 2. Standard 2 focuses on competence and the boundaries of competence. It is essential that practitioners provide services within their competence based on their "education, training, supervision, consultation, study or professional experience" (APA, 2017, p. 5). Standard 2:01 specifies that "psychologists planning to provide services in an area that is new to them must engage in the appropriate education, training, supervision, and consultation to do so" (APA, 2017, p. 5). For this standard, the code notes that for emerging areas, where recognized standards do not yet exist, "psychologists must take reasonable steps to ensure competence in their work and protect clients" (APA, 2017, p. 5). This is critical for equine-assisted clinicians, as animal-assisted therapies are an emerging sub-specialty in the mental health field. While there has been great movement in the field, there is still a paucity of research with sound methodological basis to support its use (Anestis, Anestis, Zawilinski, Hopkins, & Lilienfeld, 2014). Standard 2.05 also held relevance when considering that a mental health professional may need to partner with and delegate aspects of the equine-assisted intervention to others (Allen & Colbert, 2016). For example, if working on a team of four (the animal, the animal handler/trainer, the client, the therapist), the therapist is delegating some of the aspects of the work to the both the animal and the animal's handler (Allen & Colbert, 2016). The latter model is often used when working with horses (Allen & Colbert, 2016).

Standard 3. Standard 3 focuses on human relations and Standard 3.05 highlights the significance of multiple relationships that can occur when working in a team of three in delivering animal-assisted interventions (APA, 2017). A triad model exists (animal, therapist, and client) wherein the therapist is both the expert on the human and the expert on the animal (Allen & Colbert, 2016). Here, the therapist is serving dual roles, as both the animal handler and the clinician; balancing the needs and considering the safety of both (Allen & Colbert, 2016). This directly leads to Standard 3.06, Conflict of Interest. If the therapist has responsibility for both the human and the animal, this could prove challenging. Further, if the therapist actually owns the animal (as may be the case in equine-assisted interventions and is often the case in working with smaller animals), this may impair the objectivity and competence of the clinician (APA, 2017). For example, in no other sub-specialty of mental health service provision does the therapist share a home (or even a bed) with their co-therapist. Standard 3.05, Exploitative Relationships, may also be relevant in equine-assisted work. In the therapeutic interactions, the psychologist has responsibility for the equine co-therapist, and we must be diligent to ensure that we are not exploiting them. This is directly related to Standard 3.10, Informed Consent (APA, 2017). Forcing an animal into a client interaction without their consent is a form of exploitation.

Other Professional Associations

In 2016, the American Counseling Association's Center for Counseling Practice, Policy and Research disseminated a document entitled *Animal-Assisted Therapy in Counseling Competencies* (Stewart, Chang, Parker, & Grubbs, 2016), which provides clear guidelines for their membership on competencies in animal-assisted therapy (AAT). While a number of animal-central organizations (Eagala, PATH Intl., Opaquest) have ethical guidelines, this is one of the first official documents from a professional mental health organization to publish such guidelines.

As noted elsewhere, it is the belief of these authors, as well as Stewart et al. and many others, if professionals in the helping fields are to provide AAT services (including equine-assisted interventions) ethically and effectively, specialized knowledge and training are necessary for both the human and the animal. Using a ground theory investigation model, Stewart et al. (2016) proposed nine critical competency areas for professional counselors using animal-assisted therapy practices. Stewart et al. break down those nine overarching competencies into three domains: knowledge, skills, and attitudes. A summary of these is provided below, but for a more in depth examination of this framework, please see www.counseling.org/docs/default-source/competencies/animal-assisted-therapy-competencies-june-2016.pdf?sfvrsn=6.

We suggest that Stewart et al.'s framework can be used as a set of guidelines to help you build your competent and ethical practice as it relates to equine-assisted interventions. Stewart and her team outlined the following three areas:

> 1. Knowledge: Formal training In-depth animal knowledge, and knowledge of existing ethical requirements.
> 2. Skills: mastery of basic counseling skills, intentionality, and specialized skill set.
> 3. Attitudes: animal advocacy, professional development and professional values.
>
> (Stewart et al., 2016, p. 4)

This framework offers readers the opportunity to consider their strengths and areas for growth relative to the three domains of competency. Self-awareness and guidance from mentors and supervisors in evaluating one's competencies is a critical aspect of becoming an ethical service provider.

While the original authors note that the guidelines are intended only for counselors who incorporate their animals into their work, we would suggest that these guidelines can be used for equine-assisted clinicians who are working with horses who do not belong to them. However, it is important to note that Stewart (2017) had raised worthwhile questions regarding the welfare of animals living in institutional settings: do they have someone advocating for them to the same extent the owner of a therapy animal would, and who ensures that they receive adequate downtime given that they reside within the therapeutic setting and do not get to go home with their handler at the end of the day?

In addition to general frameworks like the one offered by the American Counseling Association above, there are a number of existing organizations that have also outlined a set of ethical guidelines and principles for their organizations. Two of the most well-known equine-based therapeutic organizations are Eagala and PATH Intl. We strongly encourage readers to access and review both Eagala and PATH Intl.'s guidelines on Ethical Standards for additional considerations (see Eagala, 2015).

International Institute for Animal Assisted Play Therapy™

One additional organization is notable for the holistic and robust approach they take to training mental health professionals and considering the needs of animals in therapeutic work. The International Institute for Animal Assisted Play Therapy™ (Van Fleet & Faa-Thompson, 2017), documented an entire philosophy and set of guiding principles that considered the needs of both humans and animals. All too often in the AAT field, the animal's needs, suitability, and appropriateness are not taken into consideration and when there is a poor fit or an animal is stressed, anxious or otherwise ill-suited to the work, both the human client and animal partner are at risk (Wycoff, 2014). The Animal Assisted Play Therapy™ model shares these concerns and addresses these in the training of future Animal-Assisted Play Therapists (Van Fleet, 2014; Van Fleet, & Faa-Thompson, 2010, 2017). These authors noted that many therapy animals are exposed to emotional distress and physical stress in therapeutic interactions (Van Fleet & Faa-Thompson, 2017). They noted the importance of overall animal welfare in working with animals in a therapeutic setting. One of the first guidelines noted is respect, which is defined as "Equal and reciprocal respect of clients and animals. The needs of humans and nonhuman animals are considered equally" (Van Fleet & Faa-Thompson, 2017). Here, the focus on balance and reciprocity is highlighted. The principles further expanded when considering things such as enjoyment and acceptance. The authors noted that the therapeutic interactions should indeed be enjoyable and pleasant for both the human and the animal, with *both* always having an option to not participate in the interaction. This is a critical aspect to consider because it highlights the importance of voluntary involvement in therapeutic interactions for all involved. How we evaluate things such as enjoyment and acceptance will be expanded below. In discussing acceptance as a guiding principle, the authors noted that the "therapist accepts the clients and the animals for who they are" and focus on meeting both client and animal in the here and now and accepting and appreciating the attributes and skills that the individuals bring to the setting (Van Fleet & Faa-Thompson, 2017).

ETHICAL DECISION-MAKING AND SELF-AWARENESS

With the formal ethics codes in mind, it is important to acknowledge the role of ethical decision-making in the provision of equine-assisted interventions. Ethical decision-making is one way that ethics is integrated into our everyday experience. Corey, Corey, and Callahan (2014) noted a number of key aspects that are central to ethical decision-making. They noted that values (beliefs and attitudes of an individual) provided guidance and direction in everyday life (Corey et al., 2014). These value systems are essential in living an ethical life and being an ethical professional (Corey et al., 2014). Morality, as defined by our perspective, on proper conduct in any given cultural context, is also an important aspect of ethics (Corey et al., 2014). This consideration is particularly interesting in light of the historical context of the human–equine relationship. Beliefs related to animals in any given society are shaped by culture, religion, language, and historical context among any number of other things. As clinicians, we may wonder, "Are horses beasts of burden to be used by humans, or are they sentient beings that can show emotion, preference, and attachment?" For a more robust discussion on the capacity of horses to experience feelings, see the incomparable and highly influential work of neuroscientist, Dr. Jaak Panskeep, who, in his book *Affective Neuroscience: The Foundation of Human and Animal Emotions*, documented animals' abilities to experience a wide range of emotions (Panskeep, 2004). Social psychologist and equine researcher Dr. David Stang aptly summarized equines' ability to feel and perceive. He noted, "Sentience is the capacity to feel, perceive, or experience subjectively. Any species that can suffer, can feel pain, is sentient" (Stang, 2017, p. 340). While this could be construed as anthropomorphism, attributing humanlike characteristics, emotions, perceptions, intentions to non-humans, we suggest here that animals have characteristics, emotions, intentions, and perceptions that are uniquely their own yet are described with the human language system. The rich and complex conversation on anthropomorphism and humans versus non-humans is beyond the scope of this chapter, but it is important to note that

> treating agents as human versus nonhuman has a powerful impact on whether those agents are treated as moral agent's worthy of respect and concern or treated merely as objects, on how people expect those agents to behave in the future, and on people's interpretations of those agents' behavior in the present
>
> (Epley, *Waytz, & Cacioppo*, 2007, p. 864)

Considering your own experience and belief system (likely impacted by culture and religion) will encourage you to draw your own conclusions on the moral debate around humans versus non-humans.

Our personal beliefs about ourselves and the horses we partner with will intersect with our professional practice. Our obligation as ethical professionals is to have self-awareness around these issues. Corey, Anderson, Knapp, and others all noted the importance of self-awareness in the provision of ethical service provision. Being aware of the influence of one's own needs, experiences, personality, values, and beliefs is a critical aspect of the work (Corey et. al, 2014). Examining your own beliefs around issues such as sentience and the emotional experience of animals will serve you well in your ethical practice and professional identity as an equine-assisted clinician. Further, examine how your prior experience with horses, both positive and negative, may influence you as a clinician working in the EAI field. If you are reading this book, it is likely (although not guaranteed) that you feel positively toward horses. Even so, did you receive an injury from a horse in the past that still makes you somewhat tense when walking behind a horse, when working with horses during thunderstorms or other loud noises, or even when a grooming a horse on the off side? If so, how might your tension transmit to clients/horses and affect the therapy process? Conversely, would your own possible positive experiences with horses and general love of them make it more difficult for you to empathize with clients who lack experience with horses and are apprehensive about them (or those who have their own prior negative experiences with them)? Even more specifically, what are the differences between your relationships with the individual horses you and your clients work with, and how do these influence your views and actions toward both the clients and the horses? These questions are equally important for the seasoned horseperson as for the novice.

In their book *Ethics for Psychotherapists and Counselors: A Proactive Approach*, Sharon Anderson and Mitchell Handelsman call us to consider the role of positive ethics in the helping profession. Anderson and Handelsman noted that "when we involve positive ethics, we are obligated to do more than just the minimum. We need to move beyond the ethical floor (staying out of trouble) and shoot for the ethical ceiling (excellent and exemplary professional practice)" (Anderson & Handelsman, 2011, p. 17). Knapp and VandeCreek in their book *Practical Ethics for Psychologists: A Positive Approach*, guided clinicians to clarify what they value and use this to guide how they behave and what they view as appropriate professional conduct (Knapp & VandeCreek, 2006). Clinicians stress a model where clinicians strive for the highest level of ethical ideals (Handelsman, Knapp, & Gottlieb, 2009; Knapp & VandeCreek, 2006; Pomerantz, 2012). For example, it is quite clear that we should work to ensure a child is not on the receiving end of a double barrel kick from a horse during an interaction, but we should strive to do so much more than that.

In 2002, Handelsman, Knapp, and Gottlieb advocated for a shift away from an approach to ethics that simply focused on avoiding discipline but rather supported a "more balanced and integrative approach that includes encouraging psychologists to aspire to their highest ethical potential" (Handelsman & Anderson, 2002, p. 731). As we suggest here for the field of EAI, Handelsman, Knapp, and Gottlieb consider ethics from a broader perspective. They note that "ethical decision making should include a greater awareness of personal and professional values as well as social influences" (Handelsman, Knapp, & Gottlieb, 2009, p. 106).

We should aim for this criterion in selecting, training, and preparing clinicians and horses for equine-assisted interventions. Anderson and Handelsman (2011) noted that positive ethics includes moving beyond the rules of conduct into exploring the moral dimensions of the profession. This may include considering our morality and how it interacts with our role as a professional. This includes exploration of values, virtues, self-care, ethical decision-making, sensitivity, and diversity, among others (Kuther, 2003). This is what we advocate for in the provision of equine-assisted interventions as well. It is the therapist's responsibility not just to be attuned to the client's needs, but also to protect the safety and welfare of the equine partner in all interactions (MacNamara, Moga, & Pachel, 2015).

SELF-AWARENESS

Self-awareness is one central component of ethical practice. There are a number of questions here that can be used to guide your own thinking around the practice of equine-assisted interventions.

Reflect on some of these questions:

- How do I feel about the prospect of partnering with horses in therapeutic interactions?
- How do I feel about my current level of knowledge and training relative to providing services that integrate horses?

- How do I feel about horses having a choice in whether they participate in therapy sessions?
- How do I feel about horses having choices within therapy sessions? If a session is going particularly well but the horse has had enough, am I willing to stop? How do I feel about different horses having different boundaries? For example, Eli adores having his head stroked, Norman tolerates it, with Dennis it depends on the day, and Naboo would rather not be touched on her head at all. We suggest that such differences can, in fact, become the basis for rich and useful conversations with clients.)
- How do I feel about horses working at liberty (no tack, tools or equipment) with clients?
- How do I feel about horses being ridden in the context of therapy?
- How do I feel about using halters, lead ropes, lunge lines, bits, spurs, whips, saddles or other tools in the context of therapeutic interactions with horses?
- How do I feel about whether a horse is stalled for most of the day in isolation, or turned out in social groups and primarily living outdoors?
- How do I feel about equine welfare as it relates to providing therapeutic services with horses?
- How do my own values, beliefs, attitudes, and understanding of the history of the role of horses in the lives of humans impact my ability to provide services?
- What does my culture and religion say about animals in general?

This line of inquiry is a means of value confrontation. It allows clinicians to examine current values and beliefs and confront them with alternative perspectives while seeking solutions to ethical dilemmas (Abeles, 1980). Cultural self-awareness, which includes a systematic examination of one's assumptions, is critical in providing ethically sound EAI services. Dr. Brinda Jegatheheesan, who specializes in the study of early childhood anthropology and psychological anthropology at the University of Washington, noted that culture and religion play a critical role in influencing an individual's attitudes towards animals. This, in turn, has important implications for equine-assisted interventions. In equine-assisted interventions, teaching ethical principles can occur through the context of confronting and exploring current value systems. This also allows clinicians to move away from simply intellectualizing the content to critically evaluating ethical dilemmas and understanding competing values and ideologies (Balogh, 2002).

Most ethical codes for the helping professions focus on the needs of humans. Your role, as someone who is providing equine-assisted interventions, is to shift your perspective to include not only the human client, but your equine colleague as well. Traditionally, the therapist has the primary role of keeping the client's well-being as a central focus of the work. Where then, do the needs of the animal co-therapist come into play? It is essential that the professional providing the services is appropriately and fully trained, competent and licensed in his or her area of practice, but this alone is not enough.

As highlighted in the self-reflection questions above, those reading this book likely have varying opinions on the human relationship to animals in general and also to horses in particular. In the context of therapy, are horses to be viewed and treated as tools, co-therapists, or clients? Each role seems partially applicable yet not entirely accurate. The way in which we contextualize the horse in therapy has direct implications for ethics and welfare considerations. It is possible that while there is utility in considering the applicability of existing ethics codes to work with animals (including horses), ultimately it may be necessary to develop new codes that encompass the unique role of the therapy animal in practice. Moreover, although the focus of this book is on practice, it is important to note that these considerations extend equally, if not more so, to horses used in EAI research. Institutional Animal Care and Use Committees (IACUCs) were developed for the monitoring of laboratory animal welfare, and may not adequately consider the well-being of horses and other animals in AAI/EAI studies. Given that sound empirical evidence about AAI process and outcome is essential to the field, ethical aspects of research should still be front of mind for the practitioner whether s/he is directly involved in research or not.

INFORMED CONSENT FOR OUR EQUINE PARTNERS

While according to the law animals are property and their consent is not legally required, nor do they have legal rights of their own, other aspects of law (e.g., cruelty statutes and laws pertaining to the protection of animals in family violence) have treated animals more like children, deserving of protection. In fact, the early history of organized child welfare in the United States was predicated upon animal welfare laws since no child protection laws existed at the time (Myers, 2008). If animals are to be viewed as more like children than property, they are technically incapable of giving informed consent, yet an adult responsible for their well-being may consent to their involvement in therapy. Is this protection adequate, or should there be some higher standard of consent (taking into account horses' greater autonomy and what we can discern about their attitudes toward different situations)? If we are to focus as heavily as we do on informed consent for humans participating in therapeutic interactions, why would we not take the same considerations into mind when inviting our equine partners to join us?

As noted in the Therapy Animal Bill of Rights (Howie, 2015, and reprinted at the end of this chapter) the author believed that consent and voluntary participation are essential elements to partnering with animals in clinical work. This is also echoed and highlighted in Van Fleet and Faa-Thompson, (2017), who also noted the importance of voluntary participation of animals in therapeutic interactions.

Informed consent has to do with the respect we have for individuals' rights, dignity, and self-determination, including their ability to make choices for themselves. It implies respect for the overall worth and value of all individuals and their capacity for making decisions that they believe are in their best interest. The APA Ethics Code notes that "Obtaining informed consent respects a client's right to self-determination by informing the client about central aspects of the relationship and obtaining from the client, consent to proceed" (APA, 2017). Informed consent for humans participating in therapeutic interactions integrates both an "informed" aspect and a "consent" aspect of entering into a therapeutic relationship. The term "informed" indicates providing thorough information about the potential interaction. It includes providing both the potential benefits and potential risks of the activity, information about the course of treatment including length of treatment, proposed outcomes of treatment and why the clinician believes this is a good choice for the client. It also included allowing the human to choose whether or not to participate in any given activity, experience, therapeutic program or treatment (see APA, 2017, Standard 3.10: Informed Consent). Informed consent means allowing the client to explore the parameters of the potential therapeutic interaction and make educated decisions about whether to proceed. At the heart of it, informed consent is about relationship building and information sharing. The APA ethics codes noted that clinicians must "provide sufficient opportunity for the client/patient to ask questions and receive answers" (APA, 2017). Building on the work of Handelsman and Galvin (1988), Pomerantz and Handelsman (2004) also focused on the importance of allowing clients to ask questions and truly hearing their answers.

Read the APA's statement on Informed Consent again. Take out the word "client/person" and enter the word "animal." If we are to engage in the highest level (remember not the floor, but the ceiling) of ethical practice, then there is no reason why we would not give our animal co-therapists the same opportunity for consent to participate in therapeutic interactions as we do our human clients. We will note again that it is in the space between "a human in need" and "an animal to serve" where the possibility exists that animals can be exploited (Wycoff, 2014; see also APA, 2017, Standard 3:08: Exploitative Relationships). It is our role in equine-assisted interventions to ensure this does not happen.

RELATIONSHIPS IN EQUINE-ASSISTED INTERVENTIONS

One critical aspect of partnering with horses in therapeutic interactions is the significance of building and maintaining positive horse–human relationships (Hausberger, Roche, Henry, & Visser., 2008). Understanding the horse's worldview, respecting him/her for who they are, and truly hearing what they are telling us are foundational to relationship building.

Using a multi-species animal-assisted therapy intervention (horses, cows, goats) with a group of high-risk teenagers, the Relationship Building Triangle© (RBT) was developed. This framework offers one perspective to the therapeutic work that holds equality and reciprocity as the foundation of the clinical work (Wycoff & Teske, 2012). Co-developed by clinicians Wycoff and Teske and teenage clients, the RBT placed three cornerstones as the foundation of any relationship (humans or animal). The three cornerstones—empathy, communication, and trust—became a metaphorical model for a 12-week therapeutic group and ultimately guided all interventions and interactions between clients and animals. The relationship between each corner of the triangle is bi-directional and each element of the RBT is foundational to engaging in healthy relationships. Interesting and dynamic themes emerged including trust, boundaries, and choices, all of which were central in helping clients build relationships with the clinician, the animals, and each other and potentially repair broken relationships in their own lives. This model suggested that change occurs in the context of the relationship. We can access the client through the relationship with the animal. The clinician's relationship with the animal and the client's relationship with the animal lay the foundation for the clinician and client to build a relationship together, and for the clinician to access the client through the relationship with the animal. The RBT provides a useful framework for considering the provision of ethically sound equine-assisted interventions.

In researching the human–horse relationship, Hausberger and colleagues suggested the Hinde theoretical framework as an important tool in understanding these relationships (Hausberger et al., 2008). Hinde's model suggested that a "relationship is an emerging bond from a series of interactions; partners have expectations on the next interaction by the previous ones" (Hausberger et al., 2008, p. 1). Hausberger and colleagues further noted that a relationship is built on a series of interactions. Whether those interactions are negative or positive affects all subsequent interactions (Hausberger et al., 2008). While seemingly obvious in human–human relationships, this may be less so in human–animal relationships. When discussing the role of building positive relationships with horses, Hausberger et al. noted that emotional cues from humans might be carried through voice, posture, expression, and pheromones (Hausberger et al., 2008). Hama, Yogo, and Matsuyama (1996) noted that an "affectional interaction" exists between humans and animals. In this research, heart rates for both horses and humans were measured. A separate group of human participants was used to measure heart rate, these participants had either a positive or negative attitudes towards animals using the Pet Attitude Scale and they stroked the horse for 90 seconds. The team discovered that when the person who has a negative attitude towards the horse is stroking the horse, there is an increase in the horse's heart rate during the interaction (Hama et al., 1996).

As clinicians, we need to regularly assess our equine partners' experience of the therapeutic interaction when seeking positive relationships. The clinician needs to use their skills of observation to assess if and how our animal partners want to do the work. In the same way, we would continually ask and look for answers from our clients about how they are doing in any given situation, we can do the same with our animal partners. In the same way that we would observe the body language of a child who is engaging in or approaching a therapeutic situation, and provide support or relief as needed, we can and should do the same for our equine partners. While the questions are often straightforward, the results are crucial to the success of the animal/client report, and they are: How are you doing? Are you OK with this? Does this feel safe to you? Do you want to proceed? Do you want to stop? Is this too much? Is this not enough? Are you distressed? Are you enjoying this? How can I support you? The listening to and seeing the results (responses) as answers can be much more challenging but we must continue to ask these questions and look for the answers.

One final note on informed consent as it pertains to EAI: we have focused on the issue of informed consent for our equine co-therapists, but consider also that human participants (and those giving consent on behalf of underage participants) may lack an understanding of what EAI entails. To the extent that EAI differs from traditional therapy or education approaches, it is important (over and above "regular" informed consent) to inform participants thoroughly about those unique aspects of what will be involved. This could include, but is not limited to: explaining the nature of the interaction with the horses; information on the horses who will be used in the interactions; outlining whether other people such as horse handlers will be present, and their identities and roles; and explaining the clinician's commitment to ensuring the well-being of all participants including the health and welfare of the horses. As always, adequate documentation of informed consent is necessary not only for ethical reasons but also legal ones. If you are new to EAI, we recommend seeking guidance from an experienced practitioner regarding consent forms and other documentation.

ANIMAL ABUSE: BEFORE AND DURING EAI

A particularly contentious subject in the field of AAI as a whole is whether individuals who have harmed animals should be allowed to participate in interventions involving animals. Some programs screen out for animal cruelty, either as a charged/convicted offense or as a self-reported behavior; some do not; others do not ask the question. On one hand, for ethical and safety reasons, interventions targeted at perpetrators of other forms of violence do not typically recommend contact with the victim (or with potential other victims) as part of the offender's rehabilitation: someone convicted of child abuse is unlikely to be sentenced to work at a children's home without public outrage, and couples therapy is controversial and largely eschewed in the field of domestic violence intervention. On the other hand, just as with individuals who have not harmed animals, the use of animals in therapy has promise as a potent means of teaching boundaries, empathy, prosocial behavior, and attachment skills. If interventions with animals can be delivered in a carefully structured, supervised setting that minimizes risk to the animal while allowing the individual to practice developing more positive relationships and behaviors with animals, perhaps these serve as a valuable step toward individuals eventually interacting with animals in less supervised settings. A major challenge of "no animal contact" orders in sentencing is that they are very difficult to enforce, given the general lack of enforcement resources for animal protection and the ease for most people of obtaining access to animals, including horses. We therefore adopt the assumption that individuals who have abused animals are likely to have opportunities to interact with and/or acquire animals again in future without the supervision or perhaps even the knowledge of the justice/intervention system. The most influential question may be: What is the likelihood that a client who has previously harmed animals will harm a horse during EAI? Unfortunately, the literature on animal abuse prediction, as with prediction of violence risk more generally, is insufficiently precise to allow us to make an accurate determination on this topic in all cases. However, as in all clinical work, we cannot overstate the importance of *individualized assessment* that recognizes that a behavior (in this case, harming an animal) can result from many different motivational, attitudinal, situational, and other factors. The assessment process seeks to clarify the function of the behavior for the client, which allows the clinician to select an appropriate intervention. If a clinician does not feel comfortable or competent making such an assessment, ethical principles suggest that s/he should consider making a referral. However, we contend that:

1. All EAI programs should already be incorporating individualized assessment into intake and treatment planning.
2. The process of asking clients about their less-than-positive interactions with animals, including animal maltreatment, need not be as challenging or nerve-racking as it may seem.
3. This process can and should be situated in the larger framework of exploring the client's relationships with animals as a whole, which is an important part of assessment for any purpose and often yields rich information. The Boat Inventory on Animal-Related Experiences (Boat, 1994) serves as an excellent guide for this purpose.

As in all aspects of this chapter, we emphasize the importance of considering the safety and well-being of the animal rather than solely the potential benefit to the human participant. In an appeal to parsimony, we also challenge the field to grow its evidence base, investigating whether EAIs do in fact provide unique benefits to animal abuse perpetrators that could not be achieved without the presence of the animal in the intervention (Gupta, Lunghofer, & Shapiro, 2017). With these observations, we leave the choice of whether to proactively extend EAI to animal abuse offenders (and/or to screen out individuals who have previously harmed animals) to the individual clinician, with recommendations on these questions to consider: What about animal maltreatment that occurs during the course of a session, even if the client has no known history of harming animals of any kind? First, how is maltreatment defined: according to the law, which varies widely among states and countries, or according to some other standard? Is maltreatment only physical (hitting, kicking) or do other behaviors such as yelling qualify? Either way, how will the ground rules of what constitutes acceptable behavior with horses be laid out in advance so that no confusion occurs? Be aware that clients, as do all people, come with different levels of experience with horses and different attitudes about what constitutes acceptable treatment. Assuming you have specified acceptable conduct and a client has crossed the line, how will you handle the situation in a way that respects the best interests of both the horse and the client—and if those two sets of interests diverge, which one should take priority?

SUITABILITY AND PREPARATION IN EQUINE-ASSISTED INTERVENTIONS

As the field of animal-assisted interventions has advanced, increasing care has been given to understanding and protecting the rights and needs of both human clients and animal co-therapists. Dr. Cynthia Chandler, in her book *Animal-Assisted Therapy in Counseling and School Settings*, highlights the importance of risk management and ethics when working with animals in a therapeutic setting. Chandler highlights in her writing that working with animals in a mental health setting is defined as the incorporation of a specially trained and evaluated animal. The animal becomes a therapeutic agent in the counseling process, and clinicians use the human–animal bond as part of the treatment (Chandler, 2001). With the advancement and popularity of AAI as a possible treatment option for a wide range of clinical presentations, there is a growing need for highly qualified animals to serve in a wide range of capacities. One of the ways that we ensure an animal is qualified for specific work is in the appropriate selection and preparation of a specific animal for a specific job. The human needs, human wishes, human hopes, and desires often cloud the judgement of the human and get in the way of our ability to truly see the animal. If the animal is part of the healing team in any capacity, there is always a possibility that the animal can be exploited (Wycoff, 2014). In considering suitability in EAI, a general framework that follows a needs assessment model can be useful (Maher, 2012; Wycoff, 2014; please see Maher for a robust discussion and protocol on the needs assessment process).

In order to assess the extent to which we can reasonably (fairly and humanely) expect that a specific animal can do a specific job, we need to consider the unique characteristics of the job and the animal. It would be wildly presumptuous to assume that any arbitrarily selected animal could or would be qualified for a job in an animal-assisted intervention (MacNamara & MacLean, 2017; MacNamara et al., 2015). The first "Standards of Practice" for selection were published in 1996 by the Delta Society. Fredrickson et al. suggested four broad criteria to guide the development of selection procedures (Fredrickson et al., 2010). Prior to this, early efforts at selection focused almost exclusively on risk management. We suggest that far beyond risk management alone, considering the actual, underlying suitability of an animal for therapeutic work is critical.

In all professional helping organizations, there are guidelines for training, supervision, licensing and ongoing professional development to maintain the highest level of service. Interestingly, (and of concern) is that there is often less care given in selecting and training our equine therapy partners than there is the human therapist. All too often aged horses, who are thought to be "quiet" and "tolerant," are retired into therapeutic programs, with little thought given to the more nuanced aspects of temperament and behavior that might indicate goodness of fit for a particular line of work. Retiring a horse into an EAI program may even be seen by the horse's owner/caretaker as a proactive ethical decision to avoid sending the horse to auction, slaughter, or other unforeseen futures. However, if inadequate consideration is given to the suitability of the horse for EAI work, such futures may ensue regardless. MacNamara and MacLean (2017) note the importance of selecting appropriate and effective animal participants in animal-assisted interactions, with a focus on considering both the goodness of fit for the human and animal. They note a four-step model that can be used when selecting the right horse for the right job. They focus on ensuring that the animal is selected "based on how well their natural and trained skills, and capabilities, fit what they are expected to do with, and for the students with whom they interact" (McNamara & McLean, 2017, p. 183). Their four-step process includes:

1. The goal of the lesson or activity.
2. Delivery method.
3. Animal qualifications.
4. Considerations for selecting individual animals.

The selection of horses requires a systematic approach, and training alone is not sufficient for assessing suitability and equine temperament (Sian-Lloyd, Martin, Bornett-Gauci, & George, 2008; Wycoff, 2014). Moisa, Barabasi, and Papuc (2012) discussed a detailed approach to the selection of equines for hippotherapy by considering aspects of both temperament and personality, as well as reactivity. Equine temperament was defined by some to include fear reaction, social motivation, reactivity to people, perseverance/distractibility, and locomotive activity (Hausberger et al., 2002). Others characterized six features: dominance, anxiety, excitability, protection, sociability, and curiosity/inquisitiveness (Sian-Lloyd et al., 2008).

A research team from Japan assessed equine temperament via caretaker questionnaire and examined reliability with a simultaneous behavior test. Momosawa and team surveyed caretakers through the Japan Racing Association inquiring on the horses' behaviors and tendencies in everyday interactions. The research team then exposed the horse to a novel situation and observed the horse's behavioral response. In an unfamiliar, indoor arena, each horse (individually) was exposed to two, slowly revolving balloons in the center of the arena over the course of a five-minute period (Momosawa et al., 2003). The results did demonstrate that the horses whose caretakers reported them as more anxious, in fact, did defecate more and have a higher heart rate during the exposure to novel stimuli than the other horses. This suggests that caretakers are likely useful partners in considering the appropriateness of a specific horse for participation in equine-assisted interventions.

Caregiver report alone, however, may not be sufficient. Caretaker assessment may misrepresent a horse's suitability for EAI. Direct assessment and behavioral observation are critical in truly understanding an animal's underlying suitability (not just trained skills) for participating in equine-assisted interventions. In developing a temperament test for donkeys specifically for use in animal-assisted therapy, Dr. Carlos Antonio Gonzalez-De Cara from the Department of Animal Medicine at the University of Cordoba considered the significance of sensory stimuli as well as temperament (Gonzalez-De Cara, Perez-Ecija, Aguilera-Aguilera, Rodero-Serrano, & Mendoza, 2017). The specific aim of the research was to characterize a donkey's sensory reactions (tactile and sound) and temperament (fearfulness and reactivity to human) in order to assess appropriateness for the animal to engage in therapeutic activities. In evaluating 36 Andalusian donkeys, the team concluded that these particular donkeys demonstrated more reactivity to visual than auditory stimulation. The team was meticulous in their evaluation and observation of these donkeys. When considering their reactivity to humans and novel objects and spaces, they considered variables such as: attentive to other stimuli, glances to stimuli, glances to human, sniffing stimuli, sniffing the human, licking/nibbling the stimulus, licking/nibbling the human, time near stimulus, startled response, alert position, vocalizing, defecating, trotting, galloping, ambling, time spent near object, length of time to put one foot on the novel area (Gonzalez-De Cara et al., 2017). For assessment of tactile tolerance, the team used a previously developed scale (Lansade & Bouissou, 2008), and moved a 3cm wide instrument (of varying hardness: wood, plastic, and rubber) along the stifle and haunches of the donkey (Gonzalez-De Cara et al., 2017). The reaction was assessed using a modified scale related to the intensity of the response of the donkey (Lansade, Bouissou, & Erhard, 2008). The range of responses went from no reaction to the donkey directing attention to stimulus with ears and eyes, standing and trembling of a stimulated area to changes in moving the leg moving the entire body laterally and finally engaging in aggressive reactions or movement (Gonzalez-De Cara et al., 2017).

This highlights the importance of assessing not only emotionality or temperament with novel objects but also tolerance to various aspects of handling (Wolff, Hausberger, & LeScolan, 1997). It is important to note that this research tells us information about a group of donkeys, but for EAI, we need to assess a specific equine for a specific job. Specificity in assessment is just as critical as validity. While extrapolation from a donkey to horse behavior may be inappropriate, the approach that the team used can help us frame the importance of very fine-tuned, specific assessments when considering the suitability and traits of a specific animal for a specific job.

Training the EAI Horse

Beyond the selection of a horse suitable for EAI, what (if any) specific training of the horse should take place, and how does this question relate to ethics? The question of how much and what training is appropriate/optimal for horses in EAI programs remains the subject of much debate. Should EAI horses be "bomb-proof" for safety? Does "bomb-proofing" a horse through traditional desensitization methods (e.g., "sacking out") constitute maltreatment? Do we harbor different definitions of these terms, such that we might see tying a horse's legs together and throw him on the ground as abuse, but view rubbing plastic bags across him and tying them to his tail as a normal and healthy procedure? If we do make a differentiation there, in what scientific basis (not opinion) are we grounding our judgments? Knowing that the horses' personalities and responses to stimuli/stressors vary greatly, can we logically adopt a one-size-fits-all approach in determining what is humane training? Is a "bomb-proof" horse even desirable for EAI work, or (in certain applications, at least) is it important for the therapeutic purpose that a horse be able to demonstrate natural fears and other responses to stimuli? Do certain desensitization practices risk numbing a horse in a self-protective way that mimics human trauma? What about programs that deliberately use mustangs or off-the-track thoroughbreds in their work for purposes of helping clients identify with the "wild" instincts of these animals, helping place these often-unwanted horses into useful settings, or both? How do we conceptualize "training" of horses for these applications compared to therapeutic riding or other endeavors? We have asked a great many questions in a row here, and have done so deliberately. Similar to the debate over suitable training methods for horses in any work, we do not purport to identify a single preferred approach. Nevertheless, we encourage clinicians to be aware of these issues and to be proactive in identifying methods and programs that align with their views on training—as well as being open to adapting their views on training to new information as experience and science accumulate.

The International Association of Human–Animal Interaction Organizations released a set of guidelines for welfare of animals involved in human–animal interactions. The taskforce noted that animals that are being considered for participation should be carefully evaluated by animal behaviorists, veterinary behaviorists, or others who are experts on the behavior of a given species (Jegatheesan et al., 2014). They highlighted the importance of the appropriate disposition and training for animals participating in AAI as well as the regular (ongoing) evaluations to ensure the animal continues to demonstrate the appropriate suitability. The guidelines further noted, as we have noted here, that professionals who are working with these animals absolutely must receive training and have knowledge of the animals' suitability and needs (Jegatheesan et al., 2013).

EQUINE WELFARE AND HUSBANDRY

Animal welfare and husbandry are two critical components of providing ethical services in equine-assisted interventions. Overall welfare and health management are essentials aspects of partnering with horses in therapeutic settings. While a full discussion on this topic is beyond the scope of this chapter, we direct readers to the following researchers for additional information: Dr. Temple Grandin, Dr. Claudia Feh, Dr. Sue McDonnell, among others. Useful resources include *The Domestic Horse: The Origins, Development and Management of Its Behaviour and Relationships and Communication in Socially Natural Horse Herds* (Mills & McDonnell, 2005). What is important to mention here is the natural needs of horses for social relationships (herd mates), regular and free choice grazing, ample turn out space and time, minimization of small living quarters for extended periods of time, and adequate and ongoing access to forage and grazing. Whether you are responsible for the care of the horses in your EAI work or you partner with an equine facility, consider whether the husbandry of the horses upon whom you rely is optimized for their own needs, or for those of the human clients. Does the need for horses to be readily accessible for sessions result in increased stall time and reduced turnout compared to what would be possible without the EAI program? Does the scheduling of sessions permit horses to have ample breaks for their mental and physical health? These issues of equine husbandry and welfare are often de-prioritized in light of the needs of the human and we would suggest that these tradeoffs require our serious attention.

Ethical equine-assisted clinicians will both educate themselves and partner with others to deepen their knowledge and understanding of their equine co-therapists. One additional resource for improving equine education is the text *Horse Science, Horse Sense*, by social psychologist Dr. David Stang (2017). This is an exhaustive volume that covers everything, including equine behavior, social relationships, consciousness and sentience, grooming behaviors, eating, drinking, procreating, and everything in between. The text has been meticulously researched and cites more than 1,000 peer-reviewed, scientific resources. This is an absolute must-read for anyone who wants to include equines in their practice.

There are a number of useful learning activities that can be useful for improving your understanding of horses and their needs. One exercise for the ethical equine-assisted clinician is to increase your knowledge around what the horse's physical body can tell you. Researchers at the Animal Health Trust Center for Equine Studies in England, led by Dr. Sue Dyson (Head of Clinical Orthopedics) have been researching horses' facial expressions and pain manifestation. Dyson and her team completed a systematic, blind assessment of facial expressions (mouth, eye, ears, nose, muzzle, head position) and Dyson is developing an equine ethogram (similar to the Henneke Body Condition Scoring System, which is another tool that the equine-assisted clinician should be familiar with) to evaluate pain and distress. She and her team are trying to educate owners around understanding physical pain in the horse and understanding that "bad behavior" isn't necessarily behavioral alone (Dyson, Berger, Ellis, & Mullard, 2017; Mullard, Berger, Ellis, & Dyson, 2017). Dyson and her team note a number of facial markers that distinguish between a lame and sound horse, solely from reviewing images of the head. Lameness is a basic expression of pain and discomfort and while equine-assisted clinicians might not need high-level equine athletes for their work, we can use this information to guide ethical decision-making around understanding the needs of our equine partners. Dyson's study categorized 519 photos of horses as either clinically lame or sound. The team identified and recorded a total of 27,407 facial markers. (For a more detailed accounting of the ethogram please see Table 1 of Dyson et al., 2017). Dyson's systematic review of pictures of horse's heads suggests that facial expressions alone can provide information on soundness and presumably pain levels. This type of research can provide excellent insights into the needs of our equine-assisted intervention partners.

Dyson and her team have a number of excellent videos on their research that can be found here in an edited press release at www.thehorse.com/articles/39285/an-ethogram-for-ridden-horse-facial-expressions-of-pain.

Finally, the best teachers on animals are the animals themselves. Observe horses living in a variety of settings: turned out full-time in social groups, stalled full-time in isolation, grazing on grass, getting fed in stalls, in regular physical work, out of regular physical work, blanketed in the winter, not blanketed in the winter, shod, unshod, and every combination in between. This is not an exercise is identifying "right" or "wrong," but rather increasing your awareness. You will see horses with a wide range of stress levels, physical and mental soundness, and can learn quite a bit by simple observation. To be ethical clinicians in equine-assisted interactions, we need to educate ourselves on the social, emotional, and physical needs of horses. Providing feeding, housing, social and living situations that mimic the natural propensity of the horse as closely as possible will result in the least amount of stress for the animal. If we are to provide the highest level of ethical practice in equine-assisted work, we absolutely must become students of the horse.

SELF-CARE AND BURNOUT MANAGEMENT

No chapter on ethics in the helping profession would be complete without a discussion on burnout and self-care. Throughout the mental health field, the issue of self-care is prevalent. Knapp and VandeCreek (2006) highlighted self-care as including self-regulation, emotional competence and understanding the occupational challenges and hazards of the. Charles R. Figley, of the School of Social Work, Traumatology Institute, at Florida State University, noted that compassion fatigue is multi-factorial and involves the cost of caring, as well as empathy and emotional investment in the clients and the work. He noted:

> The very act of being compassionate and empathic extracts a cost under most circumstances. In our effort to view the world from the perspective of the suffering we suffer. The meaning of compassion is to bear suffering. Compassion fatigue, like any other kind of fatigue, reduces our capacity or our interest in bearing the suffering of others.
>
> (Figley, 2002, p. 1434)

While originally developed around working with clients who have a trauma history, it is likely that compassion fatigue can occur in clinicians across a wide range of client populations. Pines and Aronson note that "burnout is a state of physical, emotional and mental exhaustion caused by long term involvement in emotionally demanding situations" (Pines & Aronson, 1988, p. 9). We would suggest that both human clinicians and our equine co-therapists can experience burnout and compassion fatigue when working with clients. Ethical clinicians and providers will work hard to manage their stress and burnout related to their role as helpers and do the same for the horses that they work.

CLOSING

There is no doubt that equine-assisted interactions have the potential to provide a number of benefits to our human clients. While researchers are continuously working to improve methodology in researching those effects, those of us who do this work see the impact regularly. Even with the incredible benefits that humans experience in the presence of horses, it is our ethical obligation to also consider the needs of the horses. Remember, they were drafted into these roles. Humans put them there; they did not make that choice. Their general willingness to respond to humans and human demands is what makes them both wonderful therapeutic partners and vulnerable to exploitation in work. Consider a terrible—yet, we contend, informative—comparison: the selection of pit bull terriers for dogfighting. Contrary to popular notion, what makes the pit bull breed valuable for fighting is not its thirst for blood, but its loyalty and desire to please its owner. Dogs in the pit often continue fighting not because of their desire to win, but because their handlers are egging them on. Horses, while a different animal, work with us not because of their natural instincts (which are to flee), but because we ask them to. If we are going to ask our horses to partner with us in the EAI endeavor, we owe it to them and our clients to consider not only the humans' needs, but the horses' as well.

In closing, one final note on ethical considerations in equine-assisted therapy. In her seminal work *Teaming with your Therapy Dog*, author Ann Howie, LICSW, ACSW, developed a bill of rights for any animal engaging in animal-assisted interventions. While initially developed for therapy dogs, Howie noted that this framework applies to any animal that is being used in service of humans in a therapeutic interaction. She thoughtfully integrated the animal's perspective here and notes the importance of addressing the animals' needs in the interaction. We encourage you to review these below and consider how many of these are true for your equine co-therapist.

THE THERAPY ANIMAL'S BILL OF RIGHTS©

As a therapy animal, I have the right to a handler who:

- Obtains my consent to participate in the work
- Provides gentle training to help me understand what I'm supposed to do
- Is considerate of my perception of the world
- Helps me adapt to the work environment
- Guides the client, staff, and visitors to interact with me appropriately
- Focuses on me as much as the client, staff, and visitors
- Pays attention to my non-verbal cues
- Takes action to reduce my stress
- Supports me during interactions with the client
- Protects me from overwork by limiting the length of sessions
- Gives me ways to relax after sessions
- Provides a well-rounded life with nutritious food, physical and intellectual exercise, social time, and activities beyond work
- Respects my desire to retire from work when I think it is time.

REFERENCES

Abeles, N. (1980). Teaching ethical principles by means of value confrontations. *Psychotherapy: Theory, Research and Practice, 17*, 384–391.

Allen, K. & Colbert, L. (2016). Ethical and safety considerations for use of animals in a therapeutic setting. *Psychotherapy Bulletin, 51*(1), 35–45. Retrieved from http://societyforpsychotherapy.org/ethical-safety-considerations-use-animals-therapeutic-setting.

American Association for Marriage and Family Therapy. (2017). *Code of Ethics*. Retrieved from www.aamft.org/Legal_Ethics/Code_of_Ethics.aspx.

American Psychological Association (APA). (2017). *Ethical Principles of Psychologists and Code of Conduct*. Retrieved from www.apa.org/ethics/code/index.aspx.

Anderson, S. K., & Handelman, M. M. (2011). *Ethics for Psychotherapists and Counselors: A Proactive Approach*. New York: John Wiley & Sons.

Anestis, M. D., Anestis, J. C., Zawilinski, L. L., Hopkins, T. A., & Lilienfeld, S. O. (2014). Equine-related treatments for mental disorders lack empirical support: A systematic review of empirical investigations. *Journal of Clinical Psychology, 70*(12), 1115–1132.

Balogh, D. W. (2002). Teaching ethics across the psychology curriculum. *APS Observer.* Retrieved from www.psychologicalscience.org/teaching/tips/tips_0902.html.

Boat, B. (1994). *Boat Inventory on Animal-Related Experiences*. Cincinnati, OH: University of Cincinnati, Department of Psychiatry.

Chandler, C. (2001). *Animal-Assisted Therapy in Counseling and School Settings.* ERIC/CASS Digest.

Corey, G., Corey, M. S., Corey, C., & Callanan, P. (2014). *Issues and Ethics in the Helping Professions with 2014 ACA Codes.* New York: Nelson Education.

Dyson, S., Berger, J. M., Ellis, A. D., & Mullard, J. (2017). Can the presence of musculoskeletal pain be determined from the facial expressions of ridden horses (FEReq)? *Journal of Veterinary Behavior: Clinical Applications and Research, 19,* 78–89.

Eagala. (2015). *The Global Standard for Equine Assisted Psychotherapy and Personal Development. Code of Ethics.* 8th edition. Retrieved from http://home.eagala.org/sites/default/files/attachments/EAGALA%20Code%20of%20Ethics1.pdf.

Epley, N., Waytz, A., & Cacioppo, J. T. (2007). On seeing human: a three-factor theory of anthropomorphism. *Psychological Review, 114*(4), 864–886.

Figley, C. R. (2002). Compassion fatigue: Psychotherapists' chronic lack of self-care. *Journal of Clinical Psychology, 58*(11), 1433–1441.

Fredrickson-MacNamara, M., & Butler, K. (2010). Animal selection procedures in animal assisted interaction programs. In A. Fine (Ed.), *Handbook on Animal-Assisted Therapy: Theoretical Foundations and Guidelines for Practice* (3rd edition, pp. 111–134). Academic Press.

Gonzalez-De Cara, C. A., Perez-Ecija, A., Aguilera-Aguilera, R., Rodero-Serrano, E., & Mendoza, F. J. (2017). Temperament test for donkeys to be used in assisted therapy. *Applied Animal Behaviour Science, 186,* 64–71.

Gupta, M., Lunghofer, L., & Shapiro, K. (2017). Interventions with animal abuse offenders. In J. Maher, H. Pierpoint, & P. Beirne (Eds.), *The Palgrave International Handbook of Animal Abuse Studies* (pp. 497–518). London: Palgrave Macmillan.

Hama, H., Yogo, M., & Matsuyama, Y. (1996). Effects of stroking horses on both humans' and horses' heart rate responses. *Japanese Psychological Research, 38*(2), 66–73.

Handelsman, M. M. & Galvin, M. D. (1988). Facilitating informed consent for outpatient psychotherapy: A suggested written format. *Professional Psychology: Research and Practice, 19*(2), 223–225.

Handelsman, M. M., Knapp, S., & Gottlieb, M. C. (2009). Positive ethics: Themes and variations. In S. J. Lopez & C. R. Snyder (Eds.), *The Oxford Handbook of Positive Psychology* (pp. 105–113). New York: Oxford University Press.

Hausberger, M., Roche, H., Henry, S., & Visser, K., (2008). A review of the human–horse relationship. *Applied Animal Behavior Science, 109*(1), 1–24. Retrieved from www.sciencedirect.com/science/article/pii/S0168159107001414.

Howie, A. R. (2015). *Teaming with Your Therapy Dog.* West Lafayette, IN: Purdue University Press.

Jegatheesan, B., Beetz, A., Choi, G., Dudzik, C., Fine, A. H., Garcia, R. M., Johnson, R., Ormerod, E., Winkle, M., & Yamazaki, K., (2014). *The IAHAIO Definitions for Animal Assisted Intervention and Animal Assisted Activity and Guidelines for Wellness of Animals Involved: Final Report.* White paper. International Association of Human-Animal Interaction Organizations. Retrieved from https://petpartners.org/wp-content/uploads/2015/07/8000IAHAIO-WHITE-PAPER-TASK-FORCE-FINAL-REPORT-070714.pdf.

Knapp, S. J. & VandeCreek, L. D. (2006). *Practical Ethics for Psychologists: A Positive Approach.* Washington, DC: American Psychological Association.

Kuther, T. L. (2003). Promoting positive ethics: An interview with Mitchel M. Handelsman. *Teaching of Psychology, 30,* 339–343.

Lansade, L. & Bouissou, M. (2008). Reactivity to humans: A temperament trait of horses which is stable across time and situations. *Applied Animal Behaviour Science, 114,* 492–508.

Lansade, L., Bouissou, M., & Erhard, H. (2008). Fearfulness in horses: a temperament trait stable across time and situations. *Applied Animal Behaviour Science, 115,* 182–200.

MacNamara, M. & MacLean, E. (2017). Selecting animals for education environments. In N. R. Gee, A. H. Fine, & P. McCardle (Eds.), *How Animals Help Students Learn: Research and Practice for Educators and Mental-Health Professionals.* New York: Routledge.

Maher, C. A. (2012). *Planning and Evaluating Human Services Programs: A Resource Guide for Practitioners.* New York: AuthorHouse.

MacNamara, M., Moga, J., & Pachel, C. (2015). What's love got to do with it? Selecting animals for animal-assisted mental health interventions. In A. H. Fine (Ed.), *Handbook on Animal-Assisted Therapy: Foundations and Guidelines for Animal-Assisted Interventions* (4th edition, pp. 91–101). San Diego, CA: Elsevier Academic Press.

Mills, D. S. & McDonnell, S. M. (Eds.). (2005). *The Domestic Horse: The Origins, Development and Management of its Behavior.* Cambridge: Cambridge University Press.

Moisa, C., M., Barabasi, J., & Papuc, I. (2012). Selection methods for horses used in hippotherapy. *Bulletin of the University of Agricultural Science and Veterinary Medicine, 69*(1–2), 131–138.

Mullard, J., Berger, J. M., Ellis, A. D., & Dyson, S. (2017). Development of an ethogram to describe facial expressions in ridden horses (FEReq). *Journal of Veterinary Behavior: Clinical Applications and Research, 18,* 7–12.

Panskeep, J. (2004). *Affective Neuroscience: The Foundation of Human and Animal Emotions.* New York: Oxford University Press.

Pomerantz, A. M. (2012). Informed consent to psychotherapy (empowered collaboration). In S. J. Knapp, M. C. Gottlieb, M. M. Handelsman, & L. D. VandeCreek (Eds.), *APA Handbook of Ethics in Psychology, Vol. 1. Moral Foundations and Common Themes* (pp. 311–332). Washington, DC: American Psychological Association.

Sian-Lloyd, A., Martin, J., Bornett-Gauci, H., & George, R. (2008). Horse personality: Variation between breeds. *Applied Animal Behaviour Science, 112*(3–4), 369–383.

Stang, D. (2017) *Horse Science, Horse Sense.* Middletown, DE: Independently published.

Stewart, L. (2017). *Creating a Competent, Cross Disciplinary Future: Provider Competencies.* Presented at the 2nd annual Conference on Animal Assisted Interventions, Rochester, MI.

Stewart, L. A., Chang, C. Y., Parker, L. K., & Grubbs, N. (2016). *Animal-Assisted Therapy in Counseling Competencies.* Alexandria, VA: American Counseling Association. Retrieved from www.counseling.org/docs/default-source/competencies/animal-assisted-therapy-competencies-june-2016.pdf?sfvrsn=6.

Van Fleet, R. & Faa-Thompson, T. (2017). *Animal Assisted Play Therapy.* Sarasota, FL: Professional Resource Press.

Wycoff, K. (2014) *Ethical Considerations in Animal Assisted Therapy.* St Johnsville, NY: Elemental Animal, Inc.

Wycoff, K. & Teske, D. (2012) *Animal Assisted Therapy in Clinical Residential Settings.* Psychological Staff Training and Annual Retreat, Harrisburg, PA.

2

What Science Says About Equine–Human Interaction in Equine-Assisted Therapy

An Outline to a Theoretical Framework

Katarina Felicia Lundgren

INTRODUCTION

If you are as amazed as I am about the results and effects of equine-assisted therapy (EAT), you will have asked yourself the same questions as I have. What happens between horses and humans in EAT? How come we get these results? What is this interaction about? What is it in the interaction that is so effectual? How does the horse know what to do? What is it that the horse does? What does the equine specialist add to EAT?

In this chapter I will outline a theory, based on research on intersubjectivity, that looks upon horse–human interaction in EAT from a cognitive science point of view. I did not invent the theory of intersubjectivity, it is widely used and maybe most known in research describing what goes on between parents, mostly mothers, and infants as well as between offspring of other primates (and other animals) and their mothers and other caretakers. It is also used to describe interactions between subjects in general, and specifically interactions involving individuals with autism spectrum disorder (ASD) and different kinds of attachment and developmental disorders.

Intersubjectivity also plays a prominent role and is used in intersubjective (and relational) psychoanalysis/psychotherapy, which states that all interactions must be considered contextually; interactions between the client and therapist or the child and parent cannot be seen as separate from each other, but must be considered always as mutually influencing each other. The theory of intersubjectivity describes basic phenomena going on in different kinds of relationships. Basic, but not simple. It describes how we experience emotional engagement with social partners and/or objects and how the outcomes from these socio-emotional engagements impact our socio-emotional (both intra- and interpersonal) cognition (Bard, 2017). What I will do in this chapter is to apply the theory of intersubjectivity to the relationship between horse and client. Also, I build and expand on Sheldon Siporin's proposal to use intersubjectivity as a theoretical framework to explain what is going on in EAT (Siporin, 2012).

Asking the question of what is going on in EAT will not yield one simple answer. It cannot be brought down to one explanation, like the horse's ability to read body language, or the mirror neuron (system) theory (Hickok, 2014). These kinds of answers will give us an undifferentiated and simplistic answer. EAT gives room for complex interaction with meanings on many levels. To answer what is going on warrants complex answers. Even if the theory of intersubjectivity looks deceptively simple, it builds on research and knowledge from many academic fields and from many practitioners' experiences. It will be able to contain the complexities.

We need to start connecting the dots between what we already know about what is going on in EAT and how we can start asking the questions necessary to find more in-depth answers and expand our knowledge and understanding further. For this we need a common theoretical framework, which can form a basis for further research, to serve the fast-growing field of EAT and its clients. To be able to use the presence of a horse to its full potential in EAT, intersubjectivity needs to be explored. To explore what intersubjectivity brings with it means we must assume that the horse is as much a subject as the human, which means deep knowledge of both humans and horses is necessary.

INTERSUBJECTIVITY, PSYCHOTHERAPY, AND HORSE–HUMAN INTERACTION

Non-verbal communication, conscious or not, is important in all therapies, even strictly talk therapies, as is the relationship between client and therapist. This relationship has been compared to the relationship between infant and parent (often the mother). Between an infant and a mother (also in non-human animals) coordinated joint engagement takes place, with gestural behaviors, body orientation, visual attention, and facial and body expressiveness. It is a reciprocal interaction with turn-taking and includes similarity and symmetry in behavior (but also sometimes asymmetry and compensatory actions (Brinck, Vasudevi, & Zahavi, 2017). The infant expresses his emotions by intensity, timing, and shape—which are communicated with rhythmic patterns, vocal tones, and behavioral forcefulness (Siporin, 2012). This is also the language of the horse. The way of communicating between mother and infant and horse and client is similar. This way of communicating is present in all communication between individuals, but the older we get, the more unaware we usually become of it. Apart from when we interact with infants, then we sometimes use it a bit more consciously, as often also with animals, knowing that neither of them use verbal language. It is also used by the therapist in both understanding the client and in conveying calmness to the client. This often-implicit communication between client and therapist become more explicit between a horse and a client. "It urges expansion of client awareness and may evoke early parent–infant interaction patterns. Thus, with the human therapist's careful guidance and interpretations, EAP may promote emotional healing and empathetic growth" (Siporin, 2012).

The expanded intersubjectivity theory for EAT is based on the following assumptions:

1. We humans have more in common with horses than what sets us apart, from an emotional and social point of view. The similarities play the more important role, but the differences are also important. It is vital with species specific knowledge as well as knowledge of horses' and humans' common mammalian background, since we share similar brains and similar neural networks that work in similar ways. We need to be acute aware of these similarities and differences to be able to use them in EAT and to ethically let the horse be part of this work. In EAT we need to be extra aware of our own glasses. Through which lenses are we looking at the horse and his interaction with humans? Otherwise we will see similarities where there are none, and differences where there are none.
2. A horse is a subject and not an object. To be able to facilitate therapy for a client, the horse needs to be seen as a subject. This also has ethical implications concerning on what grounds and how a horse participates in EAT. "Animals are self-aware, unified subjects of a mental life" (Rowland, 2017). What goes on between a horse and a human is intersubjective inter/exchange, a sharing of experiences. The subjectivity and the intersubjectivity are in focus, the interaction that takes place between the subjects.
3. We all strive to attach, to connect. To be able to establish functioning relationships, you need to be able to attach securely to another human being or, in lack of a secure human, to or via, for example, a horse. Every individual is striving to connect to another individual, no matter how damaged the ability to attach is, and no matter how dangerous it is perceived by the individual to do so. The striving for connection can take very destructive ways, but is there nonetheless. Your way of attaching (bond with a social partner) is determined by your early experiences (or lack thereof) with intersubjectivity.
4. Intersubjectivity forms the basis for communication: for how it forms, develops, and takes place; for how a common ground for communication is established and maintained. It describes how we communicate non-verbally, use mental imagery, how language develops and how metaphors form our ways of communicating. Intersubjective sharing with a horse is immediate and external to language.
5. We are all social beings who practice and take part in social learning, imitation, mimicry, emulation, the chameleon affect, joint attention, gaze following, understanding intention, and so forth, to become socially cognitive beings able to interact with each other, within the society, culture, and context we live in. Intersubjectivity starts with

coordinated joint engagement and leads through different socio-emotional experiences, to social learning, and is critical for our development into intentional beings.

6. Intersubjectivity feeds empathy. It is only when we truly see "the other" that we can be truly empathetic. This goes for all kinds of empathy. Between humans and between a human and a horse. When you meet another human, you see him as having a mind, you do not see him merely as a body. This is the core of intersubjectivity—you choose to see the human as having a mind, not asking for proof (Aaltola, 2013). Through intersubjectivity you learn about minds. As humans, we are predisposed to look for mindedness, by our way of anthropomorphizing. Anthropomorphism is a double-edged sword. Humans look for minds as our own everywhere, humanizing our world (which also can be used in EAT). As humans, we can use our anthropomorphism to promote empathy (as practitioners in EAT still holding specie specific differences in our minds), or we can use it to gain superiority, reach objectification, instrumentalization, and dehumanization (Waytz, Epley, & Cacioppo, 2010). Empathy in its turn is linked to moral awareness.
7. Intersubjectivity is also a place/space that comes into existence between two subjects: the creation that is the shared experience that makes two minds at certain moments become a consciousness beyond one mind, to become one shared mind, "a we." In this space the categories between "I" and "the other" (or between human and horse) opens up and changes. This is where trust and mutual attunement can grow. What is important in this space is how you relate to others. Intersubjectivity marks an openness to others (horses as humans). This experience is often non-lingual and non-analytical and enhances our ability to reconfigure our understanding of ourselves and others (Aatola, 2013). This intersubjective space is applicable to all the relationships between participants in EAT, horse–client, therapist–client, therapist–equine specialist.

The theory of intersubjectivity also rests on an assumption of dualism, dialog, dynamics, and pendulations. Practiced, it uses similarities and differences, in many different ways and on many levels, to facilitate for someone to become an "I," see a "you," and take part in a "we," and know the differences. The self emerges, develops and differentiates itself in relation to "the other" (and so do a "we," and the understanding of a "you"). A healthy infant has an early ability to discriminate people as distinct, sentient, and animated entities in the world. Early affective engagement to develop this is crucial to a child. These engagements provide the infant with interpersonal experiences encompassing an interplay between similarity and difference, connectedness and differentiation (Brinck et al., 2017). This is a natural process for everybody involved (parent/caretaker and child). It occurs spontaneous when everything "works," develops as it should in early childhood relationships. It can be used consciously, in EAT, when things have "not worked" to repair gaps in socio-emotional cognition and development.

The theory of intersubjectivity in EAT is simple. This is what happens when you meet "the other," your social partner in EAT. This is what you see in "the other."

1. You see you.
2. You see the ones that you have met during your life, as a generalized idea about people, or as different people who has been significant to you.
3. You see the one you meet.

All three of the meetings/ways of seeing will take place in therapy. And all three of them get easier with a horse present, either to be the primary social partner or to be a (more or less temporary or initial) mediator between the therapist and the client. They also help to fill in all the roles you have given to other social partners in your life, based on your life experiences. The horse will be him; he will be you and he will be persons from all your former relationships; and he will be the sum of your belief systems. He will adjust to what you need, to what and whom you need to see for the moment. In this he will be very flexible. A client will be freer towards a horse than to a therapist. The therapist will also be freer with a horse present. The experiences in therapy will be less intense and less confontational and will reach deeper than the spoken word, into the body, since the spoken word is not the language of the horse.

INTERSUBJECTIVITY IN EAT: THE COGNITIVE FRAMEWORK

EAT is about a (deliberate) sharing of experience (about objects and events). By deliberate I mean that it can, in different ways, be goal directive and intentional. Intersubjectivity can either be dyadic, two subjects interact and share an experience with each other, the experience concerns the participants themselves and has an inbuilt reflexivity (mutual sharing), or one subject interacts with an object, but is socially aware of another subject (individual sharing). Or it can be triadic—you interact and share an experience with someone about something or someone (a third element). Intersubjectivity as a sharing of experience points to the interactive aspects of a relationship (Brinck, 2008).

Intersubjectivity, with pre-verbal reciprocity, is the interaction that takes place for all newborns, humans as horses, between themselves and a caretaker (several caretakers), and plays a vital role in everyone's development into social beings. This interaction is then extended into other relationships. This is true for every mammal. And every mammal is, to survive, dependent on developing these socio-emotional skills.

The intersubjective meeting is based on both the similarities between the one you meet and the differences. To recognize what is similar, you need to be able to establish what is different. The meeting with the other is based on mutual engagement and is dynamic, it presupposes a sameness and an identification but also is inherently double, because self-awareness also presupposes the awareness of another subject, who will then reflect the similarity by points of difference. With a horse this is made so much easier for a client. Both due to the similarities between a horse and human (social, emotional, cognitive, communicative beings), but also by the obvious differences. Learning intersubjectivity, a sharing of experiences, as infants (and foals) is done per-verbally, and is contextual (is, for example, culture dependent). It begins with coordinated joint engagement and is done by exchanges of gaze, bodily proximity, gaze following, joint attention, shared intentionality, imitation, social learning, etc., and is genuinely reciprocal, even if neither or one of the subjects are aware of the sharing per se (knowing together). What was missed in this development as an infant can be taught and trained by interacting with a horse who knows this (even if he doesn't know he knows).

The sharing can be mutual, but also individual, meaning that an individual gains access to another subject's experiences via observation(s). This is a one-way, distanced, and instrumental sharing, like gaze alternation, seeking out social referencing by looking at another's expression of emotions. Many states of mind are made overt by behavior. By observing posture, movement, gesture, facial expression, gaze, head and body turn, non-verbal vocalizations, etc., another's attention, emotion, attitude, interest, and perceptual knowledge can be understood. Attention reading, the recognition of goal-directed intentions in others, from observations of their behavior is a generic form of individual sharing (Brinck, 2008).

Besides being the client's socio-emotional partner in EAT, the horse offers explicit emotional behaviors for the client to see and learn to read other's attention and intentions from. As a client, you will learn that context is essential, which will help you to develop plasticity and enhance your flexibility. Several distinct behaviors in horses share the same function and can realize the same act. As one distinct behavior can be interpreted in many different ways, it can mean many different things. A behavior does not always reveal its cause (Hickok, 2014). Spending time with horses will help you learn to read others, but not to over-interpret what you see. In EAT one activity can be observing horses, whether as an introductory activity, because of human fears, for safety reasons, or other reasons. This is individual sharing, both with the horse(s), other group participants, and the therapist.

These behaviors in a horse are also what the equine specialist is looking for and uses when sharing horse observations with the client. By these observations the client learns to share, to observe, to draw conclusions from the horse's behavior about the other's attention and intentions and see patterns in his own beliefs systems.

At play between the client and the horse is also contagious attention. This can sometimes explain how the horse knows what the client needs (from the therapist's point of view) and why he attends to exactly the things the client is working on.

There is also a qualitative difference in what is intersubjectivity shared, which can be translated into measurable overt behaviors, which are looked for by the equine specialist and the therapist. These can be divided into three groups:

1. **Interaffectivity:** Simultaneous matching of affects and emotions to the affect and emotions displayed by another agent. It emerges from emotional contagion and an individual participating in interaffectivity develops skills for monitoring the emotions of self and others. Interaffectivity is dyadic.
2. **Interattentionality:** Alignment of attention to the attention displayed by another agent. This behavior can both be a result of contagion or be purposive. Attentional states spring from arousal. They reflect the agent's readiness to act, directed to a target of action. Interattentionality is often dyadic and concerns individual sharing.

3. **Interintentionality:** The sharing of information with another agent, about the intentions and beliefs of the self and other. It is first bodily based, later in development it becomes symbolic and verbal. Interintentionality is essentially triadic and allows for an allocentric (versus egocentric) or de-centered perspective (Brinck, 2008).

THE VALUE OF THE HORSE AND THE EQUINE SPECIALIST

What happens in EAT happens in other therapeutic settings as well. It is not new. The added value is the horse and the competence about horses that the equine specialist brings in. This will enhance therapy, not make it radically different. Therapy is still therapy. It is the same work that is being done, by the therapist and, of course, by the client. The horse is not a therapist; he is assisting in the therapeutic work. The horse is putting a magnifying glass onto the therapeutic process. He is making it more accessible and less confrontative. But he does more. The horse helps clients who are not able to receive help and benefit from more traditional forms of therapy. He invites the client to use both non-verbal and verbal language. The horse can be a companion in therapy, for comfort, closeness, and attachment. He brings in a natural way in bodily aspects (rhythm, touch, and other sensory experiences), which help with grounding, self-awareness, staying in the present, keeping a distant perspective, etc. The horse adds a lot to therapy, and I don't think we have even begun to understand to what extent. This is a topic of its own. But we can conclude that the horse makes the therapy more effective. Makes it richer, reach deeper when needed, and gives the therapist a possibility to reach clients otherwise not so easily reachable. To be frank, EAT saves money and time for everybody involved. There are clients whom EAT will not suit, but mostly for practical reasons.

The equine specialist has many functions, among them the more obvious ones, to secure safety for all involved, humans as horses, and to look after and ensure the horse's mental and physical wellbeing during therapy and off therapy. But also, there are some not so obvious functions. The equine specialist is a specialist in equine behavior and horse–human interaction. This means that the horse observation that is used in EAT is the equine specialist's field of expertise. The more the equine specialist knows about horses—as subjects, specie and a mammal, about differences and similarities between horses and humans, and horse–human interaction—the more the equine specialist can contribute to a therapy session. Because it is not only an intersubjective set-up, it is also an interspecies set-up. And extensive knowledge about horses is equally important as knowledge about humans in order to keep everyone safe and to get the most out of the conjoint meeting between human and horse. Because there will be mirroring and anti-mirroring, there will be seeing each other in each other and individual unrelated and related parallel behaviors, there will be common mammalian behaviors and specie-specific behaviors. It is probably possible for a skilled therapist to also be a skilled equine specialist and combine the skills so to be able to work on their own with clients. But keeping track of client behavior and horse behavior, apart from all other aspects of bringing in a horse into a therapy session, is an enormous task. And it is not so easy to be a specialist on both humans and horses, both takes years of training and a lifetime to master. The role of the equine specialist is also a topic that needs to be addressed further, to develop the field of EAT.

There is a lot of things going on in a EAT session and it can be described from many different points of views. In this chapter I am tracking it all back to a theory of intersubjectivity. I have also outlined what such a theory can incorporate. Since this chapter only allows for a brief description, much of its details are omitted, for clarity. There is more background to describe and more details to be added from different disciplines and about the theory of intersubjectivity itself. My aim in presenting it in this chapter is to point out the need of a theoretical framework for the future work of EAT and what such a framework can offer. This theory of intersubjectivity in EAT is just a starting point. It needs to be further developed. And I am looking forward to do that, in a collaborative way, in a global EAT network.

REFERENCES

Aaltola, E. (2013). *Empathy, Intersubjectivity and Animal Philosophy.* Department of Social Sciences, University of Eastern Finland.

Bard, K. (2017). Dyadic interactions, attachment and the presence of triadic interactions in chimpanzees and humans. *Infant Behavior & Development, 48*, 13–19.

Brinck, I. (2008). The role of intersubjectivity in the development of intentional communication. In J. Zlatev, T. P. Racine, C. Sinha, & E. and Itkonen (Eds.), *The Shared Mind: Perspectives on Intersubjectivity*. Amsterdam: John Benjamins Publishing Company.

Brinck, I., Vasudevi, R. & Zahavi, D. (2017). The primacy of the "we"? In C. Durt, C. Fuchs, & C. Tewes (Eds.), *Embodiment, Enaction, and Culture: Investigating the Constitution of the Shared World*. Cambridge, MA: MIT Press.

Hickok, G. (2014). *The Myth of Mirror Neurons: The Real Neuroscience of Communication and Cognition*. New York: W. W. Norton & Company.

Rowland, M. (2017). Beyond the looking glass: Self-awareness in animals. *The Philosopher's Magazine*, February.

Siporin, S. (2012). Talking horses: Equine psychotherapy and intersubjectivity. *Psychodynamic Practice, 18*(4).

Waytz, A., Epley, N., & Cacioppo, J. T. (2010). Social cognition unbound: Insight into anthropomorphism and dehumanization. *Current Directions in Psychological Science, 19*(1), 58–62.

Section 2

DEPRESSION

3

EQUINE-FACILITATED PSYCHOTHERAPY FOR THE TREATMENT OF DEPRESSION

Molly DePrekel and Natalie Runge

INTRODUCTION

In this chapter the authors discuss treating clients with depression with an equine-facilitated psychotherapy (EFP) approach. The authors have training and experience conducting EFP sessions from a client-centered perspective, building a framework that includes interventions such as cognitive reframing and restructuring, neurobiological interventions, sensorimotor approaches, competency-based interventions, mindfulness techniques, and relational attunement work. We have found this framework to be effective in EFP and working with individuals as it helps build self-efficacy, increase attunement, rewires negative thinking patterns, and helps the client build connection with them self and the world around them. In this chapter the authors will provide statistics on depression, rationale of utilizing EFP with clients with depression, and provides theoretical approaches to EFP. By explaining guidelines for implementing EFP, the authors address ethical issues that may arise in EFP programs and explain guidelines for implementing EFP. The authors illustrate an EFP session through transcript analysis and a case example and describe techniques for therapy goals and objectives.

DESCRIPTION OF PROBLEM

Depression is one of the most common mental health disorders experienced among adults and youth in the United States (US) (retrieved from National Institute of Mental Health (NIMH), 2017a, 2017b). The American Psychological Association (2016) states that individuals suffering from depression experience symptoms such as feelings of sadness, helplessness, and hopelessness, anger or irritability, concentration issues, sleep and appetite changes, social isolation, low energy, loss of interest in previously enjoyed activities, and suicidal thoughts or gestures. A survey administered to adults in 2016 by the NIMH found "an estimated 16.2 million adults in the United States had at least one major depressive episode. This number represented 6.7% of all U.S. adults" (NIMH, 2017a). The same year, the NIMH also administered a survey to adolescents (12 to 17 years old) and found that within the US 3.1 million adolescents (representing 12.8% of the population of adolescents) had experienced at least one major depressive episode within the past year (NIMH, 2017b). The NIMH states 10.3 million adults (representing 4.3% of the U.S. population aged 18 and older) and 2.2 million adolescents (representing 9.0% of the U.S. population aged 12 to 17) have experienced a major depressive episode with "severe impairment" in regards to the impact of the major depressive episode on the individuals overall daily functioning (NIMH, 2017a, 2017b).

In 2017, Mental Health America administered a survey to collect data on various mental health issues including the prevalence and impact of depression within the U.S. The survey found that depression among youth in the U.S. has increased 1.2% between 2010 through 2013 and that "11.01% of youth (age 12–17) report suffering from at least one major depressive episode (MDE) in the past year" and "7.4% (1.8 million youth) experienced severe depression" (Mental Health America, 2017). Furthermore, a total of 62.6% (or six out of ten) youth with depression do not receive any type of outpatient treatment services and "only 22% of youth with severe depression receive any kind of consistent outpatient treatment (7–25+ visits in a year)" (Mental Health America, 2017).

ANIMAL-ASSISTED THERAPY AND INTERVENTIONS

As the data from the above surveys has shown, the number of youth and adults in the US suffering from depression is significantly high and the prevalence, recurrence, and pervasiveness of depression is increasing. Schramm, Hediger, and Lang (2015, p. 193) state that "prevention of relapse and recurrence" of depressive episodes "presents one of the most important goals in the treatment of depression" and that animal-assisted therapy and interventions may be viable therapeutic options to help treat individuals suffering from depression and to prevent relapse of depressive symptoms. In a meta-analysis conducted by Souter and Miller (2007), they found that four out of five empirically supported research studies showed that exposure to animal-assisted therapy and/or animal-assisted interventions significantly reduced depressive symptoms. In an open pilot study, Schramm, Hediger, and Lang (2015) found that utilizing mindfulness techniques in conjunction with animal-assisted therapy (nature and animal-assisted mindfulness training) proved to be an effective therapeutic intervention in treating traumatized individuals with depressive symptoms and preventing relapse of depressive symptoms. Equine-facilitated psychotherapy can be an effective approach for clients with depression.

In her dissertation titled *National Survey on Equine-Assisted Therapy: An Exploratory Study of Current Practitioners and Programs*, McConnell notes that in her survey of mental health practitioners and programs conducting equine-facilitated psychotherapy therapy, 150 participants (100%) reported that the horse was the catalyst for clients (McConnell, 2010). Furthermore, significant themes came from the survey of programs about how practitioners related to client sessions, these included attachment, self-efficacy, confidence and the manner in which the therapist treats the horse (McConnell, 2010). The last theme listed above is illustrated in one therapy session conducted by one of the authors. In this equine-facilitated therapy session, an adult client reported she knew she could trust the clinician by the way the clinician interacted with the equines. The client went on to say the clinician talked calmly to the equines, asked permission, and said please and thank you. For a client struggling with depression to observe and comment on interactions demonstrates an ability to move beyond one's own despair and hopelessness. Also, this client was working at trusting the clinician and the equine interactions increased this perceived trust of the clinician.

A RELATIONAL MODEL

In equine-facilitated psychotherapy, it is the belief of the authors that it is important to work from a relational model. Asking clients to work with a large animal they often don't have any experience with requires open dialog, relational attunement, and rapport with a clinician. Individuals suffering from depression oftentimes have strained relationships as depressive symptoms cause them to socially isolate. Building a relationship with an equine as well as with the clinician may be beneficial in helping individuals suffering from depression as it allows them to interact and connect with another being and decreases their social isolation. Working from the basis of a relational model, one approach to utilize as a framework for EFP is Attachment Theory. John Bowlby, the father of Attachment Theory, emphasized that individuals are born with an innate desire to attach to another species and that our brains are hardwired with an attachment system that begins to develop at birth and is malleable throughout life (Bowlby, 1998). The human–animal bond (HAB) refers to the types of attachments and relationships that exist between people and animals, the emotional tie between two beings, and the relational connection or association between two or more beings based on need, benefit, and value (Lagoni, Butler & Hetts, 1994).

Clinicians can also promote a relational approach in EFP by employing Natural Lifemanship principles and their model of trauma-informed equine-assisted psychotherapy (TF-EAP) where the overarching goal is to develop healthy relationships with oneself and others (Jobe, Shultz-Jobe, & McFarland, 2016). The TF-EAP model is based upon medical research of the brain and "treats psychological and behavioral disorders through a trauma lens by intentionally using horse physiology to regulate human physiology and horse psychology to heal human psychology" (Jobe et al., 2016). Many symptoms resulting from trauma are also characteristic of symptoms of depression and traumatic experiences can oftentimes lead to depressive symptoms in some individuals. The TF-EAP model proposes that it can address these symptoms by helping individuals build a connected relationship with an equine while reforming and creating new neuropathways that help individuals build healthy, attuned, connected, and lasting relationships with themselves and others.

It is also important that clients with depression not only transform their cognitions, they can also benefit from movement and interacting with the natural world. In his book, *The Depression Cure: The 6-Step Program to Beat Depression without Drugs*, author Stephen Llardi argues that "the rate of depression among Americans is roughly ten times higher today than it was just two generations ago, and he points the blame to our modern lifestyle" (Borchard, n.d.). Of the six steps, the following four can be utilized in equine-facilitated psychotherapy: sunlight exposure, physical activity, increased social support, and engaged activity that keeps one from ruminating (Borchard, n.d.).

Clients with depression are often unmotivated to move their bodies and at times just walking out to the pasture or arena can assist in healing. As we understand more about brain neurology and the positive effects that exercise, nature, and mindfulness can have on the brain, clinicians can prove psychoeducation on these concepts and apply them in equine sessions giving clients a first-hand experience by noticing any relief they may feel from their symptoms. In traditional talk therapy, clinicians can educate clients and ask them to go outside, move their bodies, and be in nature, yet clients with depression may find this overwhelming as they often report having low energy or feeling fatigued. On the other hand, a clinician walking with a client into a barn might suggest trying these concepts of nature, exercise, and mindfulness with the equines, which can be more powerful and experiential than just asking a client to go outside on their own. A client can experiment with movement with an equine through leading, they can try mindful grooming exercises, and they can observe the equines in their natural habitat. After interactions with equines, getting a self-report on what clients noticed can provide assessment and treatment planning information on what they liked and how they can bring this into their daily life. For example, a client who achieved mindfulness and felt calmer while grooming could be asked to find ways in their everyday life to create other mindful moments. Another client who liked being outside and walking with a horse could practice every day going for a walk and watching other animals such as dogs, squirrels, or birds and attempt to find joy in a nature walk.

The following are some examples of how to implement a few techniques treating clients with depression.

GUIDELINES AND PROCEDURES

An Insider's Look at EFP Sessions

An intake is done at the office first without equine interaction. This gives the client a chance to meet the clinician and the clinician can go over paperwork, answer any questions, and talk about the approaches of equine-assisted interventions and other approaches used, such as Cognitive Behavior Therapy, Eye Movement Desensitization Reprocessing, Sensorimotor Psychotherapy, Faster Emotional Freedom Technique, Adaptive Internal Regulation Model, Tellington Ttouch, Yoga Calm, and Trauma Focused Equine-Assisted Psychotherapy.

One way we start working with clients is to have them observe each equine, ask questions, and then allow them to meet the equines. This is done in whatever way the client states they feel comfortable. For example, some may want to have a barrier of the fence between them and the equine, others may want to go in the paddock with each equine or others may want the equine in crossties. The clinician or equine specialist if there is one present will go over safety and other information about equines so the client can begin to relax and feel comfortable interacting with the equines. This may be all that happens in the first session.

In a subsequent session, clients may learn mindfulness grooming, this exercise allows clients to notice how they feel as they groom the equine. Discussion can occur about equines being masters at noticing if one's body and mind are not attuned and if words and feelings don't match. Clients may report they are not afraid and yet they will hesitate or jump if the equine moves or makes a big snort or breath sound. The equine may get fidgety or move away from the client and we can then ask the client to check in and see if they are really feeling calm internally. Often clients will report they are nervous or they might shut down and then the clinician can intervene and teach some self-regulation and calming techniques such as breathing a bit deeper, slowing down movements, talking out loud to the equine, and just building a connection.

For clients with depression, this idea of slowing down and allowing a relationship to develop may be foreign, as clients have stated "well he won't like me if he knows me," or "I know he walked away because he doesn't like me."

This gives fodder to the clinician to work with as they can wonder out loud if the client feels that in other relationships and how that can add to depression. Another important aspect of relationship development is working with the client to change their behavior based on the needs of another and building relational attunement. We will often say to a client "try another way." We are building capacity for clients to attune and notice maybe what they are doing isn't working so they can be flexible and try something new or different. In a session, this may look like an equine moving away from a client who is brushing him/her. The client may interpret this as rejection and the clinician can reframe this to "try it another way," i.e., brush softer, use another brush, try just touching with your hand and see what the equine may like and also what feels good to you. The clinician can stress the interaction and mutual connection in the relationship. If clients become more flexible in relationships and attune to themselves and others they may begin to sense mood improvement and thus become more interactive with others.

Another technique we utilize in treatment with depression is Tellington Ttouch (Tellington-Jones, 2010) for self-regulation and client equine attunement. The ones most often taught are hair and ear slides that clients do on the equines and watch how and where the equines like to be touched. Once a client tries these slides and notices the equine licking and chewing, dropping their head, and eyes slightly closing or relaxing the clinician can ask the client what they notice with the equine and what they notice inside themselves also. The next step is this technique is to have clients try ear and hair slides on themselves and notice if they can self-soothe and feel more relaxed. We will have clients try this in session and then ask them to do this as homework each day for mindful self-calming. One note is that is a client or even equines don't like direct touch they can do Ttouch off the body and still feel some relief and calming. It is interesting to have clients try ear and hair slides on different equines and notice what each equine likes, how the client may feel different with each equine and again have them work to shift their behavior based on their own needs and the needs of another living being. More information on how to do ear and hair slides can be found at ttouch.com or there are YouTube videos online.

Resourcing and grounding in present-moment experiences can aid clients who feel sad and overwhelmed with their depression. Teaching clients to store a felt sense of calm, appreciation, and small bits of joy in their body can be restorative. Building a capacity for joy is often the work of therapy when a client feels depressed. Resourcing and allowing for happy or relaxed feelings can be the focus of sessions for clients, and adding movement experiences with animals often may enhance resourcing.

Family EFP Sessions

When conducting family sessions, observation of herd dynamics can be a valuable resource in bringing healing to family systems that are being negatively impacted by the effects of depression. Through observation of equine behaviors within a herd, family members can identify the role each equine is serving within the herd in the given moment, which can serve as a metaphor of the roles each family member plays in given moments within their own family system. The clinician can facilitate conversation regarding how each family member's behaviors impact one another and contribute to the overall family system and cohesiveness or breakdown in communication and relationship. Recognizing and analyzing ineffective behavior patterns can help the family learn how to problem-solve and navigate through family conflict by each family member taking responsibility for how their behaviors impact one another. Clinicians should be mindful when a family member recognizes an equine behavior and misinterprets what it means rather than stating what they observe the behavior is. For example, a family member might recognize an equine's ears back and state "look at how angry that horse is with his ears back"; however, the horse's ears were back because the equine heard the sound of a tractor in the field directly behind the equine. In this case, the equine ears back had nothing to do with anger at all, rather it was the equine being aware of the happenings in its surroundings. Another example is if a depressed family member appears sad, isn't talking as much as they typically do, and they are isolating themselves from other family members, it can be easy to take their behaviors personally and think they are acting standoffish and upset with you; however, it may be that the depressed family member doesn't feel like interacting due to the extreme sadness they are feeling and it feels easier to isolate rather than be around others. Misinterpreting one another's actions and behaviors can lead to breakdown in communication and lack of connection with one another. The clinician can assist the family in identifying how symptoms of depression impact each family member and how each family member's response to the behaviors of the depressed family member impact them. Bringing awareness to the behaviors and non-verbal signs each family member exhibits towards one another can help improve communication between family members and bring support to the family member suffering from depression, who may find it difficult to verbalize how the depression is impacting them or what it feels like. Furthermore, this intervention can help the depressed family member identify their depressive symptoms and more effectively manage their symptoms instead of their symptoms dictating their life.

Clinicians must also have awareness of multicultural issues when implementing EFP. Some cultural factors that may affect the process of EFP include gender, socio-economic status, age, religious beliefs, family dynamics, and how the client views equines. It's important that clinicians work on understanding the individual experiences that each client brings into the therapy session as this can enhance the therapeutic alliance, build trust and rapport, and help determine if EFP is the best course of treatment for the specific client.

Animal Welfare Considerations

Animal-assisted therapy (AAT) and the implementation of animal-assisted interventions (AAI) in clinical work have grown immensely over the past 20 years. With this growth, more research studies have been established studying the efficacy of AAT in treating mental health disorders; however, there continues to be a lack of empirically supported research that proves the benefits of utilizing AAT to treat mental health disorders. Additionally, there is a lack of research based upon how AAT is impacting the animals and how the animal's health and welfare is being monitored and addressed. Iannuzzi and Rowan (1991) are two of the first researchers referenced in literature whom studied animal welfare and the level of exploitation found within animal programs in the US. They discovered that some animal programs upheld animal welfare while others had evidence of neglect, abuse, and in some cases death of an animal. A study conducted by Kaiser, Heleski, Siegford, and Smith (2006) examined stress-related behaviors among horses used in therapeutic riding programs by utilizing an ethogram of equine behaviors. They found no significant increase in stress in the horses when ridden by recreational riders, physically handicapped riders, nor psychologically handicapped riders; however, they found a significant increase in stress among the horses when at-risk children rode them. In recent years, more attention has been given to the welfare of animals within animal therapy programming and standards of practice have been developed to assist clinicians in the ethical treatment of the therapy animals. When clinicians choose to implement an AAT program or intervention into their practice, it is of vital importance that clinicians consider the ethical guidelines that accompany partnering with the specific animal species they have chosen to partner with in their clinical work. In doing so, the ethical principles can aid clinicians by helping ensure the welfare and health of the animal(s) involved.

Ethical Considerations

When partnering with an equine, a clinician might consider ascribing to the ethical codes set forth by the Professional Association of Therapeutic Horsemanship International (PATH Intl.). PATH Intl. has established ethical standards that provide clinicians' best practice and procedures for equine-assisted activities and therapies. PATH Intl. has also established an equine welfare committee made up of several components to aid in serving as an accountability factor to help professionals maintain the welfare of the equines being partnered with. Although there are no standards of best practice that everyone in the field of equine-facilitated psychotherapy agrees upon and there are few empirically based studies that show the efficacy of treating specific DSM diagnoses with this type of therapy, clinicians and clients often report clients feeling better. During sessions the authors observe clients to exhibit more humor and smiles, and clients report decreased stress.

In addition to ascribing to ethical principles, it is imperative that clinicians consider the capabilities of the animal they are choosing to partner with and if the animal is the best choice given the therapeutic treatment goals. The MacNamara Animal Capability Assessment Model (MACAM) is a useful assessment model to aid clinicians in determining the goodness of fit of the specific animal with the specific client population being worked with. MacNamara, Moga, and Pachel (2015) state the MACAM

> identifies the critical components of animal capability for work with any particular clinical population/setting, resulting in an individualized working animal job description that accounts for contingencies of intervention delivery and specifies 'goodness of fit' between an animal and a mental health intervention method.
>
> (MacNamara et al., 2015, p. 96)

The MACAM examines the animal's responsiveness, "how an animal responds to stimuli from clients or within the clinical setting as well as the degree to which the animal displays transitional behaviors"; capacity, "degree to which the animal interacts with all elements of the environment"; skills, "trained behaviors and equipment familiarity"; and attributes, "physical characteristics that may contribute to intervention category" (MacNamara et al., 2015, pp. 96–97). By utilizing the MACAM, clinicians can gain more understanding in relation to how the animal experiences the client they come in contact with, which can aid the clinician in refining client goals and optimizing the overall AAI.

CASE EXAMPLE AND SAMPLE CASE TRANSCRIPT

Brief Description of Client and Case History

The case example that follows is an illustration of how you can incorporate self-regulation and resourcing into an equine therapy session. Resources are used to help a client feel calmer, less stressed, more present, and these resources can be used after sessions for clients to bring themselves back to a calm, grounded, safe state. When we add animal-assisted work with resourcing exercises it can offer more opportunities for kinesthetic and somatic opportunities.

Allowing clients to use all their senses to integrate a resource can deepen the experience somatically. Clients can use a word or image to bring up that felt sense of calm that is stored in their body. In sensorimotor resourcing, often clients are working with internal resources such as freezing, or submit behavior they may have not seen in the past as a good thing. For example, a client who is depressed and blames themselves for not defending themselves from an attack in their past can begin to work somatically with their body and see that freezing and not defending themselves but submitting was a lifesaving technique.

This automatic behavior was used to stay safe in the initial attack and when they work with this in session often the shame and blame dissipates. In a session with equines, a client can practice moving their body to literally stay safe in the presence of a large animal. Often we talk with clients about how their body automatically moves to a safer place when they are with the equines and it is unconscious or the brain just does it without a lot of thought that comes from the prefrontal cortex.

The below examples represent a compilation of client work from 28 years in the field of animal-assisted interactions.

Table 3.1

Transcript and Analysis of Case Example

Transcript	*Analysis*
Psychologist: Notice what happens in your body as you meet each equine.	Working with client to get an internal somatic focus.
Client: I notice I am breathing deeper.	Client is starting to recognize internal systems.
Psychologist: Does that feel OK to you?	Not assuming deeper breathing is a positive.
Client: Yes. I feel less tension in my head.	Client observes positive sensation.
Psychologist: Stay with that sensation.	Expansion of a positive resource.
Client: I am not sure how to do that.	Client not judging themselves as right or wrong.
Psychologist: Well let's do an experiment and notice what happens with the equine when you take some deeper breaths and let the tension go in your head.	With an experiment, there is no right or wrong answer—stay away from judgment.
Client: I notice Whisper [horse] walking toward me. *Client smiling*	Interaction can happen when we calm our own system.
Psychologist: Nice. Can you feel your smile? That was kind of a fun experiment, huh?	Asking client to notice felt sense of smile, the "huh" allows for feedback from client.
Client: Can I say hi and pet Whisper?	Relational experience is asked for.

Transcript	*Analysis*
Psychologist: Ask Whisper.	Allows for connection and attunement.
Client: Hi Whisper I am [name]. *Psychologist is quiet and allows for mindful moment*	Client socially engages. Allowing relationship with equine.
Client: I like touching him.	Reports on self.
Psychologist: Just notice inside what good feeling feels like.	Reflection.
Client: *Tearful.* It's been a long time since I smiled and actually noticed it. **Client:** I mean I spend so much time focusing on what's wrong with me I forget about smiling.	Starting to connect with internal world in positive way. Again, re-engaging with positive feelings.
Psychologist: Oh wow, a different connection with yourself huh?	Staying with positive and getting client to notice.
Client: It feels weird like I don't want to focus on it to much as it might go away.	Depression thinking comes up.
Psychologist: Well it might, and you still have it in this moment.	Not go back to negative cognitions staying mindful in moment.
Client: Uh-huh.	Recognition.
Psychologist: We could see if we can work with this feeling to be a resource for you to take out of session.	Generalize resource to everyday life.
Client: That would be nice but I don't know I don't want to ruin it, I like Whisper and he feels soft.	Anxiety comes up and depression thinking takes over, limbic brain of overwhelm kicks in.
Psychologist: Well OK to try it and see what happens, and Whisper and I know about resourcing and can help.	Offering suggestion and interactive regulation.
Client: Sure.	Willingness to try.
Psychologist: OK, so you keep your hand on Whisper even feel him breathing and breath a bit deeper yourself see if you can find your smile again.	Somatic resourcing.
Client: I got it, it's easy with the horses right here.	Engaging.
Psychologist: In your mind's eye take a picture of this for yourself, let me know when you got it.	Working to get client to take resource image with them.
Client: Um, I think so.	Trying to stay with image.
Psychologist: So now see if you can store that feeling in your body as a felt sense, and that picture of you touching Whisper, smiling, less tension in your head and deeper breathes.	Somatic and visual together.
Client: That's a lot and I can see it inside just a bit.	Overwhelm yet staying with small piece.
Psychologist: Stay with that bit.	Bite-sizing.
Client: *Loses smile.* This is hard, my head gets busy.	Depression and limbic overwhelm.
Psychologist: OK just notice and let the ANTS [automatic negative thoughts] go.	Reframe
Client: Oh yeah, don't invite ants to the picnic, I forgot, and if they come just see them go by. *Client takes breath, horse lowers his head.*	Re-engaging.
Client: Did you teach him to do that?	Amazed and unsure at same time.
Psychologist: Um, no, he is responding to your calm and letting go of negative thoughts, horses live in the right now.	Mindfulness.
Client: So awesome.	Staying grounded and good feeling.
Psychologist: So can you think of a word that can bring you back to this feeling? Let's get the rightist word with the most juice.	Utilizing experience to take home.
Client: Breathe.	Using inner resource and trying something new.
Psychologist: OK so way that out loud and see if it fits. **Client:** Breathe [pauses]. Whisper, yeah that's it, whisper. *Horse's ears come forward.*	Engaging client in own healing. Client finds own resource word.

(*Continued*)

Transcript	*Analysis*
Psychologist: OK what tells you that works?	Having client decide what works best for them.
Client: "I feel it, the calm, no tension in my head." *Horse takes a couple steps.* "Can I still pet him?"	Notices internal somatic feelings and is in now as notices outside world also.
Psychologist: Yes, walk with him and OK great, stay with that and where it your body do you want to store that felt sense, the word Whisper, your smile and deep breath?	Bringing all senses in.
Client: It's in my stomach and even my head.	Noticing where can put felt sense.
Psychologist: Grand, let's play with that and you practice bringing in that felt sense with your hand on Whisper and smile.	Practice.
Client: OK. Does this and then pets horse. Horse walks away	Completing exercise for grounding and resourcing.
Client: It's OK, Whisper, I know you are done.	Client not judging self or horse, allowing horse to disengage.
Psychologist: That was nice can you thank him for his time?	Gratitude.
Client: Thanks you are so sweet.	Relational connection and gratitude.
Psychologist: OK almost done, can you take that resource and practice every day coming back to this image, felt sense, smile and take a deep breath?	Homework to carry good feelings into everyday life.
Client: Yep, and next time will you take a picture of Whisper and I together, with my phone?	Client willing to try new behavior and wants tangible reminder.
Psychologist: Sure, and today how about I give you Whisper's card to help you when you are not here? I want you to practice this resource everyday so when you need it as you feel bummed or anxious you can use it. Deal?	Visual and transitional object.
Client: Deal.	Agreement.

Completed Case Note Example

Type of therapy

☑ *Feminist-Multicultural*	☑ *Competency based*
☑ *Trauma focused*	☐ *Ego-State*
☐ *Bilateral Stimulation*	☑ *Expressive/experiential*
☑ *EMDR*	☐ *Couples/family*
☐ *Cognitive/Skills*	☑ *Sensorimotor*
☐ *Play therapy*	☑ *Resiliency/resource development*

Notes:

In Session Observation: Neurological/Arousal

☐ *Hyper-Vigilance*	☐ *Rapid Blinking*
☑ *Hand/Body Tremors*	☐ *Eye Rolling*
☐ *Exaggerated Startle Response*	☑ *Distressed Breathing*
☐ *Pupil Dilation*	

Notes:

Somatic/Physical

☑ *Fixed Gaze*	☑ *Stiff Limbs/Body*
☐ *Lack of Speech*	☐ *Numbing*
☑ *Muscle Rigidity*	☑ *Psychomotor Agitation*
☐ *Sweating*	☐ *Intrusive Sensory Experience*
☐ *Flushing*	

Notes:

Cognitive

☐ *Repetitive Speech*	☐ *Re-Experiencing Traumatic Event*
☑ *Repetitive Thoughts*	☐ *Confusion*
☐ *Difficulty Concentrating*	☐ *Space/time Orientation*
☐ *Dissociative Episodes*	☐ *Developmental Regression*
☑ *Intrusive Images/Thoughts/Sensory*	☑ *Changes in Voice Tone/Rate/Volume*

Notes:

FIG. 3.1. Sample Client Session Note.

Emotional/Affect

- [x] *Depressed*
- [ ] *Pleading*
- [ ] *Rage*
- [ ] *Agitation*
- [x] *Laughing*
- [ ] *Irritable*
- [ ] *Flat*
- [ ] *Euthymic*
- [ ] *Anxious*
- [ ] *Crying*
- [ ] *Anger*
- [ ] *Regulated*
- [x] *Smiling*
- [ ] *Sadness*
- [ ] *Happy*
- [x] *Affect Appropriate to Content*
- [ ] *Congruent with Mood*

Notes: -After time with equine was smiling and laughing and reported less depression.

Progress Reported by Client Since Last Session

- [x] *Used Skills*
- [x] *Improved Self-Regulation*
- [ ] *Decrease Harmful Behaviors*
- [ ] *Improved Appetite*
- [ ] *Maintained Safety Plan*
- [x] *Improved Mood*
- [x] *Improved Relationship with Self*
- [ ] *Improved Quality of Sleep*
- [ ] *Reduction in Symptoms*
- [x] *Used somatic/cognitive/emotional regulation*

Notes: -Client reported practicing smiling at people when at work and not looking down as much.

Between Session Client Report

- [ ] *Self-Injury*
- [ ] *Binge Eating*
- [ ] *Sleep Difficulty*
- [x] *Intrusive Thoughts and Feelings*
- [x] *Difficulty Functioning at Work/School*
- [ ] *Personal Hygiene Impairment*
- [ ] *Engaging in Self-Care*
- [ ] *Compulsive Behaviors*
- [ ] *Appetite/Food Issues*
- [ ] *Nightmares*
- [ ] *Isolation/Withdrawal*
- [ ] *Relational Conflict*
- [x] *Difficulty with Emotional Regulation*
- [ ] *Using Skills Learned in Therapy*
- [x] *Impact of Animal Present in Sessions on Daily Functioning*

Notes: -Client reported missing one day of work due to feeling depressed, difficulty with rebooting and emotional regulation. -Stated excited to come to barn today and noticed felt cheerful when woke up.

FIG. 3.1. ***(Continued)***

Risk and Safety Assessment

- ☐ *Life Threatening Thoughts Towards Self* ☐ *Has Plan* ☐ *Has Means*
- ☐ *Life Threatening Thoughts Towards Others* ☐ *Has Plan* ☐ *Has Means*

Intervention:

- ☐ *Developed Collaborative Safety Plan* ☐ *Will Check in Within 24 Hours*
- ☐ *Agrees to Talk with Therapist/Crisis Line Before Taking Life-Threatening Action*

Notes: No thoughts of self-harm. Denied any life-threatening thoughts.

In Session Intervention/Focus of Therapy

- ☑ *EMDR Resourcing*
- ☐ *EMDR Reprocessing*
- ☑ *Adaptive Internal Relational (AIR)*
- ☑ *Sensorimotor Psychotherapy*
- ☑ *Relaxation*
- ☐ *Alpha Stim*
- ☐ *Ttouch Self-Regulation*
- ☐ *Cognitive Skills*
- ☑ *Relationship with Self/Others*
- ☑ *Psychoeducation*
- ☑ *Experiential*
- ☐ *Yoga Calm*
- ☐ *Heart Math*
- ☐ *Adult Awareness/Most Resourced Self*

Notes:

Recommended Plan of Care Between Sessions

Practicing resource worked on in session today, use horse card to assist with self-regulation. Continue making attempts at work to connect with co-workers.

Recommendations Made

- ☑ *Continued Therapy*
- ☐ *Medication Consultation*
- ☐ *Specialty Care*
- ☐ *Seek Medical Advice*
- ☐ *Nutritional Counseling*

Notes: Will continue with individual therapy at barn, and skills group for self-regulation.

Subjective Report by Client:

Psychotherapy Note:

FIG. 3.1. *(Continued)*

Blank Template of Case Note Example

Type of Therapy

- ☐ *Feminist-Multicultural*
- ☐ *Trauma focused*
- ☐ *Bilateral Stimulation*
- ☐ *EMDR*
- ☐ *Cognitive/Skills*
- ☐ *Play therapy*
- ☐ *Competency based*
- ☐ *Ego-State*
- ☐ *Expressive/experiential*
- ☐ *Couples/family*
- ☐ *Sensorimotor*
- ☐ *Resiliency/resource development*

Notes:

____

____

In Session Observation: Neurological/Arousal

- ☐ *Hyper-Vigilance*
- ☐ *Hand/Body Tremors*
- ☐ *Exaggerated Startle Response*
- ☐ *Pupil Dilation*
- ☐ *Rapid Blinking*
- ☐ *Eye Rolling*
- ☐ *Distressed Breathing*

Notes:

____

____

Somatic/Physical

- ☐ *Fixed Gaze*
- ☐ *Lack of Speech*
- ☐ *Muscle Rigidity*
- ☐ *Sweating*
- ☐ *Flushing*
- ☐ *Stiff Limbs/Body*
- ☐ *Numbing*
- ☐ *Psychomotor Agitation*
- ☐ *Intrusive Sensory Experience*

Notes:

____

____

Cognitive

- ☐ *Repetitive Speech*
- ☐ *Repetitive Thoughts*
- ☐ *Difficulty Concentrating*
- ☐ *Dissociative Episodes*
- ☐ *Intrusive Images/Thoughts/Sensory*
- ☐ *Re-Experiencing Traumatic Event*
- ☐ *Confusion*
- ☐ *Space/time Orientation*
- ☐ *Developmental Regression*
- ☐ *Changes in Voice Tone/Rate/Volume*

Notes:

____

FIG. 3.2. Blank Sample Client Session Note.

Emotional/Affect

- ☐ *Depressed*
- ☐ *Pleading*
- ☐ *Rage*
- ☐ *Agitation*
- ☐ *Laughing*
- ☐ *Irritable*
- ☐ *Flat*
- ☐ *Euthymic*
- ☐ *Anxious*
- ☐ *Crying*
- ☐ *Anger*
- ☐ *Regulated*
- ☐ *Smiling*
- ☐ *Sadness*
- ☐ *Happy*
- ☐ *Affect Appropriate to Content*
- ☐ *Congruent with Mood*

Notes:

Progress Reported by Client Since Last Session

- ☐ *Used Skills*
- ☐ *Improved Self-Regulation*
- ☐ *Decrease Harmful Behaviors*
- ☐ *Improved Appetite*
- ☐ *Maintained Safety Plan*
- ☐ *Improved Mood*
- ☐ *Improved Relationship with Self*
- ☐ *Improved Quality of Sleep*
- ☐ *Reduction in Symptoms*
- ☐ *Used somatic/cognitive/emotional regulation*

Notes:

Between Session Client Report

- ☐ *Self-Injury*
- ☐ *Binge Eating*
- ☐ *Sleep Difficulty*
- ☐ *Intrusive Thoughts and Feelings*
- ☐ *Difficulty Functioning at Work/School*
- ☐ *Personal Hygiene Impairment*
- ☐ *Engaging in Self-Care*
- ☐ *Compulsive Behaviors*
- ☐ *Appetite/Food Issues*
- ☐ *Nightmares*
- ☐ *Isolation/Withdrawal*
- ☐ *Relational Conflict*
- ☐ *Difficulty with Emotional Regulation*
- ☐ *Using Skills Learned in Therapy*
- ☐ *Impact of Animal Present in Sessions on Daily Functioning*

Notes:

FIG. 3.2. (Continued)

Risk and Safety Assessment

☐ *Life Threatening Thoughts Towards Self* ☐ *Has Plan* ☐ *Has Means*

☐ *Life Threatening Thoughts Towards Others* ☐ *Has Plan* ☐ *Has Means*

Intervention:

☐ *Developed Collaborative Safety Plan* ☐ *Will Check in Within 24 Hours*

☐ *Agrees to Talk with Therapist/Crisis Line Before Taking Life-Threatening Action*

Notes:

In Session Intervention/Focus of Therapy

☐ *EMDR Resourcing* ☐ *Cognitive Skills*

☐ *EMDR Reprocessing* ☐ *Relationship with Self/Others*

☐ *Adaptive Internal Relational (AIR)* ☐ *Psychoeducation*

☐ *Sensorimotor Psychotherapy* ☐ *Experiential*

☐ *Relaxation* ☐ *Yoga Calm*

☐ *Alpha Stim* ☐ *Heart Math*

☐ *Ttouch Self Regulation* ☐ *Adult Awareness/Most Resourced Self*

Notes:

Recommended Plan of Care Between Sessions

Recommendations Made

☐ *Continued Therapy* ☐ *Seek Medical Advice*

☐ *Medication Consultation* ☐ *Nutritional Counseling*

☐ *Specialty Care*

Notes:

Subjective Report by Client:

Psychotherapy Note:

FIG. 3.2. *(Continued)*

REFERENCES

American Psychological Association (2016). *Overcoming Depression: How Psychologists Help with Depressive Disorders-Understanding Depression*. Retrieved from www.apa.org/helpcenter/depression.aspx.

Borchard, T. (n.d.). *6 Steps to Beating Depression*. Retrieved from https://psychcentral.com/blog/archives/2009/07/09/6-steps-for-beating-depression.

Bowlby, J. (1988). *A Secure Base*. New York: Basic Books.

Iannuzzi, D. & Rowan, A. N. (1991). Ethical issues in animal-assisted therapy programs. *Anthrozoos, 4*(3), 154–163.

Jobe, T., Shultz-Jobe, B., & McFarland (2016). Fundamentals of Natural Lifemanship: Trauma-Focused Equine Assisted Psychotherapy (TF-EAP). Independently published.

Kaiser, L., Heleski, C. R., Siegford, J., & Smith, K. A. (2006). Stress-related behaviors among horses used in therapeutic riding program. *Journal of American Veterinary Medical Association, 228*(1), 39–45.

Lagoni, L., Butler, C., & Hetts, S. (1994). *The Human–Animal Bond and Grief*. Philadelphia, PA: W. B. Saunders Co.

MacNamara, M., Moga, J., & Pachel, C. (2015). What's love got to do with it? Selecting animals for animal-assisted mental health interventions. In A. H. Fine (Ed.), *Handbook on Animal-Assisted Therapy: Foundations and Guidelines for Animal-Assisted Interventions* (4th edition, pp. 91–101). San Diego, CA: Elsevier Academic Press.

McConnell, P. (2010). *National Survey on Equine Assisted Therapy: An Exploratory Study of Current Practitioners and Programs*. Doctoral Dissertation. Retrieved from Scholar Works-Walden University (UMI No. 3412302).

Mental Health in America. (2017). *Youth Data*. Retrieved from www.mentalhealthamerica.net/issues/mental-health-america-youth-data.

National Institute of Mental Health (NIMH). (2017a). *Major Depression Among Adults*. Retrieved from www.nimh.nih.gov/health/statistics/prevalence/major-depression-among-adults.shtml.

National Institute of Mental Health (NIMH). (2017b). *Major Depression with Severe Impairment Among Adolescents*. Retrieved from www.nimh.nih.gov/health/statistics/prevalence/major-depression-with-severe-impairment-among-adolescents.shtml.

Schram, E., Hediger, K., & Lang, U.E. (2015). From animal behavior to human health. An animal-assisted mindfulness intervention for recurrent depression. *Zeitschrift fur Psychologie, 223*(3), 192–200.

Souter, M. A. and Miller, M. D. (2007). Do animal-assisted activities effectively treat depression? A meta-analysis. *Anthrozoos, 20*(2), 167–180.

State of Mental Health in America Report Overview Historical Data. (2016). Retrieved from www.mentalhealthamerica.net/issues/2016-state-mental-health-america-report-overview-historical-data#Overview.

Tellington-Jones, L. (2010). *Ttouch for your Horse*. Retrieved from www.ttouch.com.

4

An Eagala Model Approach to Using Equine-Assisted Counseling with Teens Suffering from Depression

Karen Frederick

INTRODUCTION

Depression is one of the most common mental disorders in adolescents. According to the National Institute for Mental Health (NIMH, 2017), in 2016, an estimated 3.1 million adolescents in the United States (US) had at least one major depressive episode. The 12-month prevalence rate of major depression was 12.8% of U.S. adolescents overall with 19.4% of females and 6.4% of males experiencing it. While no one cause can be identified, research suggests that depression can result from a combination of factors including genetic, biological, environment, and psychological concerns (NIMH, 2017). Some of these factors might include a family history of depression; adverse life events or trauma; life changes; and physical illness or medications.

When an adolescent struggles with depression, the symptoms may differ from the symptoms in adults experiencing depression (Smith & Segal, 2017). While adults experience sadness, fatigue, and lethargy, many adolescents do not necessarily appear sad. Teen symptoms of depression often include irritability, angry outbursts, and agitation. Other common signs include withdrawal from friends and family, loss of interest in activities that were previously enjoyed, changes in eating or sleeping habits, poor school performance, and feelings of worthlessness (NIMH, 2017).

The general expectations for teens include attending school, applying themselves to learning, and growing up to become good citizens who contribute to society. Yet, when a teen is experiencing depression, it becomes nearly impossible for them to meet these expectations. Just getting through the day can be a monumental task. From the perspective of Maslow's (1970) theory of motivation, teens who have depression have not fulfilled their basic level need for emotional safety, so progression to higher needs of a sense of belonging, self-esteem, and self-actualization cannot be met. Thus, when an adolescent's mental health needs are not met, the adolescent cannot be expected to meet the educational and other expectations placed on them.

Traditional methods of treating depression in adolescents have been twofold. First, antidepressants are often prescribed but there is a risk that this may increase suicidal thoughts and behaviors in adolescents (NIMH, 2017). Second, cognitive behavior therapy is also prominent but some adolescents do not respond well to this approach, up to 20% in one study (Goodyer et al., 2008). Some adolescents may prefer a more kinesthetic, natural treatment approach. Equine-assisted counseling (EAC) has shown some positive results in treating adolescents with depression (Frederick, Ivey-Hatz, & Lanning, 2015).

DESCRIPTION OF INTERVENTION

There are many techniques available in the modality of equine-assisted interventions. The simple act of putting oneself outdoors with nature and animals can be emotionally healing. Yet, one classic Equine-Assisted Growth and Learning Association (Eagala, 2017) activity that seems to be helpful to teens with depression is learning to create or stop movement of the horse. Emotionally, teens often feel incapable of controlling events or people in their lives. For example, they have no control over their parents' relationship with each other (or divorce) and no control over other people's actions, attitudes, etc. In the activities described below, teens learn how to control a horse's movement, which can be very empowering. In actuality, teens have more control than they might believe. These activities help teens realize that they control the responses they get from horses and people when they control their tone of voice, attitude, and choice of words.

Activity 1: Ground Tie

The goal of Activity 1, Ground Tie, is for the client to be able to stop the movement of the horse and discuss the metaphor of stopping movement in life. The materials needed for this activity are one or more horses; an enclosed arena or space for the horse(s) to choose how close they wish to be to the humans in the arena; one halter; and a long lunge line. The first step is for the client to catch and halter a horse. After catching and haltering the horse, the client should walk the horse to the activity facilitators. The counselor should hand the client the long lunge line and say, "You should now attach this lunge line to the horse's halter. After that step, has been completed, you will drop the lunge line and walk completely around the horse. The horse should not move, but should stay put in the place to which you have 'ground tied' it. The goal is for you to move and the horse to stay still. Ready? OK, go for it!"

After Activity 1 is completed, it is up to the facilitation team to decide, based on observations, how much discussion should take place at this point. Potential discussion questions are as follows:

1. What was it like trying to stop the movement of the horse?
2. What areas of their life that are moving that they wish would either slow down or stop moving?
3. How can they work to slow or stop the undesired movement?
4. What made it difficult?
5. What helped?
6. How is depression impacting their ability to stop the undesired movement?

Activity 2: Lunge

After Activity 1 is completed and any needed processing has occurred, it's time for Activity 2. The goal of Activity 2, Lunge, is for the client to create and direct the movement of the horse and to discuss the metaphor of creating/directing movement in life. The counselor says to the client, "This time, you get to stand still while the horse goes around you. So, go ahead and pick up the lunge line and see if you can get the horse moving in a circle around you. Remember, you stand still, the horse moves."

With clients who are unfamiliar with horses, this can be a challenging task. Creating movement while standing still is not easy for those who are not familiar with horses and lunge lines. Clients will generally ask lots of questions with this activity. The facilitator's task is not to teach them how to do it, but rather to encourage them to problem-solve. For example, if the client asks, "How do I do this? He's not moving!", an appropriate reply might be, "What have you tried? Do you have any other thoughts of things that might work?" It is important for teens to learn to problem-solve on their own. This can be a struggle, but it can also be quite a victory that brings confidence and hope to move on to face new challenges.

After Activity 2 is completed, potential discussion questions are as follows:

1. What was it like trying to create movement in the horse?
2. What areas of the client's life need movement?

3. How can they create the desired movement?
4. What made it difficult to move the horse?
5. What helped?
6. How is depression impacting the client's ability to create and direct the desired movement in their life?

In equine-assisted interventions, the facilitation team's role while the client is completing the activities is to observe. It is important to watch and pay attention to the words, actions, responses, emotional expressions, body language, etc., of both the client and the horse(s). All of these provide the facilitation team with information about what the client is feeling and experiencing, which can guide the processing and wrap-up discussion. The mental health and the equine professional should ask questions, express their observations, and confront or clarify based upon these observations.

It is of utmost important for counselors to be culturally sensitive to their clients. This sensitivity includes awareness of ethnicity, language, values, and family of origin concerns that may impact counseling outcomes. The counseling team's job is not to be directive, but to be sensitive and help clients find answers that are personally and culturally appropriate for the clients.

CASE EXAMPLE

Mindy (pseudonym) was a 13-year-old African-American girl who struggled with depression. Her parents were divorcing and she was living with her mother most of the time, staying with dad only on occasional weekends. However, home life was unhappy. Mom was struggling emotionally and financially. Mom was angry most evenings. Mindy tried to help out and keep her two little brothers out of mom's hair so they would not upset mom. Oftentimes, Mindy's parents would talk on the phone in the evening. Mindy's mom would usually get angry on the phone and Mindy frequently heard language that was not appropriate for a 13-year-old girl. Mindy had a hard time sleeping at night because she felt so bad about what her mom and dad were going through. This made focusing at school very hard. She often felt very sleepy at school and just wanted to put her head down and sleep. But, the teacher started calling her lazy and yelling at her. Mindy's anger became uncontrollable. Mindy started having trouble getting along with other children in her class. She was sent to the principal's office twice for hitting people. Mindy's doctor diagnosed her with depression.

Mindy came to Hope Unbridled, Inc. (HUI) for equine-assisted counseling. HUI provides Eagala model equine-assisted counseling. Mindy was invited into the very large arena where she could see five horses. We took some time to have her tell us about her observations of the horses. After discussing her observations, she went on to complete the activities. The following is a synopsis of some of the key moments of the session with Mindy.

Mindy had some trouble catching the horse she chose. In fact, the catching took about 30 minutes. This horse happened to be a rescue that had been abused. This horse would much rather run than be caught.

The following transcript analysis are about a pseudonym client.

Table 4.1
Transcript Analysis of Case Example

Transcript	*Analysis*
Client: What's that one's name?	Client seems to be drawn to a specific horse and would like to know about the horse.
Counselor: What would you name her if you could name her?	The horse's name is not revealed because we want information about what the client is seeing in the horse.
Client: Hmmm... I'd call her Freedom. She seems to really want to be free.	The horse was difficult to catch; the client sees this as a positive and names her Freedom. This provides the mental health team with interesting information.

Mindy caught Freedom and got the halter on her after quite an ordeal. Mindy expressed some frustration at the difficulty of the task and appeared to consider choosing a different horse, but persisted in her attempts until she finally caught her horse. The first activity was to Ground Tie the horse. For this activity, Mindy had chosen a challenging horse indeed.

During the course of Activity 1, facilitators realized that they had forgotten to state in the instructions that touching the horse while going around it was not allowed. However, Mindy had chosen such a difficult horse that the facilitators decided to let it go and allow Mindy to touch. Here is an abbreviated transcript of Mindy trying to "Ground Tie" Freedom.

Table 4.2

Transcript Analysis of Case Example Continued

Transcript	*Analysis*
Client: Why won't she stand still?	Client seems to be experiencing some frustration.
Counselor: What do you think she's feeling right now?	This question points the client to focus on the other individual in the relationship. What is the "other" feeling? How are those feelings impacting their behavior?
Client: I think she's scared. She wants to run away.	Client is now focusing on the horse's perspective.
Counselor: You think she's scared and her fear makes her want to leave?	Counselor paraphrases client's words to affirm her analysis and not disturb her thoughts.

Mindy spent some time talking in a soothing voice to Freedom. She verbally reassured her that everything was OK. Mindy stroked the horse to help calm the horse. Mindy walked around the horse touching the horse and pushing back and saying "Whoa," whenever the horse seemed to want to move. Mindy seemed quite pleased with herself when she completed the circle. Due to the horse Mindy had selected, Activity 1 was most likely the more difficult task. Therefore, the facilitators decided to process Activity 1 on the spot.

Table 4.3

Transcript Analysis of Case Example Continued

Transcript	*Analysis*
Client: I did it! That was *hard*! She wanted to git, but I got her to stand still and stay!	Client is very pleased at having completed the task.
Counselor: What do you think made the difference for her?	This question asks the client to reflect on what happened in the activity.
Client: I think I made her feel safe by talking soft and petting her.	Client is now focusing on the horse's perspective.
Counselor: What were you feeling while you were doing this?	Counselor asks client to focus on her emotional experience.
Client: I was kind of afraid that I wasn't going to be able to do it. But, I really wanted to do it.	Client is reflecting on her experience and openly expressing her self-doubt.
Counselor: What made it so important to you to be able to do it?	Counselor explores client values/motivation.
Client: *After some avoidant words and behaviors.* Cuz it seems lately like I can't do anything right. I try at school and fail; I try to help my mom, but she gets mad and yells at me anyway... I really wanted this horse to trust me.	Client expresses awareness of her "failures" and expresses a desire for trust.
Counselor: As I watched you doing this, I saw that you are seemed to change or soften your body language. What was going on there?	Counselor wants to see how self-aware client is of the techniques she used to calm the horse.

(Continued)

Transcript	*Analysis*
Client: I wanted to not be scary to her.	Client expresses self-awareness.
Counselor: Are you ready to try the next activity?	Transition to second activity.
Client: I think so. That was fun.	Client joins in whole-heartedly.

Activity 2 was expected to be much easier. The horse had already expressed a desire to move. Directing that movement would be the new challenge. Mindy seemed to be somewhat soft-spoken and physically timid. Based on observations of Mindy's posture and body language, self-confidence appeared to be lacking. Mindy frequently hesitated in her movements—for example, beginning to take a step one direction, then hesitating, or starting to reach out to touch the horse, then pulling her hand back as if she's worried that she'll frighten the horse. The shortened transcript of Activity 2 follows.

Table 4.4

Transcript Analysis of Case Example Continued

Transcript	*Analysis*
Client: I don't want to pull on her head! But she just wants to run *away* from me, not in the direction I want her to go.	Client expresses frustration over things not working as she hoped. Client is also expressing concern for the feelings and desires of the horse.
Counselor: Hmmm... what have you tried?	This question asks the client to reflect on what they've tried, what they haven't tried, and begin problem-solving on her own.
Client: I just let the line out and when she started going, I pulled it back tight.	Client reflects on her technique.
Counselor: What else could you try?	Counselor encourages client to problem-solve.
Client: Maybe talking to her again? That worked last time.	Client comes up with a new plan and instigates it. The horse indeed, turns and focuses her eyes on the speaker, but stops.
Client: Now she *stopped!*	Awareness of a new problem.
Counselor: Hmmm... now that's a new problem, isn't it? What would you like to try next?	Returning responsibility to the client.
Client: Hmmm... I don't want to scare her, or be bossy... dang... *Client intent on thinking about how to solve the problem.*	Client ponders the problem, options, past techniques, etc. Continues talking to the horse and using her body language to try to get the horse moving, but in a circle, not away from her. Takes her left arm and points left... saying, "Go this way!"

After some time, the horse went around Mindy. Not in the perfect arc of a compass—but around Mindy. Mindy was again pleased with completing the task. As the time was approaching the end of the session, the processing was a bit short, but Mindy left with lots to think about.

Table 4.5
Transcript Analysis of Case Example Continued

Transcript	*Analysis*
Counselor: You did it! What was that like for you?	Probing into the client's reaction to completing the task.
Client: That was kind of easier and kind of harder.	Client's reaction is a bit confused.
Counselor: What do you mean by that?	Asking for clarification.
Client: Well, easier cuz she wanted to move. Harder cuz she wanted to *leave*, not go in the circle. So...I *did* it, but it wasn't really a very nice circle.	Client expresses a desire to do a "nice" circle. Counselor makes a note to pursue "perfectionism" in the next session.
Counselor: Does Freedom care what your circle looked like?	Counselor wants client to leave on a positive note.
Client: She doesn't even know what a circle is! *Laughing*.	Client reframes something that was frustrating her.
Counselor: Why don't you spend some alone-time with Freedom until your mom gets here? Here's a brush, you can brush her and talk to her, and maybe you can find her "special spot" where she really loves to be scratched!	Alone-time is an important part of EAC—allowing clients to share deep secrets with a confidante who will never reveal what they are told.

This was Mindy's first session of EAC. When Mindy arrived, she seemed happy to be at the farm. She grinned happily upon seeing the horses. Her body language expressed some hesitation and uncertainty in how to behave in this new setting. This session allowed Mindy to gain knowledge and experience in creating and stopping movement. This session also increased levels of hope in Mindy as measured by the Adolescent Domain Specific Hope Scale (ADSHS, Frederick, 2011). Hope has been found to be negatively associated with depression (Chang, 2003). Researchers have found a significant inverse relationship between hope and depression with depression decreasing as hope increases (Ashby, Dickinson, Gnilka, & Noble, 2011). Future sessions with Mindy noted several references to this specific session. Mindy later stated that success in these activities had given her hope and made her feel as though the depression could not hold her down any more. These activities have proven to be great starter activities in a series of equine-assisted growth activities because successful completion of difficult tasks builds hope. Even if just one session is provided, these activities provide positive outcomes in combatting depression by building hope in adolescents and in adults.

REFERENCES

Ashby, J. S., Dickinson, W. L., Gnilka, P. B., & Noble, C. L. (2011). Hope as a mediator and moderator of multidimensional perfectionism and depression in middle school students. Journal of Counseling & Development, 89, 131–139.

Chang, E. C. (2003). A critical appraisal and extension of hope theory in middle-aged men and women: Is it important to distinguish agency and pathways components? Journal of Social and Clinical Psychology, 22, 121–143.

Equine-Assisted Growth and Learning Association (2017). Eagala. Retrieved from http://home.eagala.org/works.

Frederick, K. (2011). Adolescent Domain-Specific Hope Scale. Unpublished manuscript.

Frederick, K., Ivey-Hatz, J., & Lanning, B. (2015). Not just horsing around: The impact of equine-assisted learning on levels of hope and depression in at-risk adolescents. Community Mental Health Journal, 51, 809–817.

Goodyer, I. M., Dubicka, B., Wilkinson, P., Kelvin, R., Roberts, C., Byford, S., et al. (2008). A randomized controlled trial of cognitive behavior therapy in adolescents with major depression treated by selective serotonin reuptake inhibitors. The ADAPT trial. Health Technology Assess, 12(14).

Maslow, A. H. (1970). Motivation and Personality. Revised edition. New York: Harper & Row.

National Institute of Mental Health (2017). Major Depression Among Adolescents. Retrieved from www.nimh.nih.gov/health/statistics/prevalence/major-depression-among-adolescents.shtml.

Smith, M. & Segal, J. (2017) Parent's Guide to Teen Depression: Recognizing the Signs and Helping Your Child. Retrieved from www.helpguide.org/articles/depression/parents-guide-to-teen-depression.htm.

Section 3
ANXIETY

5

The Transitioning Families Equine-Assisted Model for the Treatment of Anxiety

Rebecca F. Bailey and Elizabeth Bailey

INTRODUCTION—DESCRIPTION OF THE PROBLEM

Anxiety: it can be helpful to improve performance, but it can also be devastating and disabling. Social anxiety and agoraphobia create a life where the sufferer lives isolated and afraid; post-traumatic stress response is exhausting, keeping one in a state of hyper-vigilance always; and panic attacks might have a person running to the emergency room, sure that, this time, it is a real heart attack. The individual is living in a state of fear, never sure what is really happening. Danger is misinterpreted, and the body goes into fight, flight, or freeze mode to protect itself. This physiological response may be "excessive" related to the actual danger of the stressor, and the individual becomes exhausted and unable to rationally perceive the surrounding environment.

The National Institute of Mental Health (2017), states that the 12-month prevalence for any anxiety within adults is 19.1% and that the lifetime prevalence is 31.9%. But who among us has not experienced anxiety? Anxiety disorders cost the U.S. more than $42 billion a year, almost one-third of the country's $148 billion total mental health bill, according to a study commissioned by the Anxiety and Depression Association of America, entitled "The Economic Burden of Anxiety Disorders" (Greenberg et al., 1999). More than $22.84 billion of those costs are associated with the repeated use of health care services as people with anxiety disorders seek relief for symptoms that mimic physical illnesses (Anxiety and Depression Association of America, 2010–2016).

TREATMENT OF ANXIETY

Anxiety disorders are different than the everyday normal anxiety that is a common experience in modern life. Anxiety disorders come in all shapes and sizes, from generalized anxiety, to post-traumatic stress syndrome, to full-blown panic attacks, all usually disabling. Treating anxiety is not a one-size-fits-all proposition. Treatments can include: psychoeducation; teaching skills and techniques such as coping strategies, self-regulation, and methods to address automatic thoughts and core beliefs; encouraging insight into cognitive distortions and mindfulness; psycho-dynamically oriented talk therapy, exploring history, family of origin, emotional triggers and reactions and much more. These treatments derive from evidence-based techniques from theories based on Cognitive Behavioral Therapy, Behavioral Therapy and Dialectical Behavioral Therapy, and from the theoretical influences of Psychodynamic Therapy (akin to brief Psychoanalytic therapy), Solution Focused Therapy, Client Centered Therapy, and others.

The medical model for managing anxiety can be effective but may be limited, treatment usually includes medications such as benzodiazepines or antidepressants with an antianxiety component: Ativan, Xanax, Valium, Effexor or Wellbutrin, among others. These are medications typically prescribed to manage the challenging symptoms of anxiety, but most of them are reported to be ineffective in the long term. In addition, all medications carry side-effects; patients often complain about the way these medications make them feel. The talk therapy model can be successful in teaching coping strategies, providing ways to manage dysfunctional automatic thoughts, and exploring some of the root causes. But talk and medications are not always completely useful, and may not address or provide insight into the basic triggers and interpretations that cause the physiological response of fight, flight, or freeze.

Overcoming phobia and managing responses to stress may involve retraining the autonomic nervous system and the subsequent response of the sympathetic nervous system. Often a triggering event will engage the ensuing immediate and unconscious response (i.e., increased anxiety or panic). It can be a difficult challenge to learn new ways to manage anxiety, because it is often easier for individuals to avoid the stimulus that provokes it than it is to suffer the discomfort. Another common variable in anxiety is the constant presence of negative and critical self-talk, making an important component of addressing anxiety the teaching of attainable skills for self-management of symptoms and the automatic thoughts preceding them. If the client can learn to see symptoms, perceptions, and responses a little differently, he or she could more efficiently tackle the challenges of everyday life.

Thus, we have observed that partnering with horses in a controlled therapeutic setting, and in an organic and spontaneous manner, can be an effective treatment for anxiety, post-traumatic stress, and other related issues. The client is provided with the opportunity for understanding, through the relationship with horses in a new, non-verbal way, which is then cognitively processed with the help of the clinician. Regardless of theory or model adopted, the therapeutic relationship is essential to success. It is accepted that therapeutic alliance is the most predictive of positive outcome across a range of psychotherapies (Norcross & Wampold, 2011) and it is incumbent upon the treating professionals to develop this alliance with their clients. Engaging the client in a working alliance can encourage that individual to view his or herself in a new and different way and to begin to consider perspectives other than their own (Selby & Smith-Osborne, 2013). This essential component may lead to better outcomes in the treatment of anxiety.

EQUINE-ASSISTED THERAPY

Equine-assisted psychotherapies are those that integrate equine activities within a treatment program's broader framework (Klontz, Bivens, Leinart, & Klontz, 2007), mostly through working on the ground rather than riding. Horses can be agents of therapeutic change; it is possible for them to draw out a range of emotions and responses in individuals that lead to increased insight and, eventually, to change. Observing and understanding equine behavior can assist the client in interpreting and responding appropriately to perceived threats. Horses can be excellent teachers, quick to sense and reflect influences in their environment, including human behavior. Modalities focused on somatic experience such as equine groundwork or recreational therapies may help reduce symptoms of post-traumatic stress (Cloitre et al., 2011). Learning with the help of horses is remarkably efficient given the normal short nature of intensive treatment.

Just like people, horses have their own temperaments and styles. Horses can provide immediate information about human behavior due to their acute sensitivity to their environment and the energy, and observing the equine reaction can provide the mental health professional with valuable information about the client. This innate ability to accurately read and interpret their immediate environment ensures the survival of the individual animal, and of the entire species. Horses are attuned to danger nearby, but will just as easily "let go" of their response and return to grazing; they don't hold on to the fear, and they don't hold grudges. One of the most valuable lessons learned by watching horses is their ability to regulate, relax, and return to grazing after the perceived danger has passed .

Equine-assisted therapy provides a powerful tool for the treatment and management of anxiety, grounded in the theory of experiential learning and therapy. Experiential therapy took root in the 1970s, encompassing a number of different types of therapy and therapeutic interventions designed to focus on actual involvement with various experiences, evoking emotional processing, interactions with and reactions to others (including the horses), increased insight and development of new meaning while freeing the individual from defensive or constricting behaviors (Corey, 2013). Experiential therapy goes beyond traditional talk therapy. In experiential therapy, direct experience is considered the primary agent of change (Mahrer, 1983). Change is created through experience rather than through cognition, behavior modification, or by addressing cognitive distortions. Although the data collection and research related to the treatment of anxiety with equine-assisted therapy requires further development, the suggestion is that it may be an effective way to treat this disorder Animal-assisted therapy "was associated with reduced state anxiety levels for hospitalized patients with a variety of psychiatric diagnoses" (Barker & Dawson, 1998).

EQUINE-ASSISTED THERAPY AT TRANSITIONING FAMILIES

At Transitioning Families, equine-assisted therapy is a large component of treatment. The horses, as a therapist, join with the mental health therapist and the horse professional to provide a therapeutic milieu and directed session. The trained and licensed mental health clinician will explore the client's understanding of both their own behavior and that of the horse during and after the session, with further therapy in the office at a later time. The mental health clinician works in a way that is similar to his or her role in the therapy office, acting as a guide, providing feedback, asking directed questions and *listening* to the client. The mental health professional will occasionally intervene to redirect an exercise, or to point out a behavior that cannot wait until post-exercise discussion. The trained horse professional will observe the horses' responses and behaviors and when they happened, and may intervene if necessary. During processing and discussion post-interaction, the horse professional might ask the client what he or she noticed. In this way, the mental health professional, horse professional, and the horses work together as a team in a therapeutic relationship to provide treatment to the client.

Sometimes, clients arrive at Transitioning Families carrying anxiety about working with horses. It may take some time to help them understand that the horses are essential members of the team and have equal importance as other members such as the mental health professional and the horse professional. In another twist, clients may be more comfortable interacting with the animals than with the human team members (Diane Ehrensaft, personal communication, 1990). This is not uncommon, and may require the mental health professional to work on human-to-human connection before proceeding with an exercise.

Another important component of the Transitioning Families model is the focus on normalization of symptoms. Individuals often feel "shamed" and isolated by what they think are embarrassing symptoms or ideas. Allowing clients to confront their common fears creates control and problem-solving. Confronting shame based beliefs is at the core of psychodynamic theory. At Transitioning Families, using real life experiences as well as equine therapy and other therapeutic techniques can vastly decrease the time needed for developing and problem-solving approaches to anxiety-laden responses.

ETHICAL ISSUES

The professionals must put the needs of the client first; and must remain aware of his or her own needs, personal problems, or sources of countertransference. This can be challenging when the horses participating in the exercises are owned by either the mental health professional or horse professional. In that case, the practitioners would do well to debrief after the intervention, and to explore their own countertransference. The mental health professional must abide by the ethics of his or her professional organization. In keeping with accepted ethics, all participants, including horses and humans, must be treated with the utmost respect and dignity. "Professionals are expected to exercise prudent judgment when it comes to interpreting and applying ethical principles to specific situations" (Corey, 2013, p. 38). All mental health professionals should consult regularly with others in their field. Mental health professionals should operate with a broad understanding of orientations and theories. If an area is out of the scope of the mental health professional, a consultation or referral should be made.

The client has the right to informed consent—to be informed about this therapy and "to make autonomous decisions pertaining to it" (Corey, 2013, p, 40). Sometimes, this may mean that the equine work is not yielding the expected results. Other experiential activities such as cooking, art, or music therapy may provide a better therapeutic environment for treatment. Exploration of the client's experience as the work unfolds is important so that individual needs can be met appropriately. The client also has the right to privacy—confidentiality is an abiding ethic in every care-giving profession. The Health Insurance Portability and Accountability Act of 1996 (HIPAA) exists to protect the client from having information shared electronically without their explicit knowledge or permission. Practitioners have the ethical duty to define the degree of confidentiality that can be promised and to establish the basic trust between client and provider. There are laws that mandate breaking this confidentiality in certain circumstances, such as abuse of a child, elderly person, or dependent adult.

Consideration must always be made for the safety for the horses at all times. Modeling by treating horses as an honored part of the team is imperative. Many families and individuals have never had the experience of being treated with kindness and respect. The very act of asking the horse for permission to approach during an exercise can generalize to all areas of life outside of the arena. Horses may become stressed or otherwise affected by the emotional state of a client, and vice versa. The mental health and horse professional must remain attuned to the well-being of both, and be prepared to intervene if necessary. If intervention is necessary, a discussion can follow from a variety of perspectives: psychoeducational, Cognitive Behavioral, or through insight-oriented reflection. The moment should not be ignored, and can be seen as an opportunity for growth and change.

GUIDELINES IN CONSIDERATION OF MULTICULTURAL ISSUES AND ETHICS

The professionals must consider the cultural context of the client, including clarification of cultural assumptions and differences. For some clients, exploring cultural perceptions of animals can be an important area for discussion: again, not everyone will be open to working with horses. An important concept to the Transitioning Families model is to "Meet the client where the client is." An example of this comes through a young client who had been through years of abuse and was very skeptical of working with equine therapy. She suggested that would like to brush one of the horses. This particular horse did not happen to respond well to touch. Like the woman, she too had been physically abused in the past. The girl and the horse spent numerous hours together while the client brushed the air around the horse. This was not an exercise developed by the team, but by the client. It was effective, and the horse stood, relaxed with ears forward and eyes half open. The client had broken through the horse's resistance to touch and was then able to brush the horse's coat, mane, and tail. This is an example of a client-centered, horse-centered intervention.

Occasionally clients may have medical considerations, such as allergies, that limit engagement with the animals. Creative collaboration and understanding what the point of an exercise might be, can lead to alternate interactions, such as video connections. This is not optimum, yet watching videos of equine responses can entice lively discussion.

DESCRIPTION OF INTERVENTION

A treatment plan is created from diagnosis and may address other appropriate issues or behaviors. Specific exercises are created by the entire treatment team and are derived from the treatment plan. Horses react or respond, offering information to the client, and to both the mental health professional and the horse professional. This provides material for discussion post-exercise and in the therapy office with the mental health professional. In some cases, the team will intervene actively to a response from the horse. The job of a mental health professional at Transitioning Families is to shine a light in to areas that may be otherwise avoided or missed. Individuals and families come to work with the team for assistance in moving forward in their lives, to solve problems, to reconnect with one another, or to address specific issues. Treatment is provided on a case-by-case basis with the involvement of both the client and the entire treatment team. "The overarching goal of the Transitioning Families Therapeutic Reunification Model (TFTRM) is to assist families in transitioning from crisis, challenge or conflict to connection and growth" (Judge et al., 2016, p. 235).

CASE EXAMPLE

The mother and daughter chose to attend a Transitioning Families workshop because the daughter had been previously abducted. The team designed this specific exercise for the mother and daughter, to address their ongoing issues of anxiety. Other diagnoses may have applied to both mother and daughter, but the presenting symptoms seemed more applicable to generalized anxiety interspersed with specific phobic responses; symptoms that, in both participants, seemed to be magnified and exacerbated as they faced the challenge of reconnecting to each other. This complex presentation required thoughtful planning in order to address the psychological needs appropriately.

In this case, the intervention deemed best by the clinical team was a mounted exercise. This exercise was chosen to provide an opportunity for a real-time experience of anxiety and fear, and to allow the daughter to demonstrate a proficiency the mother did not have (during her abduction, the young woman had been sequestered on a ranch with the father and had learned to ride, the mother had no prior experience of being on a horse). It was important to continue to provide opportunities for connection between mother and daughter; however, anxiety was affecting their interactions and needed to be addressed directly. This mother and daughter required some simple tools to manage their symptoms. By managing those symptoms more effectively, they could efficiently tackle the challenges of everyday life together.

Materials Needed

This is a mounted exercise involving one mental health professional and one equine professional.

- Dry erase board to list challenges that provoke anxiety
- Sharpies and note cards with tape to fasten the cards down
- Two horses
- Saddles
- Bridles
- Lead ropes
- Bareback pad (if used).

Steps

1. Using the dry erase board, the mother and daughter made a list of areas, situations, and events that might activate anxiety. The mother and daughter picked four to six anxiety-provoking areas/events/situations from the list. These were written out on note cards and fastened to the fence and various objects (e.g., jump standards) throughout the arena.
2. With the help of the equine professional, the mother and daughter chose two horses to work with. The mother and daughter were directed to place their hands on the horses' rib cage area and to notice the rhythm of their breathing. The horses were then tacked up and readied by the horse professional.
3. The first part of the exercise focused on mindful breathing. As the horses were being prepared, the mental health professional focused on mindful breathing with the mother and daughter. They stood with their hands at their sides, directed to be aware of breath and the difference between short breaths generated in the upper chest, and deep mindful breaths coming from the diaphragm, watching the stomach area expand with every inhale.
4. The exercise continued as the mother and daughter get up into the saddle, with assistance. Helmets had been placed on the fence and the mother protectively put one on her daughter's head as well as her own. Under no circumstances is anyone allowed to get on a horse without a helmet; either professional can intervene or can ask a participant what else is needed before they get on the horse.
5. The participants practiced mindful breathing as they walked around the arena, led by a horse handler or the horse professional. The mother and daughter were encouraged to hold onto, or otherwise feel the support of the saddle. They stopped, or payed attention to the marked areas of fear and anxiety as they continued mindful breathing around the arena. Both were encouraged to observe their own breathing as well as any other physiological reactions

such as "tightening, pain, or avoidance." The horses responded to the "energy" of their riders, which was noted by the horse professional for later discussion.

6. An option, depending on time, is to remove the saddles and switch to the bareback pads, noticing the difference between riding with support and without the support of the saddle.

Note. The mother and the daughter approached the horses and both agreed they were anxious by the different sizes of the horses. The mother initially encouraged the daughter to get on the smaller horse. However, because the daughter had ridden before, she convinced her mother that she would work with larger horse and the mother could take the smaller one. When the daughter raised herself up into the saddle from the mounting block the mother gasped as the horse move three steps forward. Her daughter instantly told her to stop being overprotective, she was "fine." When the mother went over to get on her horse she verbalized her own fear beginning with the mounting block which, she said, was "too high." Eventually, she asked that the mental health professional come stand next to her. The mental health professional complied and stood an arm's length away. The horse moved away from the block. Tears ran down the mother's cheeks. The mental health professional asked her what the tears were about. Mother responded by saying there were so many things she had missed when her child was away from her. Deep, mindful breathing was encouraged to ground and calm her. When mom felt able she attempted to guide the horse back to the block but the horse moved away again immediately. The mom asked the mental health professional to help. It was suggested that the mom might ask the more appropriate person: the horse professional. Once the mom had settled in the saddle, the mental health professional asked what had happened. The mother responded by saying: "It's the same crap I dealt with all those years—asking the wrong people for something they can't give me. Her father was just relentless and did not care."The daughter had not noticed her mother's tears at first, and appeared surprised when she learned what they were about. She looked directly at her mother and stated: "I wish you would understand that my dad was not as terrible as you seem to think," at which point the horse started shaking her head and began to move away. The mental health professional responded asked if they wanted to continue to discuss either the mother's topic or the daughter's statement. Both mother and daughter suggested they continue with the exercise.

The exercise proceeded without further incident, although both participants noted that they "really noticed the physical changes" when they approached the various marked areas of fear or anxiety. After the exercise was completed (time limited), further exploration of response to the exercise was discussed. Both participants verbalized increased insight into "what happens to my body" as well as the effects of mindful, deliberate breathing as a way to manage those feelings. The topics brought up by both mother and daughter were briefly discussed, with follow-up discussions continued in the context of therapy in the office.

Discussion

Diagnosing the type of anxiety seen in clients can be a challenge, and can be even more complex in families where abduction has been an issue. Diagnosis should only be made by a trained and licensed professional, and only if it falls within the professional's specific scope of practice. Amateur diagnosing is always problematic and may even be harmful.

In the case example described above, the mother had suffered from agoraphobia before her daughter's disappearance that continued during the "missing years." Evidence that agoraphobia is a hereditary disease is limited; however, it has been suggested that 15–25% of children with agoraphobia have an acrophobic parent. The daughter verbalized her own specific anxiety, that of a fear of heights coupled with an occasional "strong desire to jump from a high place." She reported that she had even gone as far as to climb to the top of a tree outside her father's home and had counted to ten in anticipation of jumping to the earth below. The daughter also expressed the feeling that she could not manage her anxiety in circumstances where she was afraid, made much worse by the threats and accusations made by each parent. What made matters worse was that the daughter's anxiety fed into the mother's anxiety, contributing to dysregulation in both.

The diagnosis of post-traumatic stress disorder is another diagnosis that could apply to both mother and daughter, but the predominant presenting symptoms fit a little better with generalized anxiety disorder, interspersed with specific phobic responses. Symptoms in both mother and daughter seemed magnified and exacerbated when faced with the challenge of reconnection. Research indicates that personality type may be inherited (Tellegen et al., 1988). Further research is needed to tease out the age-old issue of nature vs. nurture, but in this family it did appear that mother and daughter shared a genetic disposition toward anxiety, as well as a shared response reaction to stress.

This understanding of specific diagnosis and knowledge of evidence-based treatment allowed the team to create an appropriate exercise involving the horses to address the issue. Psychoeducation was provided to both mother and daughter regarding the physiological response to stress, the shared genetic factors and predisposition, and the skills and abilities to interpret triggers appropriately. This discussion, which began in the arena, continued in the office throughout the family's stay at Transitioning Families. Anecdotally, both mother and daughter reported "feeling less stress," "understanding my anxiety better," and "having improved insight and now some real tools" after this work.

REFERENCES

Anxiety and Depression Association of America (2010–2016). *Did You Know?* Retrieved from https://adaa.org: https://adaa.org/about-adaa/press-room/facts-statistics.

Barker, S. B. & Dawson, K. S. (1998). The effects of animal-assisted therapy on anxiety ratings of hospitalized psychiatric patients. *Psychiatric Services, 49*(6), 797–801.

Bourne, E. J. (2015). *The Anxiety and Phobia Workbook.* Oakland, CA: New Harbinger Publications, Inc.

Cloitre, M., Courtois, C., Charuvastra, A., Carapezza, R., Stolbach, B., & Green, B. (2011). Treatment of complex PTSD: Results of the ISTSS expert clinician survey on best practices. *Journal of Traumatic Stress, 24*(6), 615–627.

Corey, G. (2013). *Theory and Practice of Counseling and Psychotherapy.* 9th edition. Belmont, CA: Brooks And Cole.

Earles, J., Vernon, L., & Yetz, J. (2015). Equine assisted therapy for anxiety and post traumatic stress symptoms. *Journal of Trauma and Stress, 28*(2), 149–152.

Greenberg, P., Sisitsky, T., Kessler, R., Finkelstein, S., Berndt, E., Davidson, J., Ballenger, J., & Fyer, A. (1999, July). The economic burden of anxiety disorders in the 1990s. *Journal of Clinical Psychiatry, 60*(7), 427–435.

Judge, A., Bailey, R., Behrman-Lippert, J., Bailey, E., Psaila, C., & Dickel, J. (2016). The therapeutic reunification model in nonfamilial abductions. *Family Court Review: An Interdisciplinary Journal, 54*(2), 232–249.

Kahonev, L. (2013). *The Power of the Herd.* Novato, CA: New World Library.

Klontz, B., Bivens, A., Leinart, D., & Klontz, T. (2007). The effectiveness of equine-assisted experiential therapy: Results of an open clinical trial. *Sociey and Animals, 15,* 257–267.

Mahrer, A. (1983). *Experiential Psychotherapy: Basic Practices.* Ottowa, Ontario, Canada: Ottowa University Press.

National Institute of Mental Health. (2017). *Any Anxiety Disorder Among Adults.* Retrieved from www.nimh.nih.gov/health/statistics/prevalence/any-anxiety-disorder-among-adults.shtml.

Norcross, J. & Wampold, B. (2011). What works for whom: tailoring psychotherapy to the person. *Journal of Clinical Psychology, 67*(2), 127–132.

Selby, A. & Smith-Osborne, A. (2013). A systematic review of effectiveness of complementary and adjunct therapies and interventions involving equines. *Health Psychology, 32*(4), 418–432.

Tellegen, A., Lykken, D., Bouchard, T. J., Wilcox, K. J., Segal, N., & Rich, S. (1988). Personality similarity in twins reared apart and together. *Journal of Personality and Social Psychology, 54*(6), 1031–1039.

6

Natural Lifemanship's Trauma-Focused Equine-Assisted Psychotherapy and Treatment of Anxiety Disorders

Bettina Shultz-Jobe, Laura McFarland, and Tim Jobe

INTRODUCTION

Affecting nearly *one in five* American adults in any given year, and *one in eight* American children (NIMH, 2017), "anxiety disorders are the most common and pervasive mental disorders in the United States" (Anxiety and Depression Association of America, 2017). Anxiety disorders are of several types, including generalized anxiety disorder (GAD), panic disorder and panic attacks, social anxiety, separation anxiety, selective mutism, and specific phobias. It is not uncommon for anxiety to co-occur with other disorders such as post-traumatic stress disorder (PTSD), depression, attention-deficit/hyperactivity disorder (ADHD), obsessive compulsive disorder (OCD), eating disorders, and substance use disorders to name a few.

Occasional anxiety is normal, but when it is experienced as persistent and overwhelming, it can be utterly disabling to those who experience it. Anxiety disorders interfere with daily life, work, and relationships and they will often wreak havoc on physical health if left untreated, increasing a sufferer's risk for a number of chronic medical conditions (Harvard Health Publications, 2017). Disproportionately affected are women, who represent two-thirds of the estimated 40 million American adults with anxiety disorders.

In addition to being female, there are genetic and environmental risk factors for anxiety disorders, among them, exposure to stressful or traumatic life events in childhood and adulthood (NIMH, 2017).

THEORETICAL APPROACH

In Natural Lifemanship's trauma-focused equine-assisted psychotherapy (TF-EAP), we employ a trauma-informed lens that enables us to address anxiety from a neurobiological perspective. With many of the clients we serve, complex trauma and early life stress underlie diagnoses of anxiety and related disorders. The relationships between stress, anxiety and observable changes in neural systems are widely documented (Etkin & Wager, 2007; Hanson et al., 2015). By drawing on the work of leading experts on trauma and the brain, including Drs. Bruce D. Perry, Frank Putnam, Stephen Porges, Bessel van der Kolk, and Dan Siegel, we approach the treatment of anxiety through interventions targeting the client's neurophysiological response to stress.

In particular, Dr. Bruce Perry's Neurosequential Model (Perry, 2006, 2009) provides a heuristic that informs client assessment and treatment. This model takes into consideration the sequential nature of the developing brain and the neurobiological human stress response system. It is understood that trauma and early life stress interact with development in ways that result in patterns of activation of the stress response system. Anxiety is a pattern of activation involving the fear state, regulated by the amygdala, insula, and hippocampus in the limbic area of the brain (Etkin & Wager, 2007; Shah, Klumpp, Angstadt, Nathan, & Phan, 2009). A heightened fear response sensitizes the entire nervous system producing the physiological states commonly associated with anxiety such as rapid heart rate and shallow breathing. As with PTSD, which evokes similar albeit more complex neurophysiological responses (Etkin & Wager, 2007; Hanson et al., 2015), the body is essentially poised to fight, flee, or freeze in response to threat. With anxiety disorders the state of arousal persists and is easily triggered, becoming an individual trait as neural patterns are activated, frequently used, and reinforced (Perry, Pollard, Blakley, Baker, & Vigilante, 1995).

Through the practice of TF-EAP, specifically its mounted component, which we call Rhythmic Riding™, TF-EAP seeks to accomplish two therapeutic objectives simultaneously:

1. Regulate the brain's lower (sensorimotor) and middle (emotional) regions, those that are hyper-activated in anxiety and either hyper- or hypo-activated in PTSD; and
2. Integrate these regions with the prefrontal lobe to facilitate the client's ability to practice self-regulation and modulate their anxiety symptoms through learned skills and cognition.

These two types of regulation are referred to respectively as "bottom-up regulation" (BUR) and "top-down (cortical) regulation" or "self-regulation."

The TF-EAP process refers often to the regions of the brain targeted. TF-EAP terminology in this chapter is as follows: "Lower brain" refers to what is colloquially known as the survival brain or sensorimotor system, comprised of the brainstem (sensory system) and diencephalon (motor system). These are the areas of the brain involved in autonomic and reactive (flight/fight/freeze) responses. The "midbrain" is where lower and upper regions connect and is typically associated with the limbic (emotional/relational) system. Finally, the "upper brain" refers to the neocortex (thinking) region. "Bottom-up" means we target the lower regions first and progress sequentially toward the upper regions of the brain, and "top-down" means the upper region influences the functioning of the lower regions. "Top-down" regulation is what is typically thought of as self-control, which includes, for example, the ability to overcome fear through reasoning, to resist impulses, and the ability to control one's breathing (an automatic reflex) through mindful intention. "Bottom-up" regulation, on the other hand, focuses on the lower regions first by providing sensorimotor input that activates those regions in a rhythmic way. When speaking of bottom-up regulation it is often necessary to distinguish between the two regions that comprise the lower brain because they respond to different stimuli. The brainstem (lowest region) responds to sensory stimuli, which includes passive movement, or the sensation of movement a person does not need to create for him or herself. The diencephalon (low-mid region) is activated when a person moves his or her own body. To use these terms in this way is certainly an oversimplification of very complex neurological systems. However, TF-EAP does so to make elaborate and intricate processes parsimonious enough to apply to clinical practice.

RATIONALE FOR TREATING ANXIETY DISORDERS WITH TF-EAP

TF-EAP treatment emphasizes the reorganization and integration of the brain to heal trauma and related neurophysiological disorders that affect regulation and relationships. Neural integration promotes top-down (self-regulation) as well as the optimal functioning of the nervous system's regulatory networks and its resilience to stress (Siegel, 2010, 2012). Through mounted work the horse promotes neural integration by providing the rhythmic, patterned, repetitive sensory input required for regulating the brainstem (Perry et al., 1995). With the brain's lower regions activated rhythmically by the horse's movement, the therapist may facilitate neural integration by asking the client to engage in movement, relational and verbal or cognitive activities that activate the rest of the brain in a sequential fashion.

In TF-EAP, a connected relationship is always the goal. Whether the client is engaged in groundwork or mounted work, connection is essential to the healing process. From a neurobiological perspective, connected relationships with primary caregivers first begin to modulate the stress response system, creating the conditions that promote a healthy stress response and the ability for self-regulation (Perry et al., 1995; Siegel, 2012). Because of its central neuroanatomical position, the brain tissue comprising the limbic (emotional and relational) system connects the regions that surround it. Connected relationships regulate the limbic system, allowing it to serve as the hub through which communication between surrounding regions of the brain may occur.

ETHICAL ISSUES IN ANIMAL-ASSISTED THERAPY (AAT) PROGRAMS

In equine-assisted psychotherapy (EAP), given the involvement of a large animal with a stress response system of their own, there is naturally some risk for all involved, including the client. In EAP, risk is real, not perceived. Real risk actually provides therapeutic benefits by stimulating eustress, a small amount of stress within the client's window of tolerance, which is the optimal level of arousal needed for learning and growth (Ogden, Minton & Pain, 2006; Siegel, 2012). To manage this risk and ensure safety, it is imperative that the therapy team is attuned to both client and horse and able to track very subtle body cues of each that reveal when eustress approaches each being's window of tolerance. When a client is, anxious there is a risk that, when pushed outside the window of tolerance, their anxiety may significantly increase. This could start to feel unsafe for the horse. The horse needs a safe connection, and therefore the therapist or equine specialist must be able to provide a safe, calm and present connection for the horse when the client is experiencing increased arousal.

A perhaps even greater ethical concern is that the eustress inherent to mounted work may push the client toward a freeze response, characterized by dissociation, submission, and compliance. Sometimes therapists mistake this for a state of calm. If the horse has also been conditioned to be dissociative, the horse may show very little response to this and thus therapy could serve to reinforce these patterns rather than transform them. It is an ethical concern for any therapist to work with anxious clients if they are unable to discern what dissociation looks like in people and horses.

Finally, anxious clients often do not feel safe to the horse. Horses need connection. When working with an anxious client it is important that the equine specialist can attend to the emotional needs of the horse (the horse needs to be able to find connection with the equine specialist) while the therapist attends to the emotional needs of the client. Asking a horse to spend time with an anxious person (one whose body energy is high and dysregulated) is not safe. Safety, which includes *felt safety*, is a basic tenet of trauma informed care. The principles of trauma informed care must apply to the client, the therapy team, *and* the horse for the work to be effective.

DESCRIPTION OF INTERVENTION

Goals and Objectives of TF-EAP

The goal of the TF-EAP mounted session is to integrate neural networks in the brain so that the client becomes increasingly able to override anxiety through top-down cognitive strategies, such as mindful breathing and self-calming techniques. The strategy for achieving this is to first regulate the brain's lower (e.g., sensorimotor) regions under mild eustress, and gradually connect the midbrain (limbic) and upper (neocortex) regions of the brain intentionally and sequentially through various kinds of tasks while the client remains mounted.

Materials Needed

A round pen or contained space is typically used to create a boundary and increase felt and actual safety for client and horse. A lead rope and halter, bareback pad, mounting block, and helmet are recommended for the same reasons. Technology may be used if desired, including a device (e.g., smartphone) that can play music such as traditional flute and drum music. Alternatively, an actual drum may be used to provide rhythmic auditory input. Finally, when practicing self-regulation skills, a portable emWave® by the HeartMath Institute is an excellent biofeedback tool, which may be used by the client before and during mounted sessions.

Adapted from Natural Lifemanship's *Rhythmic Riding Intensive* training manual.

Table 6.1

Step-by-Step Description of a TF-EAP Mounted Session

1.	The client's horse is waiting for her in a large round pen, untacked, loose, and able to graze and move freely.
2.	If the client has already done relational work, it is also good for them to initiate connection with the horse on the ground, prior to mounting. This can include attachment, detachment, and grooming—as is appropriate.
3.	The equine professional (EP) halters the horse, and adds any other tack required (we begin with a bareback pad typically).
4.	The EP then establishes a connection with the horse on the ground through attachment/detachment/touch as is appropriate and necessary. The client is told that the EP will maintain the connection and manage the horse's movement until the client is ready and able to manage some of it with her own connection. It is important that the EP understand the difference between connection, compliance, and control. Connection can be passed to the client, so that the horse is responding more to the client than to the EP. Genuine connection that engages the limbic system is central to brain integration.
5.	The EP or therapist may ask the client, "How would you like to get on your horse?" The client may decide to use a mounting block, a mounting ramp, a leg up, or any other means for getting on the horse that fits within policies and procedures of the organization.
6.	Before the client mounts, the therapist asks her to take a big deep breath. One reason for asking this is because if they are able to do so, they have just shown that they have some level of neocortical involvement. If unable to take a deep breath, it is inappropriate to start with questioning that involves thinking. It is appropriate to help the client regulate first (through sensory input or movement). The therapist may model taking a deep breath and then take one with the client.
7.	Therapist asks questions to check in and help the client connect with herself, i.e., How does she feel? What does she notice in her body? For anxiety, the therapist will also ask the client to scale her level of anxiety from one to ten.
8.	Standing at the horse's side, the therapist takes another deep breath with the client and asks her how she would like to mount, with the EP's help if appropriate. (Client can mount in any way that feels appropriate to her, and is not unsafe or unreasonable. Process unsafe or unreasonable thinking.) The EP maintains a solid connection with the horse and holds the lead rope while the client mounts.
9.	Once client is mounted encourage her to take a deep breath and perhaps scale her anxiety again to gauge difference before and after mounting.
10.	Depending on client's regulation level and ability, we initiate movement in a variety of ways. The client may use her voice to ask the EP to begin the walk, she may squeeze the horse with her legs, or if unable to do either we may let the client know we will begin walking the horse for her. What the client is able to do in this step tells us about her current regulation/dysregulation. While it is preferred the client participate in beginning the walk, passive regulation (through the horse's movement) is sometimes necessary to help the client regulate enough in their brainstem and diencephalon. Many times, auditory input that involves simple or primitive rhythm (like drumming or traditional flute music) will help regulate the lower regions of the brain, so the client can participate in beginning the walk.
11.	While moving, the EP maintains connection with the horse, leading her around the pen at a relaxed pace. The EP role in this activity is monitoring the horse's responses to the client. She may show signs of disconnect, distress, or that she would like to be more connected to the rider. All of this is information to communicate to the therapist, as the therapist is largely focused on the client.
12.	Therapist—watch the client's body as horse and client are moving. Is there any visible tension? You may say to the client, "Safety is found when you and your horse can move together. Right now, your horse is in the lead. Your only job is to allow your body to be moved by your horse."
13.	Therapist—begin to engage the client verbally while bringing her awareness to what is occurring in her body. Ask the client, "Tell me which part of your body you notice being moved by your horse." Say, "Start noticing your hips—the way the horse is moving your hips. Show me with your hands what the movement of the hips looks like" (which is often easier than verbalizing what the movement feels like). "Use your voice to talk to me about what the movement is like" (more deeply engaging the thinking part of the brain). Through these questions, you are encouraging the client to become more cognitive, increasingly engaging the neocortex. At the same time, you are assessing whether the client can notice what is happening in her body and talk about it at the same time, an activity that requires dual attention and integration between the neocortex and the mid- and lower brain. Quite often, clients will disconnect from what they experience in their body once they start thinking and talking. It is not uncommon for the horse to stop moving when this happens and the EP will have to gently ask the horse to start moving again, keeping the rhythm going.
14.	Ask the client to notice the movement she is feeling. Notice specific parts of her body—particularly her hips. A body scan can be helpful to release tension and create more connection, particularly to self.

(Continued)

15.	Throughout this activity, the therapist and the EP both look for patterns in the dynamic between client activity and horse behavior. Notice when the horse stops, is stressed, or seeking connection elsewhere. Is it when the EP begins to internally disconnect from the horse and give more of the connection to the client? Is it when the client begins to talk? If there is a pattern of disconnection when the client is asked to think about or explain something (which is fairly common), the focus will be to integrate or create better pathways between upper (thinking) and lower (feeling/sensing) regions of the brain. This will resemble a dance, repeatedly moving between asking the client to notice sensations and explain or demonstrate those sensations. In this way, the client stays engaged at the physical, emotional, and cognitive levels, and practices directing her attention fluidly between each of those experiences. The horse's continual, rhythmic movement provides predictable, repetitive sensory input that facilitates regulation and integration. When the client becomes disconnected, you can help them reconnect by asking them to return their awareness to their hips, by placing their hands on the horse's shoulders, or noticing the horse's steps.
16.	Practice self-regulation skills and tasks engaging specific areas of the brain in a bottom-up fashion. When the client is regulated and has shown some ability to shift fluidly between sensing (lower regions of the brain), feeling (midbrain), and verbalizing or demonstrating what she is experiencing in her body (upper regions of the brain), the introduction of cognitive tasks while mounted increases constructive stress (eustress), activates the neocortex, and builds cross-brain connections throughout the entire brain. Practicing self-regulation skills while mounted and supported by the horse's rhythmic, patterned, repetitive movement promotes bottom-up regulation while practicing top-down regulation. The client will therefore more readily experience success. Being mounted thus provides a scaffold for acquiring these skills. Thirdly, the client is tasked with practicing self-regulation skills while staying connected with her body and with the horse. This increases engagement of the limbic area and facilitates connection between functionally distinct areas of the brain in a regulated, organized fashion.
17.	The skill we often start with is belly breathing. We have the client practice this and then return to it anytime she appears to hold her breath or disconnect from herself or her horse. (This should be a skill that has been practiced plenty before riding, so it is easy to recall even when slightly stressed.) When the client disconnects from her body and/or from her horse, one way to help her reconnect is to direct her attention toward her horse—"Tell me what your horse is doing." This draws her away from thinking about herself and toward noticing and connecting with the horse. Then ask her to connect with her breath, again.
18.	Body scan—this can start anywhere in the body; for example, the eyes. Sometimes we start with the hips, which are the point of connection with the horse, and move down and up the body from there. During a body scan, the therapist will ask questions to guide the client, such as: "Do you feel movement in each hip? Is there a rhythm between the left and right side? How about up and down, forward and back? The therapist may then help the client relax tension through progressive muscle relaxation. Alternatively, you can ask the client to focus on the side of the body that is more relaxed (the right hip for example) and then for a short moment notice the side with more tension (the left hip). Many times, this will help the client transfer the relaxed feeling from one side of the body to the other. Continue the body scan with the client noting any changes in his or her horse. Releasing tension and blockages in one side of the body is especially important for trauma processing.
19.	As client is more able to regulate (brainstem) and connect with her own body, ask her to attempt more controlled, intentional movements (diencephalon)—like those from Brain Gym® or yoga (reaching up tall, arms out wide, crossed over chest, reaching across body, rolling ankles and wrists, etc.).
20.	Count steps (to begin engaging the neocortex). Ask the client to notice when the horse's front left leg moves forward and to say "now" every time they notice the movement of that leg. Client may or may not be able to do this without looking at their horse's leg, and they may disconnect from their horse or themselves when they engage the neocortex. Sometimes the client will struggle to connect with the horse's movement and simultaneously with the sensations they feel in their body while they are also trying to count or talk. Each time disconnection occurs between the client and herself or her horse, help her reconnect by bringing awareness back to her body, her hips and the horse's movement. Ask the client to notice what her horse is doing to help her reconnect to her horse.
21.	What we are trying to accomplish through this process is to build connections between the brain's lower (somatosensory) regions and its mid- to upper (feeling/thinking) regions. As the brain reorganizes in this way, it becomes possible to for it to reorganize around traumatic memories. Without these pathways, it remains impossibl to think rationally about traumatic memories or feelings. While mounted, the client benefits from instantaneous feedback whenever disconnections occur. One way we help clients notice when they lose connection is to ask them to keep the horse moving, instead of relying on the EP to keep the horse moving. In this way, whenever the horse stops the client must notice it and re-establish connection, giving the horse a little squeeze.
22.	As the client progresses over time, she can be given more responsibility of the connection with her horse. The EP may hold the lead rope more loosely, allow the client to initiate starting and stopping, or turn the lead rope into reins for the client and walk alongside or stand off to the side.
23.	Practice variations with increasing challenge and complexity. Here are some variations that increase the challenge when the client has been successful at the cognitive exercises presented thus far: count forward and backward by threes; breathe in rhythm with the horse's steps; inhale and exhale over a certain number of steps; ask them to move their arms in ways that cross the midline (refer to Brain Gym® for ideas); make an infinity symbol in the air with each hand and then with both hands while the horse is moving; raise up the arms in a yoga mountain pose or warrior pose; incorporate shoulder rolls and expansive arm movements; ask clients to expand their awareness to horse, self and surroundings; learn and practice Emotional Freedom Technique (EFT), or tapping, on the ground and then on the back of the horse while moving; have clients create rhythms with handheld percussion instruments while moving on the horse's back; engage clients in any challenging cognitive tasks such as math problems, memory games and riddles.

24. As the session comes to a close, save time at the end for a few minutes of mindfulness and relaxation again, after the challenging work. This can be a few rounds of breathing, feeling the horse's movements, feeling the sun or breeze, watching trees sway in the wind, etc.
25. Bring the horse to a stop. Ask the client to scale her anxiety again to make sure client is regulated enough to end for the day. Encourage the client to breathe and thank her horse in some way.
26. Allow the client to dismount, with support from the EP and therapist as needed.

Guidelines in Consideration of Multicultural Issues and Ethics

To be culturally responsive requires insight into one's own cultural biases and perspectives as well as an awareness of the dimensions on which cultures may vary. Some of the considerations that pertain to this work include how a culture views animals and human relationships with animals, especially horses. Furthermore, cultures may vary in the valence given qualities of relationship between humans. For example, while modern, Western cultures generally understand submission to be an undesirable relationship dynamic, some traditional cultures consider it an expected norm between certain groups, classes, genders, or species in which a power differential is implicitly understood within the culture. Likewise, ideas about mental health and its treatment may vary, and also concepts about how the body and mind interact and function. There are diverse cultural norms regarding the value placed on personal autonomy and self-determination (individualism) versus group identity and cohesion (collectivism). Social norms and the expression of emotions can vary widely. How we experience connection may also vary. Because of the many dimensions across which people may vary, it is important to seek to know what triggers anxiety in our clients based on their own cultural values and beliefs. To be culturally responsive means we do not assume that our values, our ways of thinking, and our affective responses are universal. We must seek to understand our clients on their terms and be flexible in our approach to treatment.

CASE EXAMPLE AND SAMPLE CASE TRANSCRIPT

Brief Description of Client and Case History

Linda (pseudonym) is a 35-year-old female with an extensive history of complex trauma. Growing up her world was chaotic, and she has major attachment wounds. Her mother continues to struggle with severe mental health issues. Linda's earliest memories of sexual trauma begin at age 3–4, when she experienced abuse by different caretakers and nannies. Throughout childhood, Linda and her family moved in and out of international war zones. Her mother's severe depression left her unable to connect with and nurture Linda. The mother herself was sexually assaulted during her pregnancy with Linda. Once at the age of eight, when war erupted in her country, Linda was left with a neighbor who brutally raped her. Her entire life could be characterized by the experience of abusive relationships and the failure of close relationships to nurture and protect. As a teenager and young adult, she self-medicated with drugs and experienced episodes of homelessness. Despite her chaotic upbringing, Linda is now a highly educated professional with three children who are doing well.

The tragic loss of a family member is what brought Linda to therapy. The event made her think differently about her life history and she began to experience uncontrollable fear and anxiety. During the intake session Linda reported the following concerns: excessive anxiety that she can't control; feeling irritable and on edge; easily fatigued; difficulty concentrating; muscle tension; and sleep disturbance. She had started to miss work and struggle with personal and professional relationships due to her anxiety. Based on the intake and assessment process Linda was diagnosed with generalized anxiety disorder. Although she did not meet full DSM criteria for PTSD, we recognize that the life of trauma she's experienced, which includes the recent traumatic event, contributes to her anxiety. We therefore understood her anxiety as a symptom of complex trauma.

Treating anxiety through a trauma lens means we seek to understand the neurobiological patterns, which are often adaptive responses to trauma, underlying the anxiety the client experiences. We then seek to regulate the brain's neural systems sequentially while creating integration between them. The ultimate goal is sufficient neural integration so the client may begin to self-regulate and process the trauma.

The following transcript analysis are about a pseudonym client.

Table 6.2

Transcript and Analysis of Case Example

Transcript	*Analysis*
Context: By the time we began to use mounted work, the client had already completed about 15 sessions of relationship-building work with Brownie (horse) on the ground. This particular transcript represents a 1.5-hour therapy session focused on full brain integration through Rhythmic Riding Creating integration in the brain not only treats anxiety but also attachment disorders by stimulating an earned attachment pattern (Siegel, 2010).	
PREPARATION TO MOUNT	
Therapist: Before we ride today, why don't you and Brownie start with some connection?	Connection is always the goal— having the intention of riding for the day does not override this primary goal.
Client: Begins by connecting with Brownie through attachment and detachment. Client spent about five minutes asking for connection while close, as well as with distance.	Typically, sessions build on each previous session. Clients review what has already been accomplished in the relationship in order to check in with themselves and their horse—and to evaluate for areas needing more work.
Client: Once connected, client spent a couple of minutes massaging Brownie.	This helped client to connect. Because of her attachment wounds, client found connection without touch to be very difficult. Giving touch reaps many of the same physiological benefits as receiving touch, and is an important part of regulation and brain organization. The rhythmic sensory input provided by grooming Brownie provided bottom-up and co-regulation for both—because of the previously established connections.
While therapist and client step aside and prepare to mount, equine specialist does some attachment work with Brownie.	In preparation for the mounted session, which will trigger client's anxiety making it difficult for the client to connect at times, the equine specialist makes sure they can request and maintain a strong connection with the horse. This is very important for the horse's well-being, for the therapeutic process (where they horse must remain engaged and connected to provide valuable feedback), and for the client's safety.
Therapist: Why don't we take a deep breath together before you get on?	Therapist takes a couple of deep breaths with client and lets out an audible exhale. This is more co-regulation and reminds client to breathe. It engages her entire brain to have to think (neocortex) about her breath (breath is usually modulated in the brainstem) and breathe in unison with the therapist (which requires limbic connection).
Therapist: How are you feeling right now? What do you notice in your body? On a scale from one to ten, how intense is the feeling you feel right now in your body?	These questions cause the client to tune into the sensations in her body, connecting her upper and lower brain regions and finding a sense of connection; and, they offer a benchmark that will be a useful anchor for checking in with the client later in the session.
Client: I have just a little anxiety—my heart is beating kind of fast and my chest feels a little tight, but it's not too bad. I would say it's about a three right now. It was higher before I started grooming.	For client to be able to talk about what is happening in her body and even quantify the intensity of the experience means she is regulated enough to mount the horse. Her neocortex is engaged, and she is present and connected.
Therapist: I'm glad to hear connecting with Brownie helped some. How would you like to get on today?	We prefer to ask the client how they would like to mount the horse, even if options are limited. Typically, we give them their options. Choice engages the neocortex and provides valuable feedback to the therapist regarding the client's thinking.
Client: Will you give me a boost? (to the therapist)	The fact that the client chose a leg-up, which involves touch, was a sign that she was regulated enough in her limbic (emotional/relational) system to be OK with touch. She showed improvement from the previous session, where she had requested to mount from the fence, not wanting to be touched.
Therapist: Breathing calmly while standing alongside client and horse: When you're ready to get on, bend your leg at the knee and I will boost you up—with one hand on your knee and one hand on your ankle, is that ok?	Therapist will provide a leg-up while equine specialist holds the lead rope and maintains connection with the horse. This ensures safety in the event that the client experiences any fear or heightened arousal while mounting. We always ask before touching—to offer clients predictability and a choice each time.
Therapist: Take a deep breath with me, and up we go.	The therapist asks client to take another deep breath to release the pressure inside of her prior to mounting, as well as to simply practice a useful self-regulation skill. The more she practices this successfully in mildly stressful situations during therapy sessions, the more natural it is for her to use mindful breathing in situations outside of therapy sessions to regulate her anxiety.

Transcript	*Analysis*
MOUNTED—FOCUS ON BOTTOM-UP REGULATION, CONNECTION, AND INTEGRATION	
Therapist: Settle onto Brownie's back, and take another breath—let's sigh on the exhale this time.	Therapist encourages client to "arrive" on Brownie's back as regulated as possible before doing anything else. This is a good point to check in on client's dysregulation level. The equine specialist will notice if Brownie has a response to the client.
Therapist: For now, the equine specialist will be in charge of connecting with Brownie and asking her to move—all you have to do is focus on yourself.	The client is told to not worry about the horse but to start by just focusing on herself. The therapy team is very explicit about what each person's role is and what will happen next, so that the experience is predictable for the client, which helps her to regulate. This is especially important for clients who experience anxiety.
Therapist: How are you feeling right now? What number would you give your anxiety?	The therapist asks the client to check in with her body, again, and use her neocortex to rate her level of anxiety or whatever she is feeling. This provides a comparison with the previous benchmark and also attunes the client to herself while engaging upper and lower regions of her brain.
Client with wide eyes and a stiff body: I feel worse—I can't pick a number... Like a nine or ten!	Client has become much more anxious since getting on.
Therapist: Your anxiety went up a lot, didn't it? We'll get through this together. I think moving will help, can you give Brownie a little squeeze with your legs?	The therapist validates client's report (connecting) and asks client to use her body to gauge how her reported anxiety has affected her regulation. Client, with her anxiety higher, is unable to use her body to ask Brownie to walk—this tells us her diencephalon (responsible for motor regulation) is dysregulated. She will need passive sensory input/movement to regulate her brainstem and up into her diencephalon.
Therapist focuses on breathing rhythmically (with an exaggerated exhale) and starts swaying side to side: Would it be OK if we ask Brownie to start walking for you? Client: Yes, OK.	Coherence in the therapist's body provides rhythmic, regulating sensory input, and the swaying movement provides visual rhythmic input—both aid in brainstem regulation. The walking motion of the horse provides rhythmic sensory input, passively. We typically try to start the horse walking right away, even if the client is unable to articulate much, unless the client is so upset she wouldn't be able to stay on in motion, or she asks that we don't move.
Therapist: As she starts walking, just notice your breath. Maybe start to notice things with your senses—the sights and sounds, the feel of the breeze on your skin...	We start with a couple of rounds just allowing the client to relax and practice a little mindfulness of her breath and her surroundings. The movement of the horse combined with letting in sensory information is passive regulation—helping to reorganize the brainstem. After one round in the pen, both Brownie and the client take a spontaneous deep breath, indicating some regulation in the brainstem.
Therapist: Next, see if you can notice what's happening with your body. Just feel your body sitting on Brownie's back.	The objective of this instruction is for the client to bring her awareness to the repetitive sensory input of the horse's gait moving her rhythmically—regulating the lower regions and beginning to regulate the limbic system as she connects to her own body.
Therapist and equine specialist observe that as the client focuses on her body, Brownie's movements lose their rhythmic motion—she looks stiff in her walk.	The horse gives information about what is happening with the client's body—client feels some tension. Relaxation throughout the body will allow for better rhythm, and is therefore important to achieve.
Therapist: As we walk, we're going to do a body scan to see if we can help you relax as you walk, starting with the top of your head and moving all the way down to your toes. Let's start with your eyes, can you soften them so much that you can see not just what is in front of you, but on your sides, too? The therapist moves progressively through face, neck, shoulders, etc., down into feet. Helping the client notice tension and let it go.	A body scan helps the client to recognize her body tension on her own, searching for tension requires a connection to her own body, activating lower regions of the brain. Her ability to tense and relax parts of her body engage her diencephalon in an intentional way. As the client participates, Brownie shows signs of disconnection (often stopping and calling out to horses in the herd) that tells the therapy team when the client loses her ability to be connected to her horse (dysregulation in the limbic system).
As they complete the body scan, Therapist: Notice the rhythm that is between you and Brownie, notice the connection with your hips. See if you can feel the place where you and Brownie move together.	Therapist attempts to move client's attention back to the connection with Brownie by focusing on the point of contact—her hips—as she reconnects Brownie reconnects and relaxes.

(Continued)

Transcript	*Analysis*
Therapist: Let's try something else. See if you can make an infinity symbol with your left hand while the horse is moving. Follow your hand with your eyes... Next see if you can draw the symbol with your right hand, following it with your eyes... next make the movement with both hands at the same time...	When client is able, we can increase the difficulty of the movement she makes with her body, continuing to challenge and regulate her diencephalon (movement of eyes and arms). Activities like these are taken from Brain Gym© exercises.
Therapist: On this next round, I want you to try counting Brownie's steps. Why don't you start with noticing each time her left front leg moves forward? When you feel it, count each step, for one whole round. As the client begins counting, her rhythm is uneven and Brownie begins looking outside the pen, even calling to other horses. Therapist: Can you place your hands-on Brownie's shoulders and feel her muscles move with each step while you count?	When the client is able to engage in connection with her horse more consistently, she is more regulated in her limbic system. It then becomes appropriate to challenge the neocortex (reasoning and thinking part of the brain) by engaging the client's thoughts. This also increases healthy stress for new learning. If the client needs to look at her horse's leg to count the steps, this is an indication that she has disconnected from the lower regions of her brain as she activates the neocortex. It is important to help her feel the steps in her body (lower brain regions), while maintaining connection with her horse (middle brain regions), and thinking (upper brain regions) about what she is feeling. The therapy team and client notice that whenever the stress increases a little and the client begins to more deeply engage the thinking part of her brain, she and her horse tend to disconnect. It is necessary then to go back to re-establish a connection with Brownie. Increasing points of contact (touch) can support the client in staying connected with Brownie even while she engages her neocortex. This is necessary for cross-brain connections to grow throughout the brain—called integration. It is important to go back and reestablish connection each time it is lost—or we reinforce neocortex use without connection. When connection is re-established, we go back to the counting exercise.
Therapist: As we come to an end of our time here today, let's do a couple more rounds just checking in with your breath, and beginning to open your senses to all that is around you. Just allow yourself to relax.	It is important to end the session with regulation and connection after engaging in therapeutic work that is challenging. This supports integration and prepares the client to leave the session regulated.
Therapist: As we stop, for today, let's check in with your anxiety again—what number do you feel you are on now?	Final scaling of the client's anxiety to measure progress, and also make sure we do not send a client home deeply dysregulated.
Client: That was hard, but I feel lots better, maybe a one?	Client has been able to bring her "nine or ten" anxiety down to a one through her riding—she has been passively regulated through movement and mindfulness, co-regulated through her connection with her horse, therapist, and equine specialist and self-regulated through her own efforts to breathe and relax.
Therapist: Before we dismount, take a big breath and sigh it out—then tell Brownie "thank you" and "goodbye" however you would like—it could be a pat, a hug, words, whatever feels right to you.	We encourage gratitude and more connection with Brownie before the client dismounts—so she and Brownie end on a positive note.
Conclusion: The purposes of these exercises are integration of the brain, which is needed for trauma processing to begin to occur, whether deliberately in therapy sessions or spontaneously as it sometimes will. The activities will vary given that each client, horse, and relationship dynamic are unique. However, this sequence illustrates key principles for all mounted work: bottom-up regulation (regulating the lower and midbrain regions) is facilitated by the horse's movement and connection with the client. Integration and the growth of neuronal pathways between brain regions is promoted when the client engages different areas of the brain simultaneously while regulated. Rhythmic patterns of activation in the brain promote its organization and integration, which makes it possible to experience the memory of trauma in a new way. Through repetition neural pathways are formed. Each mounted session provides the opportunity to reinforce pathways that allow the client to remain connected with herself and others under somewhat stressful conditions. As she improves her connection with herself, she will become better able to override her anxiety with self-regulation. As she improves her connection with others, her relationships will become more rewarding and less triggering. She will benefit from the co-regulation within connected relationships that she never experienced as a child due to her family circumstances. We did not describe trauma processing here, but it builds on the work that was illustrated in this transcript. This is our approach to Rhythmic Riding™, which is what we call the mounted component of TF-EAP.	

The following sample session note is about a pseudonym client.

Name: Linda	**Date:** mm/dd/yyyy
Start Time: 9:30am **End Time:** 10:30am	**Diagnosis:** Generalized Anxiety Disorder (300.02)
Service Type (CPT code if billing insurance) ☐	
Average Heart Rate on EMWAVE (and observations) Emwave was not utilized this session, but in the past resting heart rate has often been over 100 bpm. Many times, as the client becomes more coherent through HRV biofeedback her heart rate will come down to 85 or 90.	
Therapeutic Goals: Facilitate integration in the brain through bottom-up regulation, co-regulation, and, ultimately, self-regulation. Reduction in generalized anxiety and anxiety related to connection in personal and professional relationships.	
Check in with client (degree to which learning in session is transferring to other areas of life) Client reports that general feeling of anxiety on a daily basis has begun to subside. She reports that she is sleeping better and is less irritable. She still, reportedly, experiences "extreme anxiety" during moments of "normal life stress" often related to some of her most intimate relationships—she continues to withdraw and disconnect in these moments.Client reports that she is beginning to recall childhood memories that she hasn't "ever really" thought about—sometimes the thoughts are intrusive (continue to r/o PTSD).	
Intervention/s used: Bottom-up and co-regulation. Mindfulness. Body Scan and progressive muscle relaxation. Notice anxiety and determine subjective units of distress. Practice sensing, feeling, connecting (to self and others), and thinking at the same time.	
Client's response to intervention/s: Client experienced high anxiety during the session (a nine or ten), but was able to regulate (one), as evidenced by soft eyes, rhythmic, deep breathing, and a relaxed posture. She was willing to participate in the interventions. Client was able to stay connected to herself (her body sensations and thoughts) and others, while experiencing and practicing interventions.	
Future plan: Continue sessions, 1 × weekly. HW: Journal as memories emerge, and practice body scan and progressive muscle relaxation before bedtime each night.	

The following scale is scored by the clinician, and is representative of the client's regulation during the session (first order outcome).

0	1	2	3	4
No self regulation; client gave up/refused to continue or was unable to change state	Client able to self-regulate with considerable intervention from therapist (e.g., co-regulation or giving step by step instructions)	Client able to self-regulate with some prompting from therapist (modeling, recalling techniques learned for breathing, muscle relaxation, mindfulness, etc.)	Child able to self-regulate with minimal prompting from therapist (e.g., asking child to recall what worked for them the last time x happened)	Child able to self-regulate with no prompting from therapist

Therapist Signature/Credentials

FIG. 6.1. Sample Client Session Note.

CONFIDENTIAL

Session Note

Name:	Date:
Start Time: End Time:	Diagnosis:
Service Type (CPT code if billing insurance)☐	
Average Heart Rate on EMWAVE (and observations)	
Therapeutic Goals:	
Check in with client (degree to which learning in session is transferring to other areas of life)	
Intervention/s used:	
Client's response to intervention/s:	
Future Plan :	

The following scale is scored by the clinician, and is representative of the client's regulation during the session (first order outcome).

0	1	2	3	4
No self-regulation; client gave up/refused to continue or was unable to change state	Client able to self-regulate with considerable intervention from therapist (e.g., co-regulation or giving step by step instructions)	Client able to self-regulate with some prompting from therapist (modeling, recalling techniques learned for breathing, muscle relaxation, mindfulness, etc.)	Child able to self-regulate with minimal prompting from therapist (e.g., asking child to recall what worked for them the last time x happened)	Child able to self-regulate with no prompting from therapist

____
Therapist Signature/Credentials and Date

FIG. 6.2 Blank Template of Client Session Note.

REFERENCES

Anxiety and Depression Association of America. (2017). Retrieved from www.adaa.org.

Etkin, A. & Wager, T. (2007). Functional neuroimaging of anxiety: A meta-analysis of emotional processing in PTSD, social anxiety disorder, and specific phobia. *American Journal of Psychiatry*, *164*(10), 1476–1488.

Hanson, J., Nacewicz, B., Sutterer, M., Cayo, A., Schaefer, S., Rudolph, K., Shirtcliff, E., Pollak, D., & Davidson, R. (2015). Behavioral problems after early life stress: Contributions of the hippocampus and amygdala. *Biological Psychiatry*, *77*(4), 314–323. Retrieved from www.health.harvard.edu/staying-healthy/anxiety_and_physical_illness.

Harvard Health Publications (2017). Retrieved from www.health.harvard.edu/staying-healthy/anxiety_and_physical_illness.

Ogden, P., Minton, K., & Pain, C. (2006). *Trauma and the Body: A Sensorimotor Approach to Psychotherapy*. New York: Norton.

Perry, B. D. (2006). The Neurosequential Model of therapeutics: Applying principles of neuroscience to clinical work with traumatized and maltreated children. In N. Boyd Webb (Ed.), *Working with Traumatized Youth in Child Welfare* (pp. 27–52). New York: Guilford Press.

Perry, B. D. (2009). Examining child maltreatment through a neurodevelopmental lens: Clinical applications of the Neurosequential Model of therapeutics. *Journal of Loss and Trauma*, *14*(4), 240–255.

Perry, B. D., Pollard, R. A., Blakley, T. L., Baker, W. L., & Vigilante, D. (1995). Childhood trauma, the neurobiology of adaptation, and "use-dependent" development of the brain: How "states" become "traits." *Infant Mental Health Journal*, *16*(4), 271–291.

National Institute of Mental Health (NIMH). (2017). Retrieved from www.nimh.nih.gov.

Shah, S. G., Klumpp, H., Angstadt, M., Nathan, P. J., & Phan, K. L. (2009). Amygdala and insula response to emotional images in patients with generalized social anxiety disorder. *Journal of Psychiatry & Neuroscience*, *34*(4), 296–302.

Siegel, D. J. (2010). *Mindsight: The New Science of Personal Transformation*. New York: Bantam.

Siegel, D. J. (2012). *The Developing Mind: How Relationships and the Brain Interact to Shape Who We Are*. 2nd edition. New York: Guilford.

7

Walking with the Wisdom of Peace

A Horse-Guided Practice to Leave Anxiety in the Dust

Sara B. Willerson

INTRODUCTION

Anxiety. It is the primary presenting issue for clients in the Horses, Heart & Soul® program. What has been fascinating to discover is that, many times, the diagnostic label of anxiety ends up being a person who is *incredibly aware* of their highly attuned sensory system, environment, and experiences that occur within their daily settings. And with that, oftentimes comes a sense of overwhelm from not having a way to create balance within themselves.

Merriam-Webster Dictionary (2017) defines anxiety as "an abnormal and overwhelming sense of apprehension and fear often marked by physical signs (such as tension, sweating, and increased pulse rate), by doubt concerning the reality and nature of the threat, and by self-doubt about one's capacity to cope with it." The National Alliance on Mental Illness (2017) reports that 18% of adults have experienced an anxiety disorder. The National Institute of Mental Health (NAMI, 2017) shared statistics that 25.1% of children between the ages of 13 and 18 have an anxiety disorder. Both of these research organizations reported that anxiety is more commonly diagnosed in women and typically begins in childhood due to environmental factors, social/peer pressures, family history of mental illness, and stressful life events.

"Anxiety affects a person emotionally, physically, mentally and spiritually" (NAMI, 2017). Societal beliefs and views on this state of being are at times harsh and unforgiving and that the presence of this physiological response is to be shamed or dishonored. Stepping into the pasture with a herd of horses quickly engages our sensory information. We may experience the physiological responses of our body (our heartbeat, our breath), sense the environmental elements coming into our awareness (the wind, sun, ground beneath our feet), and the realization that our entire being is truly present in that moment, while visually connecting with a herd of horses now looking at us with curiosity and interest. Thus, taking the first steps into attunement with ourselves through the harmonious guidance of nature and horse.

CONNECTION IN A FIELD OF THEORETICAL LENSES

> I go to nature to be soothed and healed, and to have my senses put in order.
>
> John Burroughs

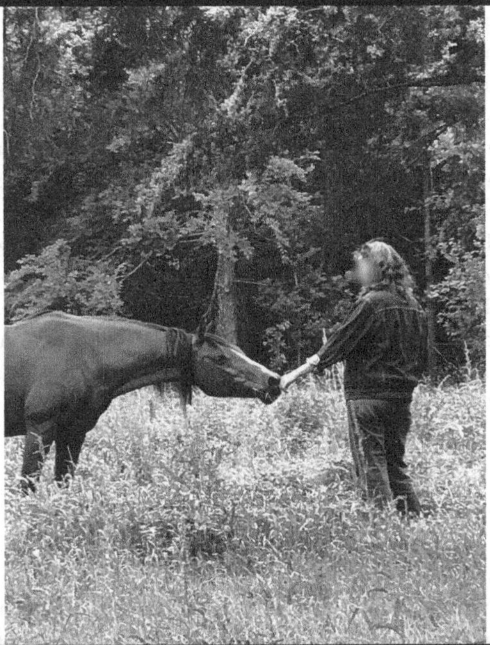

FIG. 7.1.

Equine-facilitated psychotherapy (EFP), at its core, is an experiential healing modality. It has the ability to partner with a variety of theoretical perspectives and mental health orientations. For this author, the lens that primarily resonates is Attachment Theory and the concept of Affect Attunement.

Bowlby defined attachment as a "lasting psychological connectedness between human beings" (Bowlby, 1969, p. 194). Bowlby determined that all human beings must have a safe and comforting space to return to, that our caregiver provide a secure and dependable base, that our caregiver was available to return to for safety, and when separated from the caregiver, we, the child, would experience distress until a return to our caregiver was re-established (Bowlby, 1969). In Ainsworth's work with Bowlby, Ainsworth defined attachment, "as an affectional tie that one person or animal forms between himself and another specific one—a tie that binds them together in space and endures over time" (Ainsworth, Bell, & Stayton, 1991, p. 31). As clinicians, we know that even if our clients did not have the opportunity in childhood to experience the clinical definition of a healthy, developmental attachment, it is possible for the client to re-create self-determined, healthy attachments with others in their current life. These theoretical perspectives begin to explain the deep resonance and connection that EFP clients report when partnering with a horse in a therapeutic setting. With a horse as guide, clients have the opportunity to experience a sense of attachment and reparation of past relationship interactions.

The research of Stern (1985), introduced a deeper understanding of the intricacies in Attachment Theory. Stern's quest to understand the language existing in the space between parent and child led him to define the concept of Affect Attunement.

Affect Attunement "is the performance of behaviors that express the quality of feeling of a shared affect state without imitating the exact behavioral expression of the inner state" (Stern, 1985, p. 142). This internal language involved the mother sensing and knowing the emotional state of her child and showing her feeling of this state through her actions, which related through the same intensity, temporal beat, rhythm, duration, and shape of the baby's reactions, play, and behaviors. One may argue that the mother is simply displaying empathy toward her child or even imitating the behavior she is witnessing. This display is distinctly different from empathy and imitation. Empathy is the ability to see the emotional display, cognitively understand and interpret it, and bear witness and acknowledge the emotional state through thoughts and words reciprocated back. Imitation "does not permit the partners to refer to the internal state" (Stern, 1985, p. 142). Imitation is mimicking of the behavior witnessed. "Attunement behaviors… recast the event and shift the focus of attention to what is behind the behavior, to the quality of feeling that is being shared" (Stern, 1985, p. 142). Stern recognized a state of "communion" in this deeply connected relational exchange as a "means to share in another's experience with no attempt to change what that person is doing or believing" (Stern, 1985, p.148).

The concept of Affect Attunement supports client reports of feeling seen, heard, understood, and validated on a deep internal level when connecting with horses in a therapeutic setting. This internal relational state goes beyond commonly held beliefs of horse as a mirror. It supports the validity of a horse being with their human client throughout the intensity, shape, and duration of the emotional experience, clearly sensing the ending of the experience, and allowing the client to reach the information needed at that moment in their process of healing and development.

Horses are in the moment with the client, all without attempting to change or shift the experience. Current research studies in the field of EFP support client-reported experiences of addressing attachment-related events, emotional regulation, body awareness, and non-verbal communication when partnering with horses (Lentini & Knox, 2009; Bachi, Terkel, & Teichman, 2012; Bachi, 2013; Wilson, Buultjens, Monfries, & Karmi, 2017). These evidence-based reminders strengthen the concept of horses joining with humans through the deep internal process of attunement, thus opening the door to healing previous attachment wounding and current manifestations of anxiety and distress.

PLANTING ETHICAL PASTURES

Ethics and the welfare of horses in a therapeutic setting are continuing to be developed throughout many EFP programs. They are imperative practice considerations when teaming up with horses in a therapeutic milieu. When we as professionals have a deep understanding and relationship with these sentient beings, we know and are attuned with their desires, mood, interests, healing gifts, and when, most importantly, they need and/or ask for a break. EFP healing work is intense for all parties involved, horse and human, and as the main facilitator, the horse's entire being *must* be cared for physically, emotionally, mentally, and spiritually.

EFP professional associations' codes of ethics are in place to clarify the responsibilities of their members. These codes play an important role in safeguarding the profession's autonomy and in articulating standards for the profession. Equine Facilitated Wellness-Canada has coined a succinct description when it comes to partnering with horses in a healing based professional practice:

> The equine is a sentient being, partner and co-facilitator in the equine facilitated relationship and process. The term "equine" is meant to include horses, donkeys and mules, as all of these animals have gifts to offer in the field of equine facilitated wellness. Equines have their own perceptions and emotions, and can also attune themselves to the presence and feelings of others. Through their remarkable sensitivity, perceptiveness, and intuition equines are able to offer valuable feedback and information to clients. It is crucial that they are able to express themselves spontaneously and freely through their actions and reactions when working with clients. In order to support their equine partners in this field, it is incumbent upon human facilitators to be aware of the impact that this work may have on equines, and safeguard their physical, mental and emotional well-being at all times. They must ensure that their equine partners are treated respectfully and ethically, both within and outside of client sessions. Human partners need to understand that their equine partners are completely dependent upon their stewardship, and do their utmost to meet their psychological and physical needs.
>
> (Equine Facilitated Wellness-Canada, 2015)

THE WISDOM WALK PROGRAM©

The Horses, Heart & Soul® herd has developed a five-step program centered on reducing internal disturbances that result in anxiety-related symptoms. The Wisdom Walk Program© is composed of five equine-guided steps that teach a simple practice of clearing out the clutter in order to align with the heart of who we all are! In essence, the herd of horses is teaching a process based in Affect Attunement, which supports a client in learning how to develop emotional regulation skills. This program has been taught to children, tweens, teens, and adults in both individual and group-based programming. It has been incorporated through individual sessions, weekly and monthly group programming. It is currently being developed into a curriculum-based program including video, handouts, and a journaling practice. This chapter will focus on the first step in the Wisdom Walk Program©, Peace. It is an easily used tool, in all situations, geared toward calming the internal self and clearing out anxiety-related symptoms.

Moonbeam's Peace of Wisdom

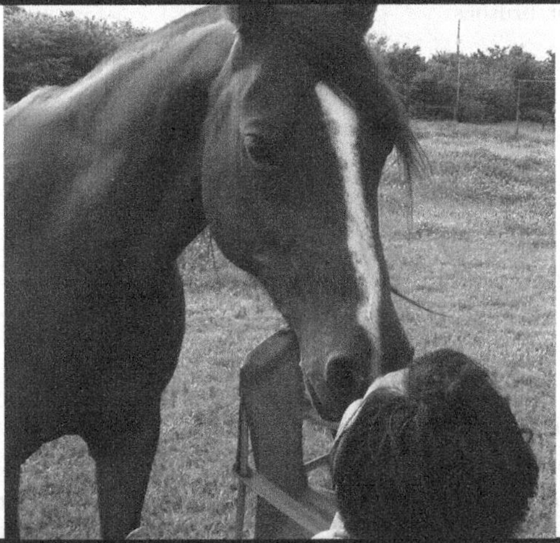

FIG. 7.2.

Step One—Peace. The first step in the Wisdom Walk Program is Peace. This program foundation is taught by a mare in the Horses, Heart & Soul herd named Moonbeam. In the Horses, Heart & Soul herd, Moonbeam is the peacemaker and the nurturer. With each of her family members, she moves in arcs and circles, always encouraging connection and movement. A previous teen client described her as "the mother in the group." Another member of a children's group shared, "She works on calming people." An adult client simply stated, "Moonbeam *is* love!"

The manner in which Moonbeam holds and manifests peace is truly mesmerizing and inspirational. This mare consistently models the core concept of this program by creating a sense of peace internally and externally, both within her herd and with her human clients. She teaches that when we are centered within our self and attuned with our heart, a sense of alignment or grounded state of being is created. It is not a thought process or mental practice of simply telling our self to "do it." It is a reminder of the importance of integrating this into practice *with* our entire being versus thinking about it and talking about it. These are very different perspectives to practice. It is a practice of the heart. It is being in connection and relationship with all aspects of the self—emotionally, mentally, physically and spiritually. This aligning attunement is harmony.

The Peace Spiral Practice

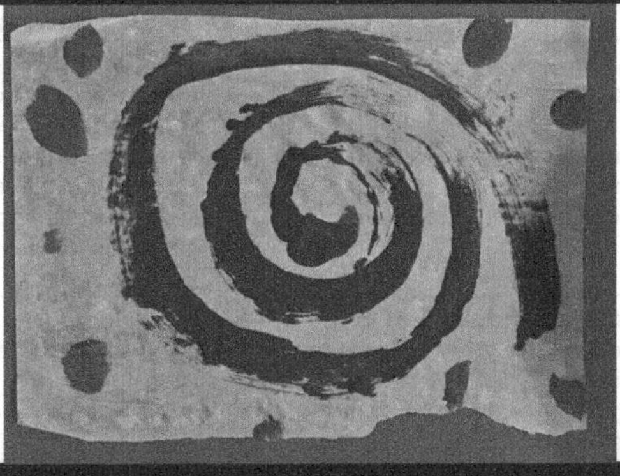

FIG. 7.3.

Supplies

- Horse to partner with—at liberty in an enclosed space or on halter with lead rope
- Imagination
- Markers, colored pencils, paint, brushes
- Tempera paint
- Paper for drawing and/or painting
- Practice journal handout
- Journal/notebook
- Thank-you carrots.

Moonbeam's Peace Spiral practice is taught through the image of a spiral. Participants are taught about the history of spirals as ancient symbols used in spiritual practice and universal signatures of growth and evolution. This pattern is found throughout nature and has been used within many cultures and beliefs to create a state of balance and centeredness. Depending on the age of the group, this symbol can be visualized through drawing/painting the image of the spiral that resonates with the participant, or even leading the client through a guided meditation of visualizing the spiral image that presents perfectly for them.

Once this concept is understood, the practice method is to visualize a spiral sitting in the center of the person's chest and spinning it in a clockwise direction while taking slow, deep breaths. Once the client settles in to the practice and gets the hang of it, they are then asked to think of something that has been bothering them, created anxiety, or even an incident that left them feeling unsettled. They are asked about the physical sensations in their body they notice in recalling this event—what they notice about their breath, are they holding it or is it short and rapid? Do they notice any areas of tightness showing up inside? Does it affect the thoughts in their head? Then they are asked to spin the spiral in the center of their chest and take some slow deep breaths.

The following transcript analysis are about a pseudonym client.

Table 7.1

Transcript Analysis of Peace Spiral

Transcript	*Analysis*
Counselor: Let's take a minute with Moonbeam [horse] to practice this technique she is sharing. She will be right here in the arena with us. She is here to support you. Before we get started, make sure you are seated comfortably in your chair with your feet flat on the ground. You are welcome to close your eyes or keep them open slightly, if that feels better for you. Take a few slow, deep breaths and just let yourself settle into your chair.	Counselor is supporting client in creating a comfortable and grounded space to step into this meditation practice. Moonbeam is grazing at liberty in the large arena space, watching her client. Counselor is ensuring safety between horse and client with horse at liberty in the arena space.
Counselor: Consider something that you have been chewing on, or that is bothering you or distracting you from where or what you want your focus to be. **Client:** My friend said some really mean things to me yesterday. I can't stop thinking about it. I have felt sick to my stomach all day.	Counselor is supporting client in mindfulness practice of bringing mental chatter to conscious awareness in order to implement the Peace Spiral tool. Client shares her current internal worries and how they are affecting her physically and mentally.
Counselor: "OK. Just take some slow, deep breaths." Client takes several deep breaths and visibly settles into her chair. She nods her head. Moonbeam walks over to client and stands at client's side with her head at client's shoulder level. Client smiles when she senses Moonbeam next to her.	Counselor is acknowledging client's vulnerable share and is supporting her in staying present and connected with her body through breath work. Client is connecting with the initial grounding/centering practice. Moonbeam is showing client she is present with her in this process and supporting her. Client is aware of Moonbeam's engaged presence.
Counselor: Out in front of you, use your imagination to see a big movie screen. On this screen, ask to see what your Peace Spiral looks like. Imagine your personal Peace Spiral now. See what it looks like, what color it is, its texture, the size of it. Notice all the unique and special qualities of your spiral.	Counselor is supporting client's creativity and imagination to be partners in this meditation space.
Client nods and continues to breathe slowly and deeply. **Client**: It's big and shiny. And it is rainbow colored. It's so cool looking!	Client is actively participating in meditation process and identifies the visual qualities of her Peace Spiral image.

Transcript	*Analysis*
Counselor: See your Peace Spiral coming off the movie screen and moving toward you. Bring that Peace Spiral into the center of your chest and center it in your heart space—right there in the middle. Now see your spiral begin to move in a clockwise direction, from your point of view. Moonbeam raises her head and rests her muzzle gently on the crown of client's head and takes several deep breaths. Client smiles and takes several deeper breaths as well.	Counselor is supporting client in the physical integration practice of Peace Spiral tool. Client becomes aware of her horse attuning with her internal experience. Client responds to Moonbeam's reminder to continue breathing.
Counselor: As your Peace Spiral moves and gets into its own perfect rhythm, continue breathing.	Counselor is guiding client in the initial practice of using the Peace Spiral tool. Counselor pauses and quietly holds space as client is practicing the basic use of this tool.
Counselor: While your Peace Spiral is turning, notice what happens to those thoughts about your friend's mean words. Notice what happens to that sick feeling in your stomach. And keep your Peace Spiral spinning. You can also envision all these things on the spiral and the spiral is spinning them all out and away from you.	Counselor is actively supporting client in putting Peace Spiral tool to use with the previously identified internal distractions.
Client scrunches her face into a grimace. Moonbeam continues to stand with her client with her nose and mouth gently resting over the top of client's head.	Client is focusing her attention on internal chatter and working with her Peace Spiral.
Counselor: Keep breathing. See all that clutter moving off, out, and away from your body as your Peace Spiral continues to spin. Allow it to spin until all that stuff is gone. It may take a minute or two. And that is OK.	Counselor is guiding client in the practice of actively using Peace Spiral tool to reduce internal disturbances. Counselor is also reminding client to take some time with this tool versus the expectation of a "quick fix."
Client continues to take deep breaths and her physical exterior noticeably relaxes. Moonbeam continues to stand quietly with her client. Client reaches her hand out and places it on Moonbeam's neck. Client smiles. **Counselor:** What are you noticing now? **Client:** All that stuff I was worrying about is gone!	Client is actively practicing the use of the Peace Spiral tool. Clear observation that client's physical body is responding to this tool. Client adds additional physical connection to the attunement process by reaching out to touch Moonbeam. Counselor is checking in with client upon observation of clients shifted physical presentation and reaching out to Moonbeam and smiling. Client is verbalizing her internal experience after integrating Peace Spiral.
Counselor: Wonderful! Now notice what you are experiencing through the rest of your body—your emotions, beliefs, awareness, and thoughts. Keep breathing while you are checking in with yourself. Counselor pauses for a moment for client to check in with herself. **Counselor:** What are you noticing now? **Client:** I feel quiet and calm inside now. And my stomach doesn't hurt anymore. **Counselor:** Just keep breathing slowly and gently. Allow that experience of calm and quiet to really settle in, all through your insides. And just keep breathing. **Client**: OK. It's like I am totally filled with calm all through me. And it's all around me on my outsides too.	Counselor is bringing client's awareness to her on going internal experience following the use of the Peace Spiral tool. It is helpful to pause and give clients a moment to check in with their internal process and awareness. Client is able to identify the real-time application of this relaxation tool. Counselor is guiding client in being with her newly attuned space and creating a holding space for this internal quiet and calm.
Counselor: Nice! Remember that you can use your Peace Spiral to bring yourself back to a place of quiet and calm whenever you need that. And that Moonbeam is right here with you. Counselor pauses for a moment **Counselor:** When you are ready, slowly let yourself come back into your chair, where you are right now. Feel your feet on the ground, here, in this arena. Let your senses hear, smell and feel all that is going on around you in this arena space. Take one more deep breath and gently open your eyes. Client opens her eyes and looks at Moonbeam who is still standing next to her with her muzzle on top of client's head, gently breathing. Client smiles at Moonbeam and gives her a pat. Moonbeam brings her head back down to eye level with client and sighs deeply. **Client:** Wow! That really works! And Moonbeam was really helping me!	Counselor is bringing meditation practice with the Peace Spiral tool to closure and supporting the client in returning to the present moment. Counselor is completing process of client returning to the present moment. Moonbeam has remained in attunement with her client throughout the practice with the Peace Spiral relaxation tool. Client verbally validates her experience with this practice and acknowledges Moonbeam's supportive, attuned presence.

Participants are then encouraged to take a few minutes to journal about their experience. Once that personal time is complete, they are invited to share their practice with the Peace Spiral. Some past clients described their experience as, "I felt calmer"; "That really helped me." One teen reported, "As it turns out, it gets all the gunk out." A child client shared, "I get mad easily. When I get mad, I don't let it go and keep it inside a long time. It feels like everything inside of me is full. When I use, the Peace Spiral it feels like everything is clean and open."

A tween-age client stated, "They've [the horses] helped me a lot because I don't have a lot of confidence and this step gives me a lot more confidence." An adult client expressed:

> I thought my heart needed my apology for all the crap that was in me and needed to be worked through. Slowly, I spun my peace spiral, putting my anxieties and self-doubts onto my spiral. Out of my palms spun my fears and pain. My spiral glowed from black, to greens, to blues. It was so serene. The spiral acted like a peace ripple that waved throughout my body. My heart felt warm and radiated.

Another adult reported, "If something negative came up, I put it on the spiral and it took it right out." Additional adult clients shared, "It made this week more bearable with all the stressors in daily living"; "Practicing it daily there was instant calm and peace."

This practice step is traditionally taught with Moonbeam present in the group setting (in the arena at liberty) or individual space with the client (in a round pen). She will typically stand next to her client and support their Affect Attunement process, or meander through the group offering the same tending if multiple people are present. After practicing the step with the client, they are invited to paint a symbol of their experience on Moonbeam using water based Tempura paint. This is a fun and powerful way to visually share their attunement experience with Moonbeam as well as showcase the creative variety of Peace Spirals that show up!

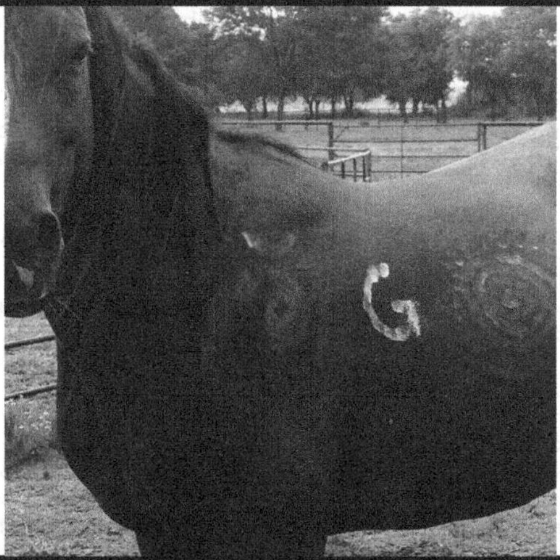

FIG. 7.4.

This program has been taught with other horses who are not members of the Horses, Heart & Soul herd. Even though these horses were stepping into a new practice, they showed up by standing next to and holding space with their client as the person practiced this Affect Attunement tool.

Weekly and monthly handouts for the Peace Spiral practice have been designed for participants to keep track of their experiences. Directions are given to create a daily practice of documenting use with Moonbeam's Peace Spiral. On their handouts, they are encouraged to write down or draw (for younger children) when, where, and why it was used. To notice what happened after using it—how they felt, did it make the situation better, did they notice a different emotion, did they notice any physical sensations and/or thoughts changing? The goal being that with daily integration of this tool, clients have a practical, hands-on approach to working with symptoms of anxiety and a way of attuning with a sense of calm and peace throughout daily life occurrences.

Handout Example for Children/Teens:

The Wisdom Walk Program©
A Five Step Program to Align With Our True Self
Horses, Heart & Soul®, LLC

Step One Peace Spiral Practice

- Time of Day I used Moonbeam's Peace Spiral:

- Why I used the Peace Spiral:

- What happened after I used the Peace Spiral:

FIG. 7.5. Peace Spiral Handout Children and Teens.

Handout Example for Adults:

The Wisdom Walk Program©
A Five Step Program to Align With Our True Self
Horses, Heart & Soul®, LLC

Practice With Step One—Peace

- Create a practice with yourself using Step One throughout the week. You might consider starting your day with it, or working with it before entering something you consider "stressful" or "worrisome." Or during a moment when you find yourself feeling "stressed," "uncertain," "flooded," or full of emotion or mental chatter.

- Keep a journal of this practice. What was happening before you worked with Moonbeam's Peace Spiral? What did you notice in your body, your thoughts, your emotions (and/or any other area) as you spun the spiral? What happened after using the spiral?

- What else did you notice about yourself, your beliefs, your actions, your choices, relationships, work, community interactions, etc in having this practice as part of your week?

- Please share your thoughts/feedback about this practice.

FIG. 7.6. Peace Spiral Handout Adults.

REFERENCES

Ainsworth, M. D. S., Bell, S. M., & Stayton, D. J. (1991). Infant-mother attachment and social development: "Socialization" as a product of reciprocal responsiveness to signals. In M. Woodhead, R. Carr, & P. Light (Eds.), *Becoming a Person: Vol. 1: Child Development in Social Context.* Florence, KY: Routledge.

Bachi, K. (2013). Application of attachment theory to equine-facilitated psychotherapy. *Journal of Contemporary Psychotherapy, 43*, 187–196.

Bachi, K., Terkel, J., & Teichman, M. (2012). Equine-facilitated psychotherapy for at-risk adolescents: The influence on self-image, self-control and trust. *Clinical Child Psychology and Psychiatry, 17*, 298–312.

Bowlby, J. (1969). *Attachment and Loss: Vol. 1. Attachment.* New York: Basic Books.

Burroughs, J. Quote retrieved from: www.brainyquote.com/quotes/quotes/j/johnburrou106918.html.

Equine Facilitated Wellness-Canada (2015). *Code of Ethics.* Retrieved from www.equinefacilitatedwellness.org/overview.

Lentini, J. A. A. & Knox, M. (2009). A qualitative and quantitative review of Equine Facilitated Psychotherapy (EFP) with children and adolescents. *The Open Complementary Medicine Journal, 1*, 51–57.

Merriam-Webster Dictionary. (2017). Anxiety. Retrieved from www.merriam-webster.com/dictionary/anxiety.

National Institute of Mental Health (NAMI). (2017). Anxiety. Retrieved from www.nimh.nih.gov.

National Alliance on Mental Illness. (2017). Anxiety. Retrieved from www.nami.org.

Stern, D. N. (1985). The Interpersonal World of the Infant: A View from Psychoanalysis and Developmental Psychology. New York: Basic Books.

Wilson, K., Buultjens, M., Monfries, M., & Karmi, L. (2017). Equine-assisted psychotherapy for adolescents experiencing depression and/or anxiety; A therapist's perspective. Clinical Child Psychology and Psychiatry, 22(1), 16–33.

Section 4

GRIEF

8

Equine-Assisted Psychotherapy, Grief, and Loss

Patti Schlough

INTRODUCTION

Often those grieving will report the following symptoms after the death of a loved one, feelings of deep sadness, loneliness, hopelessness, anger, denial of the death, crying, hyper-arousal, guilt, sleeplessness, intrusive thoughts or images about the deceased. It is important to recognize that a major shift has taken place in the life of the individual or family. Therefore, the mental health provider needs to be cautious of creating pathology around what is occurring for that client. In many cases communication, relationships, and life satisfaction are all affected by the loss. Clients are often seeking some place to grieve and process the next steps they can take as they move forward in their life's journey and honor the life that has been lost.

The two cases presented were clients who sought equine-assisted psychotherapy following a recent death of a primary member of their family system. The cases were referred to PEACE, LLC through a local non-profit, Olivia's House, which is a grief and bereavement center for children and families in York, PA. Olivia's House refers clients to PEACE, LLC when the program director feels that the child or the family might benefit from a more individualized approach or the family has identified a need that lies outside of what Olivia's House educational programs can provide.

PEACE, LLC provides traditional talk therapy, walk and talk therapy, and equine-assisted psychotherapy and learning. For equine-assisted psychotherapy services, we have two licensed mental health providers and three equine specialists. We are an Eagala model practice (Eagala, 2015); we always operate as a two-person team, which includes a licensed mental health provider and an equine specialist, all of our sessions are ground-based, no riding is involved, we provide a solution-oriented approach and we follow a code of ethics that requires continuing education for the licensed professional and continuing education for the equine specialist.

As a practitioner of mental health services, my early training was and remains very Rogerian or person-centered. Most of my professional career has been in the school system providing counseling and intervention services for adolescents with an emotional disability. Due to the need to understand the "function" of behavior, I have a heavy influence in Cognitive Behavioral therapy. In addition, I completed my post-graduate work in spiritual and existential counseling and therapy, which have a profound influence on the grief and trauma work that I have been committed to for the past 14 years. Most recently, my training in mindfulness has added a great deal to our equine-assisted work, enabling clients to practice present-moment awareness with intention through the window of attention.

The Eagala model is the "framework" where I insert the therapeutic intervention that is most appropriate for the client. Allowing the client to have an experience with the horse or horses and following the lead of the client as they interact and create a relationship with the horse will determine what theoretical direction the session may take. Planning for a session is fundamentally a great idea, but theoretically goes against the therapist as a "person-centered" clinician. In our practice, we are always thinking ahead to the next session and we often discuss what might benefit the client as we enter the next session. In the Eagala model, we move from session to session often building on what has occurred in a prior session. We consider what movement has taken place, if relationships were created, what themes emerged or become apparent, were any metaphors identified, was anything created that the client identified as part of their life landscape. All of these aspects of each session are considered but staying where the client takes us and allowing for exploration towards solution or resolution seems to have the most impact on client progress.

CASE EXAMPLE NUMBER ONE

Description

Mark (a pseudonym) was brought to PEACE, LLC due to the recent and sudden death of his 43-year-old father Bill (a pseudonym). Mark, is ten years old, in the fifth grade, he is a good student and has no identified behavior concerns in the educational setting. His mother, Mary (a pseudonym), 42 years old, is an attorney. Mary and Bill were married for 20 years and Mark is their only child. Bill was a very "hands-on and involved parent" according to Mary. Bill suffered a cerebral aneurysm, which resulted in his death. Mark was home alone with his father at the time of the incident and was able to contact emergency help but they were unable to save Bill's life. Upon intake, it had been four weeks since Bill's death and Mary was concerned about Mark's increasing concern and worry about her safety. In addition, Mark refuses to sleep in his bedroom; he is sleeping on the floor of his mother's room. Mary has noticed an increase in Mark's crying and an overall sense of sadness. Mary chose to come to equine therapy because Mary feels Mark does not talk about his father's death and she would like to "know" what he is feeling. In addition, Mark has always liked animals and when she mentioned to Mark the possibility of working with horses in a counseling setting he became excited to see what it was all about and agreed to attend sessions.

Goals

At intake, both Mark and Mary identified primary goals for their family.

1. To be able to talk about Bill (dad) without always crying.
2. For Mark to feel like he will be OK if he is not always with mom.
3. For Mark to be able to sleep in his own bed in his room again.

Intervention

The following is a transcript of the third session for Mark and Mary. Mark and Mary identified four miniature horses that they wanted to work with in session. Mark established a relationship with one that he named Carmel in the first session. Mark said he liked Carmel because he was calm and nice. Carmel stayed with Mark and Mary and seemed to "enjoy" being with them. Two others they named Butterscotch and Cocoa, however, Mark and Mary felt they were not interested in them, or that the horses didn't like them because they would walk away from them every time they tried to come near them, they responded "that's what people do when they don't want to be with you, they walk away." The fourth miniature horse they named Nips because every time they came to the horse it would either put its mouth on their shoes or pants or it would put its teeth on another horse. Both Mark and Mary discussed in the last session that "Nips had something happen to her, she nips because she is afraid." In the Eagala model we often think about session progression and creating activities based on what we observed in previous sessions, we are following the horse's behavior to help us plan for a next session.

In the first two sessions, Mark and Mary spent time introducing themselves to the horses. They had connected with one horse and felt he was calm and nice because he stayed with them. They had identified two horses that moved away from them and might not like them or were not interested. And Mark made the observation that one of the horses used its teeth on their shoes or pants or on other horses and this may be because she was afraid. The first two sessions we had the clients moving towards the horses. This session we planned to have the horses move towards the clients. The clients would create a space or spaces that would draw the horses to them. Having the clients' think of how to have something "move towards them" may help them identify things they need to do for Mark to regain his confidence in life and safety in being alone.

Set-Up and Materials

Mark and Mary are greeted in the indoor arena by the treatment team, the four miniature horses are un-haltered and walking around loose in the indoor arena. Materials needed: four miniature horses, brushes, plastic pipes of various widths and lengths, hula-hoops, and cones of various sizes.

Step-by-Step Instructions

Greet clients; ask about how things have been going in the past week. Have the clients create two spaces in the arena that they label, as "something needed" by the horses and can help build a relationship with them.

The following transcript analysis are about a pseudonym client.

Table 8.1

Blank Progress Note

Transcript	*Analysis*
Treatment Team: What do you remember from our last session? **Client, Mark:** Carmel [horse] was the nice one, she stayed with me, I think Nips isn't very nice.	Keeping in mind what the identified goals of treatment are and what the clients remember from the last session. Thinking about an activity that can encompass what is prominent about this experience now and last session. Treatment team assesses what was significant from the last session.
Treatment Team: Was there anything else you noticed about the horses? **Client, Mark:** Those two walk away when we get close, see look at them now. *Treatment team watches with clients as Butterscotch and Cocoa walk one behind the other away from the clients.*	Using a clean language question, "anything else" keeps question open-ended. More detail is provided, allows team to plan/develop activity.
Treatment Team: What do you think would keep them close? **Client, Mark:** Maybe a nice place, some place where I could brush them.	Planning activity. Client-led activity.
Treatment Team: A place that's nice and a place where you could brush. And what about Nips, what does Nips need? **Clients:** I'm not sure, maybe a place where they could eat and feel safe.	Restating client goal for session. Client-led activity, client identifies what horses need based their observations.
Treatment Team: Using anything in this arena, build those two places, one that's nice and you can brush, and another that is safe and Nips can eat; let us know when you are done.	Treatment team directs clients to activity through client-stated goal.
Clients create two spaces using PVC pipe, cones, and hula hoops. The spaces are at opposite ends of the arena and the boundaries are well defined. They have collected bits of hay and made a small pile in each space and have brushes placed in the center of one space. Total time 15 minutes. *During the time the clients are creating the two spaces. Carmel stands at one end of the arena near the door, Nips has been standing facing the clients, then moves into each space, head down, nose to ground. Nips picks up a plastic pipe that was a boundary for the safe place and moves it away from the space, she does this four times. Several times Mark fixes it but Nips moves it again. Butterscotch and Cocoa move together toward the spaces but never go "inside the spaces."*	In the Eagala model the treatment team is watching for SPUD'S (Shifts, Patterns, Uniqueness, Discrepancies and apostrophe S or our Stuff). In this example, we are watching/observing the clients' process as well as the interactions of the horses with the clients or what information the horses are providing through their movement. In this situation Nips has moved the boundary several times (a pattern is noted). Clients notice and respond to the horse's movement.
Clients: We are done.	Treatment team acknowledges by nodding and walking towards clients.

(Continued)

Transcript	*Analysis*
Treatment Team: *Moving towards clients, and gesturing towards the spaces.* What's been happening?	Gesture is made toward the space, arm sweep; eyes of team are looking at the space and the horses in or near the space. This creates a non-verbal invitation to discuss the client process.
Client, Mark: This space is a nice place where I can brush them and that place [*pointing to the other end of the arena*] is where Nips can eat. **Treatment Team:** Is there anything else about this space or that space?	Treatment team stands together and continues to watch and nod as client explains the spaces. "Anything else," open-ended, invites further description.
Client, Mark: I put hay in both of them so they would all feel comfortable.	Client stating what was observed by treatment team, client indicates reason for movement/ action.
Treatment Team: Take some time and see if you can get a horse or horses to your spaces. **Client, Mark:** OK.	Redirecting clients back to activity.
Treatment Team: moves away from clients. Mark proceeds to Carmel first and picks up a few hay pieces to try to get the horse to "follow him." Mark and Mary are seen talking and pointing towards each horse. Mark and Mary move to Carmel, petting and talking to him. The horse remains still; he does not move. Nips does move toward Mark and Mary; they then attempt to get Nips to follow. After some effort and verbalizations Nips follows Mark and soon Carmel follows Nips. Both clients move towards the space with the brushes; across the arena Butterscotch and Cocoa enter the space where there is just hay.	Moving away/out of client space allows for clients to problem-solve. Clients are observed as involved in activity, working together and discussing what each horse needs.
Client, Mark: *Turns to the treatment* "That works."	Client indicates that they are finished with the task.
Treatment Team: "What works?"	Restating, using client's words.
Client, Mark: They went to different spaces but it's still good, they have what they need.	Client responds with "what works" for the horses.
Treatment Team: They have what they need, is there anything else?	Restating, using client's words.
Client, Mary: They feel safe and they trusted us.	Clients respond with what they noticed in horses.
Treatment Team: What kind of trust is that?	Expanding on client response.
Client, Mark: We made it safe for them, we took our time.	Client states what was needed to make the space safe. (As the mental health professional, I am thinking that this might be what Mark needs, time.)
Treatment Team: What did they do to let you know that it was safe and they trusted you?	Expanding on response by directing the question through the horses' movement.
Client, Mark: They are still in the spaces we made. *Points to Butterscotch and Cocoa.* Sometimes you don't need to lead them you just have to let them go on their own.	Client stays with present moment experience, observing what is happening in the present and begins to relate to his own experience.
Client, Mark: I need to go on my own, take my time.	Client responds by stating his need.
Treatment Team: What happens when you take your time?	Restating client response.
Client, Mark: I can understand, I can trust. **Client, Mary:** When you are afraid you are better off going slow.	Client indicates what he needs. Clients are processing together
Treatment Team: And when Nips can understand and trust, is there a relationship to that kind of trust and the kind of trust that you need?	Clarifying client statement, this is a Clean Language question, relationship questions are useful but the "timing" of their use is critical. The question asks for more exploration of the self.
Client, Mark: Yeah I guess, I need time to understand, I think that's what I need to do too.	Client explaining need.
Treatment Team: Take some time with them [*gesturing to the minis*] and see if there is anything else they need. *Minis just standing in spaces, still, two in each space.* **Client, Mark:** OK.	Treatment team directing back to activity. This is important as it allows further exploration of needs.

Transcript	*Analysis*
Mark spends the last few minutes with Butterscotch and Cocoa, just petting them and picking up pieces of hay and feeding them.	Clients exploring and connecting to horses.
Treatment Team: What happened?	Final check-in.
Client, Mark: They stayed with us, they didn't walk away, I think they trust us.	Client stating what they observed while petting and feeding hay.
Treatment Team: Would this be a good place to stop for today?	Treatment team sensing closure of session.
Clients, Mark and Mary: Sure, I like them. *Reaching over and petting Butterscotch.*	Clients return to herd and pet each horse before leaving.
Client, Mary: They worked together and we worked together.	End of session. Note: Homework was given to the family: discuss with each other a plan for getting Mark back to his own room/bed. Mark has to indicate his "needs" and "time" needed to accomplish task.

CASE EXAMPLE NUMBER TWO

Description

Tara (a pseudonym) is a 23-year-old female who is employed full-time as an administrative assistant for a local IT company. She is seeking equine-assisted psychotherapy following the sudden death of her father, Allen (a pseudonym). Her father's death occurred one month prior to intake. Allen's death occurred because of a cardiac arrest; he did not have any prior notable medical history; he was 59 years old at the time of death. Tara describes her relationship with her father as often being strained and distant. Her parents were divorced when she was 14 years old and she remained in the primary care of her mother. Tara has one older brother who is married and has a young family. Tara describes her relationship with her mother as "off and on," she reports being "closer to mom than dad" but feels that she has never been supported by either of her parents since their divorce. Tara lives alone but has a few close "work friends" who have really helped her since her father's death. Her direct boss, Alice, has been a "very big support" and was the person who suggested that Tara seek counseling after several very tearful and difficult conversations. Tara felt that the "experiential aspect" of equine-assisted psychotherapy would be more suitable for her than talk therapy.

Goals

1. To accept her father's death.
2. To "let go" of all of the unfinished business she had with her dad.
3. To "move on" without feeling guilty.

Intervention

This is Tara's fifth session. She reports improvement in her mood, being less tearful and engaging more with others. Tara has chosen to work with the same three horses that she started with from her first session. The horses are located in a large pasture next to the barn. All three horses are geldings, a large bay draft she named Strength, a large chestnut draft cross she calls Calm, and a gray quarter horse she calls Spirit. In Tara's last session, she recalled that Spirit would not come to her. At the time, she reported, "That is what Spirit needed; to be free, and to do what he wants."

Set-Up and Materials

All three horses are loose, un-haltered, roaming freely around the field. The treatment team greets Tara. Materials needed: three horses in the field, halters, and lead ropes.

The following transcript analysis are about a pseudonym client.

Table 8.2

Transcript Analysis of Case Example

Transcript	*Analysis*
Treatment Team: Hi Tara, how have things been going? Is there anything that has come up for you since our last session?	Greeting and checking in with client about anything that has been prominent.
Client: Things are pretty good; my boss, just got a promotion, she will probably have to move to a different office and that's really upsetting. I mean I am happy for her but it feels like I'm going to be left alone. **Treatment Team:** Your boss was promoted and might be leaving, you're feeling left alone?	Client states mood and then indicates a "change" that has just occurred and what her feelings are about this new situation. Restating/ reflective client response.
Client: Yes, she really wanted this promotion, it's more money, more responsibility but I feel like she's leaving me behind. I know that it has nothing to do with me, I'm happy for her, I just want to be able to feel that and I want to trust we can still be close. **Treatment Team:** You want to feel happy for Alice and still be close? **Client:** Yes.	Client stated her "desired outcome" as it relates to her boss. This can also be viewed through the struggle she has with the death of her father. The desire to "accept what happened and to let go." Using the client's words to get a desired outcome.
Treatment Team: *Directing client's attention to the herd.* Is there one horse that you would feel happy with if you could get close? **Client:** Yes, Spirit is the one that I can't seem to get close to, he does his own thing.	Client and treatment team are watching herd graze, client nods and smiles. Client points to Spirit.
Equine Specialist: *Hands client a halter and a lead rope.* Take these and take Spirit for a walk to each of the four corners of the field and let us know when you are done.	Treatment team's process is to have client explore "connection" and "relationship." How does the client connect to Spirit and how will she create a relationship?
Client spends the first ten minutes just being near Spirit, touching, talking and walking around Spirit. *The other horses come near Spirit and then move away. Two other herd members move in and out of space.* *As soon as client brings the halter to Spirit the horse turns away. Client tries several times. Spirit never leaves her but moves away from the halter when it is presented.* *This goes on for the next 15–20 minutes.* *Client puts halter down on ground, goes again to Spirit, petting him, begins talking to him, stretches hand out, motions to Spirit. Spirit lifts head, moves to halter on ground, puts nose on halter, grabs halter with teeth, lifts off the ground and lets go, halter drops to ground.* *Spirit moves toward client and begins to follow. Client now walks next to Spirit towards corner of pasture, places hand on horse's neck, both walk together. They reach corner, client pets and talks to Spirit.* **Client**: I think I'm done.	Treatment team discusses SPUD'S, and the "pattern of halter presented and horse turns away." Treatment team notes that "moving away" may be a theme. Treatment team discusses what "halter might represent" to client. Treatment team notes uniqueness of Spirit picking up halter dropping it and then moving towards Tara.
Treatment Team: What happened out there? **Client:** I think he is beginning to trust me; he didn't need me to hold on to him, he let me lead him to where I wanted to go.	Waiting for client response, treatment team moves towards client who is still with Spirit. Treatment team is moving towards client rather than have client move out of her experience. Client places hand on Spirit's back, Spirit stands with treatment team and client.
Treatment Team: He is beginning to trust, he let you lead him. **Client:** Yeah, I just let go of the rope and leash and he let me know that he knew what I wanted.	Restating client's words. Clarifying what happened.
Treatment Team: When let go of the rope and leash, what happened next? **Client:** He picked them up and dropped them, just like I need to drop what holds me back from moving forward. I need to trust that I can get where I need to be without having to have a visible sign all the time.	Using client's words, exploring more about client's experience.
Treatment Team: Is there anything else about need to drop? **Client**: I need to drop the guilt, I need to trust that things will work out the way they are supposed to, I can have what I want without holding on to anything.	Using client's words. Spirit moves closer to client, and blocks the treatment team's view of client. Treatment team stays in place, sensing that the movement of the horse was assisting the client with her felt experience.

Transcript	*Analysis*
Client: Just like that. *Acknowledging Spirit moving closer to her.* I don't always need an answer; I can just trust that things are the way they should be.	Client puts her hands on Spirit, stroking his neck as she discusses trust. Client is "connected" to what she is talking about. Horse leans into client.
Treatment Team: When you can trust that things are the way they should be, what happens next? **Client:** No, nothing else needs to happen I just need to be here and be OK with that.	Treatment team is turned towards client and Spirit, gestures towards client and horse.
Treatment Team: Take the last few minutes and just be OK with being here. We will meet you at the gate when you are done. *Ending session, client meets treatment team at the gate, brief discussion of experience. Treatment team suggests homework for client is to "notice" what she is holding on to when she thinks about her boss's promotion.*	Treatment team moves away from client and Spirit. This gives client time to stay in space and have closure with Spirit. Homework will begin a process of "mindfully allowing and letting go." The first step is to "notice" that she is holding onto something. Introducing simple mindfulness skills to a client's daily experience can help the client to realize that they are not their thoughts. The practice of "noticing" what is being held onto builds self-awareness.

PEACE, LLC Counseling Services
PROGRESS NOTE

Date: ____________
Time:____________
Client: ______________________________**Session#**______ **Modality:**_________________

Mood: WNL, euthymic, anxious, depressed, elevated, irritable
Affect: WNL, labile, expansive, flat, blunted, inappropriate
Motor: WNL, lethargic, hyperactive, agitated, tremors/tics
Speech: WNL, loud, soft, pressured, incoherent
Presentation: WNL, silly, guarded, angry, apathetic, confused, tired

Symptom presentation:

____

____

Issues addressed:

____

____

Goals targeted:

____

____

Homework:

____

____

____

Counselor signature and date: ______________________________

Equine session:
Brief description of session activity.
Draw or write a description of session use SPUD framework, identify any metaphors and themes

FIG. 8.1. Blank Progress Note.

REFERENCE

Equine Assisted Growth and Learning Association (2015). *Fundamentals of the Eagala Model: Practice Untraining Manual.* 8th edition. Santaquin, UT: Eagala.

Section 5

ADHD

9

"Combing" through ADHD Symptoms Utilizing Mindful Grooming

Carlene Taylor

INTRODUCTION

Applications for equine-facilitated psychotherapy (EFP) techniques are as varied as the differences in providers that are now coming from around the world as EFP has gained in popularity. Over the past 25 years since EFP was first formally introduced as a dynamic model of mental health treatment, it has been utilized for many different symptom profiles and disorders for varying populations. This segment will address the use of the cognitive therapy (CT) technique of mindfulness combined in the context of a process experiential theoretical (PET) orientation to the practice of EFP to treat the symptoms of attention deficit/hyperactivity disorder (ADHD) in the farm-based treatment setting. Additionally, application of learning from the experiential setting to the client's lived experience in their "real world" will be addressed. The techniques to be discussed have been applied to client populations of people ranging in age from eight into young adulthood with modifications for age-appropriate attending behaviors based upon normal developmental considerations or developmental impairments. A composite client case example has been provided to illuminate the application and process of the specific interventions recommended. However, let's begin with a discussion of the specific signs and symptoms of ADHD, its prevalence, and the ethical application of EFP as a treatment modality.

ADHD: SIGNS, SYMPTOMS, PREVALENCE, AND TREATMENT CONSIDERATIONS

Prevalence

In 1999, Green, Wong, Atkins Taylor, and Feinleib reported that the prevalence of ADHD in the school-aged population of children ranged from 4% to 12%. These authors also found that up to half of children diagnosed with ADHD also had one of five common co-morbid diagnoses: oppositional defiant disorder, conduct disorder, anxiety disorder, depressive disorder, or a learning disability. Green et al. addressed how accuracy of reporting measures, geographic region, and other psycho-social factors appears to impact prevalence rates, which might indicate a higher degree of subjectivity in the diagnosis of this condition. This is confirmed in a 2014 meta-analysis in which Polanczyk, Willcut, Salum, Kielig, and Rohde noted that extraneous factors were better able to account for findings reporting dramatic increase in ADHD prevalence over the previous decade. The authors concluded actual rates of ADHD prevalence had not dramatically increased when administration and geographical regional differences were factored into prevalence rates. Thus, we can conclude that the prevalence of ADHD is stable within our population, but not quite the "epidemic" that may have been portrayed in pop culture in recent years.

Signs, Symptoms, and Diagnosis

Clients with ADHD often experience great social difficulties, emotional dysregulation and difficulty succeeding in academic and work settings. ADHD is often present with co-morbid conditions of depression and anxiety. Persons with ADHD often experience social isolation, feelings of rejection, and report being bullied more often than individuals without a mental health diagnosis (Sonuga-Barke et al., 2013). According to the *Diagnostic and Statistical Manual of Mental Disorders* (DSM-V), people with ADHD have persistent patterns of inattention and/or hyperactivity-impulsivity that impairs functioning and/or development. There are three primary presentations that can make ADHD look very different depending upon the presentation type (APA, 2013).

1. **Combined presentation**: Both criteria inattention and hyperactivity-impulsivity present for six months.
2. **Predominantly inattentive presentation**: Inattention, but not hyperactivity-impulsivity for six months.
3. **Predominantly hyperactive-impulsive presentation**: Hyperactivity-impulsivity only for six months.

Symptoms include:

Inattention: Lack of attention to detail, careless mistakes. Difficulty attending to tasks or play. Seems not to be listening. No follow through, fails to finish tasks. Trouble organizing tasks and activities. Avoids tasks that require mental effort. Loses things necessary for activities. Easily distracted and forgetful (APA, 2013).

Hyperactivity and impulsivity: Fidgets, taps hands or feet, or squirms in seat. Moves around, cannot sit still. Restless, runs or climbs at inappropriate times. Unable to play or take part in events quietly. "On the go" acting as if "driven by a motor." Talks excessively. Blurts out an answer. Trouble waiting for a turn. Interrupts or intrudes on others (APA, 2013).

Treatment Considerations

The symptoms of ADHD impact the social, emotional, and cognitive development of children particularly during the critical developmental years of elementary school and can have lasting effects impacting outcomes into adulthood (Wong, Hall, Justice & Wong, 2015). Wong et al. (2015) also noted that ADHD is a biologically based illness that often requires psychopharmacological treatment, which includes the use of stimulants. Stimulant medications can have significant side-effects including appetite suppression, sleeplessness, and increased emotionality. Sonuga-Barke et al. (2013) explored a meta-analysis of ADHD studies. Their findings revealed that relative to specific ADHD symptoms, targeted pharmacological intervention was the most effective and that Cognitive-Behavioral/psychotherapeutic interventions were not as effective as medication. In fact, their findings suggested that combined pharmacotherapy and psychotherapy was not any more effective that pharmacotherapy alone. When taken by themselves, this could suggest that psychotherapy/behavioral therapies are not effective for ADHD. However, Chronis-Tuscano (2013) noted that ADHD is a complex disorder with functional effects reaching far beyond the individual ADHD symptoms alone, and psychotherapeutic/behavioral approaches are effective in the development of coping mechanisms that assist clients in improved overall functioning even if the non-medicine-related treatments do not significantly reduce the ADHD symptoms directly.

In effect, it seems the literature suggests that psychotherapeutic and behavioral treatment efforts are best focused on the development of functioning adaptations so that clients can cope with the life challenges that ADHD symptoms bring. To that end, we present an integrative technique that combines a traditional Cognitive-Behavioral technique—mindfulness meditation—with the therapeutic horsemanship activity of grooming, allowing the client to experience symptom management and task completion in the therapeutic moment. Processing following the activity assists clients in translation of this technique into task behaviors for activities of daily living outside of the therapeutic environment. The following is a discussion regarding the creation of the necessary therapeutic container and the implementation of the technique.

PROCESS EXPERIENTIAL AND MINDFULNESS: AN INTEGRATIVE APPROACH

Process Experiential-Emotion Focused Theory

A key component to a therapeutic outcome is building the necessary container of therapeutic relationship or any technique, no matter how innovative, is destined to fail for lack of therapeutic alliance. To be clear about this component, we will address the theoretical orientation of the overall program in which the example is provided. The program at LightHorse Healing, Inc. is grounded in a process experiential-emotion focused theoretical approach. Process experiential theory, also known as emotion-focused therapy (PE-EFT) is an evidence based, neo-humanistic theory integrating person-centered, Gestalt and existential therapies (Elliot & Greenberg, 2007). The founding theorists, Elliot and Greenberg, identify six primary therapist behaviors integral to the application of this theory: achieving empathic attunement, fostering an empathic/caring therapeutic bond, facilitating task collaboration, helping the client process the experience appropriately to the task, supporting completion of key tasks and fostering client development and empowerment are keys to application of this theory.

In general, PE-EFT is an approach that seeks to help clients transform contradictions and impasses brought to light through the process of task completion into wellsprings for growth by bringing challenges experienced in the real world into the here and now of the therapeutic session. The personhood of the therapist is an integral part of the therapeutic container that makes this process possible. Techniques from other theories are often employed in the context of the PE-EFT relationship container to bring about healing and behavioral change. In essence, doing experiential work as a therapist is less about the specific model or theory techniques deployed and more of a way of being in the world. This unique perspective includes a deep belief that humans are, at their core, good, healthy, and desiring of growth. It honors every individual's innate knowledge and wisdom while supporting the importance of authenticity, congruence, relationship, and active engagement in all aspects of relationship and of life. Experiential practitioners live this philosophy. It is their orientation to the world and thus they are comfortable modeling it in every interaction. For the therapist with this worldview, the PE-EFT approach is a natural fit when integrated with equine-facilitated psychotherapy.

Mindfulness Meditation for ADHD

Smalley et al. (2009) reported that mindfulness is positively associated with self-directedness and self-transcendence, which are counterintuitive to the individual with ADHD. Their findings indicate that interventions that increase mindfulness might improve symptoms of ADHD and increase the personality traits of self-directedness and/or self-transcendence that could be considered positive coping behaviors to overcome developmental deficits caused by ADHD. Van de Weijer-Bergsma et al. (2012) identified improvement in executive functioning as noted by parental and teacher reports and improvement in actual functioning on attention tests in an adolescent population with ADHD after an eight-week mindfulness training program. The authors noted that effectiveness waned after a 16-week follow-up with no further training and suggests that long-term effectiveness may need the development of a maintenance program or regular independent practice. These two studies are representative of positive reports for the inclusion of mindfulness practice to benefit those with ADHD. There appears to be reasonable evidence to suggest inclusion of mindfulness practices can be beneficial to the client struggling with symptoms of ADHD.

Baer (2003) described mindfulness as intentionally bringing one's attention to both the internal and external experiences happening in the present moment. In keeping with traditional mindfulness practices as outlined by the "father" of mindfulness, Jon Kabat-Zinn (1990), the mindfulness practice of purposefully directing one's attention in the present moment and in a non-judgmental way, is what is deployed in the LightHorse Healing, Inc. program. Clients are invited to attend to their internal experiences occurring in each moment with focus on bodily sensations, thoughts, and emotions while staying attuned to the sights, sounds, and responses of their equine partners. Thus, the practice of mindfulness is the lived experience in the moment of non-judgmental observation of the ongoing stream of internal and external stimuli as they arise from the client as they complete their task.

CASE EXAMPLE

Client Description

Jane (a pseudonym) is a 22-year-old unmarried Caucasian woman. She identifies as Christian, but denies a regular religious practice. She lives with her parents who recently moved to the community from a southeastern city where she was home-schooled by her mother from third grade through high school. The client reportedly received a homeschool diploma equivalent to public high. She is currently enrolled in an online class/training program for canine massage therapy; however, client and parent report she is not making sufficient progress to complete the course in a timely manner. Jane reports difficulty keeping a job. She indicated having been hired three times in a field that she is highly interested in (working with animals) but states she has been "let go" from all three positions within 60 days of beginning work and seems confused as to the reasons. She stated she received positive feedback from her employers but eventually she was "dropped off" the schedule or just not called back to work without a formal evaluation or termination. Initially, the client had little insight about her potential role in the employment difficulties but with success in treatment, client could develop insight into her behaviors that may be impacting her employability. Currently, Jane works in a pet-sitting business that was developed and is supported by her mother who complains about Jane not taking the initiative to get new clients or follow through on leads/referrals. Mother reports feeling overwhelmed that she is "working harder" in Jane's business than Jane seems to be.

Jane reports being of heterosexual orientation and in a committed relationship with her boyfriend of four months. Jane indicates "I don't want to mess this up, [he] is so good for me and we are perfect together." Jane came in for counseling following a psychiatric inpatient crisis stabilization experience. The eighth in her lifetime, hospitalizations reportedly beginning as early as six years of age. Jane reportedly threatened suicide and took a bottle of thyroid medication following an incident of being "gang raped" by several men at a party. Jane reported a history of high-risk sexual behaviors with multiple partners since moving to the community following the breakup of a committed relationship of over three years with a person she describes and "emotionally, physically, and sexually abusive." Jane indicated she began dating this person at 17 with no prior sexual experiences and in retrospect she understands the relationship to have been abusive. Neither incidents of sexual abuse have received attention from legal authorities. Jane did not report the behaviors of her long-term boyfriend because she was complicit in the acts and did not understand them to be abusive until after the relationship broke up. The recent sexual assault was reported to authorities as part of a process involving her inpatient hospital stay. However, the client reported that law enforcement did not consider the incident as criminal because she was impaired (smoked marijuana and consumed high amounts of alcohol) and witnesses corroborate the men's stories that the client initiated a group sexual activity and at no time did she appear to be non-complicit in the acts. The client states she does not have a clear memory of the events that led up to the acts, but that she felt like she "would never have agreed to" sex with multiple men at the same time.

Reason for Referral

Jane is voluntarily seeking mental health treatment reporting a diagnosis of anxiety for which she takes medication and "whatever else is going on that makes me do stupid things that I regret later." She reported she has a history of mood lability and difficulty with focusing, completing tasks, keeping a job, attending to activities of daily living, providing for herself (totally dependent upon parents), repeated suicidal ideation and previous attempts, sexual promiscuity, low self-esteem, shame/guilt/remorse, and lack of direction. Client reports that she has had "horrible" experiences with psychiatry and many of her hospitalizations have been following medication changes. She stated that beginning near the last year of her longest relationship (identified as abusive) and intensifying following her recent sexual experiences, she has experienced hypervigilance, intense anxiety and periods she describes as "zoning out or losing it," which sounds like periods of disassociation and intense emotional dysregulation.

She currently is taking a medication she describes is for "anxiety" as her only psychotropic medication and does not wish to pursue medication changes until she has a better understanding of "what is wrong with me." Client was recently diagnosed with a thyroid condition similar to *Hashimoto's thyroiditis* in which thyroid supplementation involves increasing certain thyroid hormones and decreasing others. She is being followed by an endocrinologist who recommended counseling and addressed how it is possible some if not all her psychiatric symptoms could be explained or at least exacerbated by her thyroid condition that went undiagnosed until she was 21.

Diagnosis and Justification

The client stated she has received psychiatric treatment from many different providers and received many different diagnoses in the past including multiple mood disorders, personality disorders, and has been medicated with a variety of mood stabilizers, antidepressants, antianxiolytics, and antipsychotics. She denied a history of psychotherapy other than occasional attempts of a few sessions with different providers recommended by past psychiatrists. Thus, a fresh perspective was needed on determining a working diagnosis and further detailed exploration is recommended as part of an ongoing process of treatment. With review of all available medical and mental health records and in consultation with her primary care and endocrinologist as well as integrated with information gleaned from clinical interview and bio-psycho-social assessment the following working diagnosis:
hyper- and hypo-thyroidism

bipolar disorder, type I, due to general medical condition of hypo- and hyper-thyroidism

ADHD, combined presentation of inattention & hyperactivity/impulsivity post-traumatic stress disorder, dissociative subtype.

Justification

In consultation with the client's physician's current thinking concerning the client's dramatic psychiatric history, beginning at a very early age is best explained as a secondary condition to a genetic abnormality with the patient's thyroid that created intense mood swings and when combined with severe ADHD lead to impaired social, emotional, behavioral, and moral development, which over time compounded her functional challenges. A diagnosis of PTSD has been acquired by trauma that has occurred due to poor judgment, poor decision-making, and lack of self-protective factors commonly found when psycho-social development is impaired as the client fell victim to sexual predators and/or engaged in risky sexual behaviors that at the time of engagement were consensual but post-experience was traumatic. The client's identification of the symptom of anxiety and panic when explored further appears to be more related to dissociative experiences and a result of a presentation of PTSD or hyper-activity or manic presentation of mood instability. Exploration of substance use/abuse/ addiction was completed and client has had some substance use and limited periods of substance abuse, but decided quickly after beginning to use substances at 20 years of age that she could not use alcohol or drugs in excess and ceased use of marijuana completely. She reports occasional use of alcohol but not in excess.

Medication Considerations

The client is currently taking Saphris prescribed by a previous psychiatrist in her former city. Saphris is an atypical antipsychotic that the client takes daily and when she feels a "panic attack"—as she refers to them but more accurately describes an impending dissociative experience—coming on. The client's previous provider requires that she obtain a local psychiatric provider so further psychiatric follow-up is needed. At this time, she is not receiving medication to address her ADHD symptoms and is not interested in medication intervention due to potential complications with other psychiatric illnesses and medication interactions.

Goals of Intervention

This client is a complicated case with multiple issues presenting. Initial goals for treatment were defined as:

4. Complete bio-psycho-social assessment from an integrative team (medical, psychological, psychotherapeutic, and psychiatric) to explore and confirm diagnosis and to inform long-term treatment planning.

5. Involve client in life visioning to determine her desired outcome of treatment. Client identified being engaged in a safe long-term romantic relationship, productive self-supporting meaningful work, improved adult child–parent relationships as her long-term life vision.
6. Develop symptom management skills to address symptoms of mood lability, focus, attention, task completion, academic and work performance, organization, goal-directed behavior, and social/relational improvement with individuals and groups.

Rationale for Use of Equine-Facilitated Psychotherapy

The client describes herself as an "animal person" and finds animal relationships to be more successful than human relationships. She selected this provider because of the provider's expertise in animal-assisted therapy and the provider's inclusion of a canine partner in the clinical office setting and the opportunity to work in a therapeutic farm environment. In addition to client self-selection, the client's symptoms and impairment are significant enough to require a high interest activity to improve compliance with treatment recommendations. The client's high motivation to work more closely with the animals and in the therapeutic farm setting provided the necessary impetus for the client to take control and change behaviors over which she indeed did have control. Additionally, because of the client's initial low insight into her behavioral impact on others and her high number of previous psychiatric/mental health providers, the PE-EFT approach of this therapist, the therapeutic program, and the experiential nature of the work allowed the client to receive direct feedback when possible from the animals thereby lowering resistance to difficult insight that was necessary for the client to facilitate lasting change.

Contraindications, Ethical and Cultural Considerations

Due to the severity of this client's symptoms, there were many opportunities for contraindications for this client to participate in EFP to be present. Active disassociation, psychosis and behavioral dyscontrol creates an unsafe situation for the client and animals and thus is contraindicated for EFP participation. The client's culture of upper-middle class socio-economic status, previous attraction to equestrian sport without having had the opportunity to participate in equine activities in spite of a longing, and her liberal Christian spiritual background supported offering the LightHorse program to this client. However, the deep interpersonal connections with EFP and the high risk/high reward nature of EFP could present an ethical issue with this client in the event that EPF services were to be suspended due to mental/emotional/behavioral decompensation, financial support withdrawn from parents because the client is unable to pay for services on her own resources, or other unforeseen factors before client had made sufficient progress in treatment to not be emotionally harmed by the withdrawal of services.

To address these potential contraindications and ethical concerns, the client began therapy in the more highly controlled environment of the clinical office, which is not connected to the farm and is located in a professional office in a nearby town. The client's family was involved in treatment planning and rapport was established with both the client and her parents, working diagnosis, initial treatment planning, and establishment of rapport of other integrative medical and psychological team members was established before suggesting EFP sessions as part of the treatment modality. The client successfully completed the life visioning exercises in session with the therapist, demonstrated the ability to be present and control dissociative experiences. A full disclosure process was provided to the client and her parents about the risks, potential contraindications and ethical concerns if the "plan" does not go as planned for all concerned. Everyone involved agreed to the risks vs. potential benefits and agreed to do their part to prevent conditions that would lead to one of the issues of concern. The client was clear on behavioral expectations (regular compliance with therapy appointments, direct and clear communication with therapist, medication compliance, and reasonable follow-through on appropriate homework assignments necessary to ensure progress outside of session would be possible.

Finally, the client began services at the farm with a limited six-session introduction prior to being paired with an individual horse for increased depth work followed by a check-in evaluation with the client and parents to identify observed benefits and to discuss any observed risks before moving forward. At the check-in session with the client and parents, it was noted the client's mood had been more stable at home, and her compliance with therapy appointments and assignments had remained consistently positive. The client had gained some tremendous insights into her behavioral impact on others and was more receptive to receiving feedback from the experiential environment than she had been to accept feedback from the therapist in the clinical office setting. It is significant to note that the ADHD symptoms of disorganization, poor time management, lack of focus, poor attention, and poor performance on task completion has not improved significantly since beginning therapy in the office nor in interventions currently presented in the experiential setting. The client, family, and therapist agreed to proceed with EFP and to specifically target these problematic symptoms that were negatively impacting the client's life.

Additional ethical considerations had to be addressed when the client was cleared for longer-term EFP sessions that would ultimately facilitate a deeper therapeutic relationship with the equines. The program horses range in age from 15 to 28 years of age and there are three miniature donkeys whose age is unverifiable. Equine selection to work with this particular client had to be considered. Many clients are able to meet, greet, and then choose from all available equines during their particular appointment time. However, this client was not suited for the youngest of the horses due to his particular sensitivities and personality characteristics. She was not well suited for working with the oldest of the horses—although he is in good physical shape and enjoys client engagement—because her particular level of intensity, the potential that at some point he will have to retire from the program, and the fact that working with older horses can be unpredictable in terms of timing for illness or retirement meant that this therapist was not comfortable facilitating what could be an emotionally intense equine relationship between this client and a horse who has reached an advanced age of 28. The miniature donkeys were also not well suited for this client due to intensity. Thus, this client was given the choice between only two horses rather than choosing between any equine in the program, which is preferable.

EFP SESSION DISCUSSION

Equine Partner

In the previous six-week "introduction" sessions, the client was introduced to the overall program components of the LightHorse Healing, Inc. Therapeutic Horsemanship Program, which includes mindfulness practice, grounding, centering, and introduction to the Native American Spiritual philosophy. Likewise, she was also introduced to the "herd" members, both human and equine that are typically present during her session and had participated in experiential activities such as stall/pasture cleaning, composting, gardening, and the use of art or journaling for processing the experience in the moment and at home following the session.

Through this introductory experience, Jane had come to know the "stories" of the equines in the herd and which ones were available for her individual work. She elected to work with Odie. Odie is a 22-year-old American Quarter Horse. Odie and his brother Deacon have been program horses for the past two years. Prior to his program involvement, Odie was a trusted friend of his owner since birth and together they have ridden trails around Georgia for hundreds of miles. Odie's owner died three years ago and Odie's life as he knew it changed. Odie is well behaved and safe, but highly sensitive and is prone to anxiety. Jane was aware of Odie's challenges and that encouraged her to ground herself and monitor her internal responses to help Odie remain calm in their interactions.

Goals and Objectives of Session/Intervention

Three sessions into connecting Jane and Odie, Jane had previously been introduced to the primary grooming tools and learned the appropriate use of each tool. She and Odie had begun to get used to each other and were settling into familiarity in the stall. She demonstrated increased comfort at reading Odie's body language and gauging her anxiety level when in Odie's presence.

The goal of the fourth session was for Jane to demonstrate increased ability to mindfully complete a task and increase sustained focus.

The objectives for this session were:

- to practice non-judgmental focus and sustained attention in two 10-minute mindfulness periods
- identify and process her internal and external experiences with the therapist
- attend to the responses of her horse
- adjust her behavior if needed to demonstrate responsiveness to another.

Jane had previously participated in guided meditation with this therapist, but had trouble staying focused for the meditation. She reported her mind wandered during the meditation and found the process to be anxiety-producing because she could not let go of judgment that she was in someway not "meditating correctly." She previously had not been successful at participating in mindfulness meditation at home. Overall the goal and objectives of this session are working toward the overall treatment plan goal: Goal 3: Develop symptom management skills to address symptoms of mood lability, focus, attention, task completion, academic and work performance, organization, goal-directed behavior, and social/relational improvement with individuals and groups.

Session Set-Up/Materials/Process

For this session, Odie was in his stall and his halter and groom box were on hand. His stall was cleaned and he completed eating his hay so there were no food distractors in the environment. Fly control methods were deployed to limit environmental distractions. The task of this session was for Jane to engage in mindfulness practice and focus her attention for two ten-minute segments during the session while she used the curry comb on each side of Odie. In the mindfulness session, Jane was instructed to focus on her internal and external sensations without praise or blame. Additionally, she was to attend to Odie's responsiveness to her grooming. She was instructed to notice intrusive thoughts and utilize her breath to reconnect with the present moment. At the end of ten minutes of focus, this therapist processed with Jane her experience and with insight about her initial experience, she retried the exercise to improve her focus and experience progress beyond her personal expectations.

The following transcript analysis are about a pseudonym client.

Table 9.1

Transcript Analysis of Case Example

Transcript	*Analysis*
Therapist: Ready to work with Odie [horse] today? Therapist looks for eye contact, congruence and compliance with instructions. Client: Hi! Eye contact with therapist. Hi, Odie. Peeks in stall. Oh yes! I start getting excited about seeing Odie a few days before the session. He is so sweet! Odie acknowledges client over the stall door, client touches nose affectionately and reaches for halter.	Client check-in prior to encountering horse is part of safety and pre-screening to ensure contraindications for experiential therapy are not present before session begins.
Therapist: You certainly look like you are ready, let's do a quick body scan before you go in and check where you are inside. Do you think Odie is comfortable with us hanging out here in front of his stall to check in? Are you comfortable checking in here? **Client:** Takes a step back and looks at Odie, ears forward and noise hanging over the stall door. Yes, I think he is cool with it and I know I am good.	Continued check-in process.
Therapist: Great. You know the drill by now, plant your feet into the earth, soften or close your eyes, and turn your attention to your breath. Notice your breath, no praise, no blame, just notice your breath. Where is, your breath going in your body? Pause. Scan from the bottom of your feet, notice your feet connected with the earth, move your attention up your legs, notice your muscles, the joint spaces in your ankles, knees, hips. Move your awareness up your back body, and up your front body. Move your attention with your breath into your shoulders, down your arms, through your elbows, forearms, wrists and out your hands, breathe in and send your breath into your neck, throat and into your head, out the top of your head. Take one more minute and with your next breath scan your whole body from feet to head and back again. No praise, no blame, just noticing what you notice. Pause. Now, gently wiggle your fingers and toes, gently let the light come back into your eyes and bring your attention back into this space with Odie and I. Odie's head is over stall door, close to client's face. Therapist waits for client to make eye contact with therapist and connection is established. Client follows therapist's directions, and chooses to close her eyes, deepens her breathing. She reaches out with her right hand and takes hold of Odie's halter that is hanging at hand/shoulder height near her right arm. Client remains still and quiet with no obvious signs of distraction.	Use of this brief, guided meditation check in is to continue to confirm client's current level of functioning and compliance with therapist's directives before entering the horses stall. It is also to establish a base line of client's ability to focus and attend for even a brief period, which will serve as the base line in the primary task assigned for the session.

Transcript	*Analysis*
Therapist: Tell me what that experience was like for you. Client: Relaxingsmile. I could pretty well follow along, I kept feeling Odie's breath on my face, that was nice, and my mind would wander to what we were going to do next and I had to try and get back to my body. Holding the halter helped me feel by having something in my hand. My knee is sore, it does not hurt, but I feel it [prior knee surgery]. My breath was in my chest but I felt it slow down on its own. My anxiety is about a five, not in a bad way, excited. I just can't focus for long, I'm sorry.	Open ended statement allows client to explore and express her total experience and highlight what was most important/significant to her. Client answered in an open-ended way and gave therapist clues to her sensitivity to physical touch and established a base line of feelings of anxiety and focus.
Therapist: Of the two minutes that meditation took, how long, what percentage, do you think you were "in" the meditation vs. how long you were distracted? **Client:** Hmm. I think I was in it about 50% of the time. Better than last week, usually, but only about half the time. I just can't focus, I'm sorry.	Client to identify bench mark pre-intervention and client's inability to release judgment is a current issue.
Therapist: What happened to "no praise, no blame"? Smile. Remember the importance of suspending judgment on yourself. You are perfect, just the way you are. No one ever improved by shaming themselves into it. **Client:** Sheepish smile. Thank you, I'll try to remember that.	Offering client unconditional positive regard, investment in therapeutic rapport and modeling for client non-judgmental outlook.
Therapist: Let's go in with Odie. **Client:** Smile—goes in, begins to halter Odie as she has practiced in previous sessions, she greets Odie, makes eye contact, pats him on the neck, and places halter on Odie and proceeds to tie him as per procedures already learned.	Transition from pre-session to begin designated task completion
Therapist: I notice you have this haltering down pat. Nice job, you seem more confident today than four weeks ago. **Client:** He makes it so easy, he holds he head still. It's like he likes this part.	Positive reinforcement, encouragement. Client demonstrates alliance with horse, identified connection and transference.
Therapist: Why would a horse "like" to be haltered and tied in his stall with some humans? Odie haltered and tied, client stands ready for next directive. Take a moment and check in with Odie. How is Odie? **Client:** Because he likes the attention. Talking to Odie. We will do almost anything to get attention won't we Odie? Client steps back and looks at Odie's face and body. Odie is relaxed and excited, kind of like me, I guess. His ears are forward, he put his head down into the halter like he wanted to be haltered.	Challenging client to question depth of connection. Continued identification (will use this identification in later sessions when time to confront client's attention-seeking behaviors).
Therapist: Todays exercise is continuing with grooming but this time we want to add a component to the task. How comfortable do you feel you are with the curry comb and brushes thus far? **Client:** I think I am good with it, at first it was hard to know how much pressure to use and it was just weird being next to him, didn't want to get stepped on, but I feel comfortable with it now.	Set up and check in with client to ensure base of comfortability with the task before adding the component of mindfulness during the exercise.
Therapist: Great! This time, we want to slow the process down and use the mindfulness technique we have been practicing, like outside the stall, except this time follow your breath and focus your attention on what you are doing in the moment while you are grooming with the curry comb. The only goal here is to keep your head (thoughts), your heart (emotions), and your body (behavior) all doing the same thing at the same time for an extended period Client begins to get curry comb out of the groom box while instructions are being given, +for impulsivity.	Set-up of task, provide instructions and provide client with parameters and expectations for success/completion. This defines and brackets the task.
Therapist: You could focus and stay present for about a minute at check-in, right? **Client:** Yep, that was about it.	Setting base line to compare for improvement at end of task.
Therapist: Well, I am going to keep a timer and when time is about half over I will let you know. When half-time is over, hopefully you will be about halfway through that side, if you are not, just use it as a guide to adjust how quickly you work to complete the side. Take your time, there will be plenty of time to complete the task, no rush. Attend to the feel of Odie's skin, keep checking in with your eye contact with him, the goal is to keep you mind in the moment with the task, but it's OK to attend to different processes like your emotions, the actual task of currying, your assessment of how Odie is doing, etc. Got it? **Client:** Smile. Sure, this sounds like fun, are we good with Odie? Makes eye contact with Odie.	Clear instructions, parameters of the task, attending to reducing anxiety with clear instructions so client knows exactly what to expect. Purposefully did not tell her time length of task so as to not create anxiety of time limit.

(Continued)

Transcript	*Analysis*
Therapist: Remember to start by connecting with your breath and if you find yourself distracted, return to your breath and resume where you left off before the distraction occurred. **Client:** Got it. Client centers herself, closes her eyes for a moment and as she exhales and begins currying behind the horse's ears on the left side.	Gave client final directive and reminder of how to return to focus in case she loses in during the activity. Demonstrates she is engaged in the task.
Therapist moves back to a portable chair in the back corner of the stall where horse and client can be observed, therapist sets silent timer to begin exercise and engagement with client. Client engages in task; limited distractions are noted. At one point in the experience she stops, closes her eyes, breathes, and resumes.	Task begins.
At seven minutes, therapist gently reminds client time is half over. Client seems mildly started, makes eye contact with Odie, surveys the whole horse's body, re-grounds herself and resumes second half of task.	Task continues without intervention for therapist. Detail of instructions provided in beginning so that therapist can stay "out of the way" of the way during the task.
Therapist continues to monitor process and keep time for remaining eight minutes of task. Time is called at 15 minutes, with therapist saying "exercise finished." Client steps away from activity, she had completed currying the left side and was reworking/rechecking hip for last minutes of time.	Task continues with observation, not intervention.
Therapist: Moves near client and horse. How did it go? **Client:** How long was that? I sort of feel like it might have been a few moments, but then it could have been forever. I kind of lost track of time, I was so into it. Smiling.	Open-ended question inviting client to direct processing.
Therapist: Does that surprise you? **Client:** Yes, I know it was longer than the beginning but it's like I have no idea how much time passed. It was amazing. I feel so relaxed!	Continuing open-ended questions, not giving time answer to encourage depth of process
Therapist: How do you think Odie feels? **Client:** OMG, he is relaxed too. He is still propped up on his hip, his eyes were half closed. It was like he was breathing with me. I could feel him breathe, it is SO cool! His body was warm and it was like I could see the circle partners in his coat.	Allowing client to settle into her insight and assessment that she exceeded her expectations of performance.
Therapist: Did you have any trouble staying focused? Tell me a bit about what happened along the way. **Client:** At first I could feel anxiety in my chest, but I stopped, breathed and remembered "let go" to let go of my expectation. I knew if I got caught up on my worry it would upset Odie, I just didn't want to upset Odie, I wanted him to be able to relax and enjoy being with me and I know if I am anxious I will make him be anxious too. And it worked! I was shocked, it worked! I forgot about being worried and just got into the grooming. It was like I could see it with different eyes. How did you do that?	Invite client into specific processing about the experience as set up for second attempt.
Therapist: How did I do that? I didn't do anything. How did YOU do that? **Client:** Wow. I did do it didn't I? Smile.	Empowered client to claim progress rather to project progress on to therapist.
Therapist: Any other insights you have about that experience you want to share before we move on to the other side? Can't leave him only half done, right? **Client:** Wow. I am kind of tired all of a sudden. I hope I can do it again.	Moving client to second half of task, checking for any other insights not yet spoken.
Therapist: Will you approach this side any differently than you did the last one? **Client:** I think I better understand what it feels like, so I am ready to go. Odie is still just chilling, aren't you Odie? Talks to Odie directly.	Opening the client to task responsibility.
Therapist: How many times in that experience did you feel your mind wander and you had to pull yourself back into the moment? **Client:** About three times, just for a few seconds, I was really surprised.	Setting parameter for second half of task by having client identify progress initially and set goals for next round.

Transcript	*Analysis*
Therapist: Great. Get yourself and Odie ready, and I'll keep time again. Same deal as before, I will give you a gentle reminder when half-time is complete. Client picks curry comb back up, and moves to left side of horse's neck, makes eye contact. Puts comb and hand on neck, closes eyes, breathes for a moment, horse lowers head gently and client begins task.	Reset for secomd half of task, still did not disclose how much time is being measured to encourage client to just go with the process. Client observed trying her own "grounding" exercise as she puts both hands on horse as she focuses on her breath.
Note: Client completed second half of task as planned, therapist followed similar process as in the initial task. Narrative resumes with processing at the end of the second half of task completion	
Therapist: How did it go? **Client:** Awesome. I don't think I lost focus at all. I can't believe it. I have never been so focused and I am so relaxed right now. I kind of feel like Odie looks [obviously relaxed]. How did that happen?	Open-ended processing, allowing client to notice what was significant to her rather than therapist observations.
Therapist: Let's consider this segment only first. What did you experience physically in your body when you were doing the task? Client: I could feel the warmth of his body through my hand. I felt my feet in the dirt, when I finished grooming I just wanted to touch him and he let me. He let me just lay my head on him and I could feel his ribs moving when he was breathing. It was amazing.	Directing processing through physical, emotional and mental experiences to allow client to solidify processes that lead her to success in task completion. Client was very aware of her kinetic response. Kinetics may be an important coping skill to help this client be focused in the moment.
Therapist: Notice any feelings? **Client:** Peace. Just peace. I was anxious a bit the first time, which made me more distracted, but this time I knew how cool it had felt the first time, so I was comfortable just going with it. It was peaceful and now I am feeling tired, but in a good way.	Although client was not asked to compare and contrast the two experiences, she did it naturally on her own. Had she not, therapist would have directed questioning to comparison eventually.
Therapist: Now, what about thoughts? What did your thoughts do? **Client:** This time, just really kept thinking about what I was doing, watching the dirt come up off the skin and seeing the circles in his fur, wondering if he was as OK as I was and feeling happy when I looked at him and saw him relaxed. The first time, I could feel myself get distracted a couple of times, but not this time. I was in it.	Continued process, explore different avenues of experience.
Therapist: How do you feel right now, in the moment, just talking about it? **Client:** Tearful, amazed. I would have never believed I could do it, it must have been Odie that made me do it.	Lead client to present/emotion-focused processing
Therapist:: Odie? Odie stood there and enjoyed it. Who did it? **Client:** Pause. I guess I did, but I don't know how. How long did I stay focused?	Empowering client to accept her abilities so she can repeat outside of the therapeutic farm setting.
Therapist: Would you believe it if I told you a total of 20 minutes—two ten-minute periods? **Client:** NO WAY!	Previously kept time totals in the background so client to discuss experience and depth before realizing or addressing her area of challenge.
Therapist: Way. Smile. **Client:** Why was it so easy here and it is impossible at home?	Provided positive feedback and reinforcement for client's ability to be the change she wants to see. Client trying to integrate learning into real world.
Therapist: Was it so easy here? Or did you just apply yourself? I saw you try, not give up. It did not look easy, but you were successful none the less **Client:** I guess it wasn't easy. I did try.	Empowering client to not expect "easy" to be successful.
Therapist: When you break it down what did you really do? **Client:** I knew up front what I was trying to do and I tried it, I was concerned about staying cool so I did not upset Odie, so that was what guided me and kept me from freaking out and when I noticed it wasn't working, I stopped found my breath and tried again.	Client breaking down her process, therapist listening so process can be reinterpreted to her for application to other settings.

(Continued)

Transcript	*Analysis*
Therapist: How can you do that when you are trying to do something that's like, not in the barn, something you need to/want to do in the "real" world? **Client:** Oh wow, I am usually just a mess out there. I don't feel out there like I do right now here. Actually, I don't usually feel like I do now anywhere. Smile.	Directing exploration to application.
Therapist: Yes, but if you feel like it here you can feel like it out, there, right? How we do one thing is how we do all things, we just have to re-create the right conditions out there, right? Let's pick an example of something you need to do out there and want to do. Not wanting to do it is another problem, let's just work with something you "want to do" out there first. **Client:** Yes, that makes sense. Let's talk about my course, I really want to do that, but I just cannot focus. I study for five minutes and then I am done, I got to move.	Reinforcing client's ability to make changes with the right steps, empowering client to make changes in life.
Client and therapist continued to process session, addressed learning styles, coping skills for learning challenges and reinforced concepts and insights gained during equine experiential session. Client addressed her physical and emotional symptoms that continue to hinder her in forward movement. **Client:** Thank you Odie. Hug, pat on neck, snuggle at neck. You are so amazing. I could not do it without you. Offers treat.	Keeping client connected to the partnership between her and her horse, giving gratitude for her therapy partner's help and keeping the connection going.

FURTHER DISCUSSION

Client Outcome Over Time

The session above occurred a few months prior to this writing. The client and therapist continued to work with the themes uncovered in the meditation process. Client continued to work with letting go of judgment so that she could be open to learning about herself and make adaptations in her task behaviors to work with her natural tendencies while she also applied herself to learn new skills, such as mindfulness practices. The therapist worked to deepen therapeutic alliances, engender hope and impart information that allowed client to continue to learn about herself and grow.

The following sample session note are about a pseudonym client.

The following session note example is about a pseudonym client

Client Name: Jane Dough
Date of Session: 10/15/2017
Page: 1 of 2

Date of Birth: 1/1/1998
Time: 1:00 pm–1:58 pm
Billing Code: 90856

Mental Status Exam:
Client was present, on time and appropriately dressed for the experiential session. She displayed a mood congruent with her slightly anxious affect at the beginning of the session, which relaxed to euthymic throughout the process of the session. She denied any current history of suicidal or homicidal ideation since last session. She was oriented to person, place, time, and situation. No evidence of disassociation occurred during today's session and there was no evidence of formal thought disorder. Speech was somewhat rapid at the beginning but became more modulated through session. Attention was easily distractible at the beginning of the session, but improving by the end. Client reported normal appetite, sleep, and elimination with no changes in medication since previous session.

Treatment Goal Progress:

Goal 1: Complete bio-psycho-social assessment from an integrative team (medical, psychological, psychotherapeutic and psychiatric) to explore and confirm diagnosis and to inform long-term treatment planning.

Progress this session: Maintained, client awaiting medical appointment.

Goal 2: Involve client in life visioning to determine her desired outcome of treatment. Client identified being engaged in a safe, long-term romantic relationship, productive self-supporting meaningful work, improved adult child–parent relationships as her long-term life vision.

Progress this session: Progressing, client working to bring vision to reality.

Goal 3: Develop symptom management skills to address symptoms of mood lability, focus, attention, task completion, academic and work performance, organization, goal-directed behavior and social/relational improvement with individuals and groups.

Progress this session: Progressing, today's session focused on this goal.

Objectives and Interventions

- Demonstrate increased ability to mindfully complete a task and increase sustained focus.
- To practice non-judgmental focus and sustained attention.
- Identify and process her internal and external experiences with the therapist.
- Attend to the responses of her therapy animal.
- Adjust her behavior if needed to demonstrate responsiveness to another.

FIG. 9.1. Sample Client Session Note.

Situation/Subjective:
Client expressed difficulty focusing that is significantly impacting her ability to provide for herself and complete necessary tasks for activities of daily living and work/study behaviors. Current difficulty is challenging her above to obtain and sustain employment, client is concerned that she is dependent upon her parents and unable to provide for herself. Client reported difficulty following guided meditation and practicing mindfulness on her own leading to feelings of being defeated and helpless.

Observation:
Client was eager for session and engaged with writer and equine partner. She found focus difficult outside of the connection with her horse, but with clear parameters around the task, and non-judgmental encouragement client was able to develop a curiosity about herself and find methods that helped her increase her focus and ability to remain mindful throughout the exercise. Client was able to process learning and apply it to external challenges and make a plan to apply knowledge learned in session to the outside world.

Action:
Writer guided client in a guided meditation to check client's appropriateness for experiential work with equines. Client was present and cooperative with therapist; no evidence of disassociation was noted. Client followed writer's directions and engaged in two focused mindfulness exercises. Writer led client in interpersonal exploration that allowed her to transfer knowledge of learning style to create adaptations for task behaviors associated with learning for her to try between sessions. Therapist utilized process-experiential/emotional focused approach to the application of a Cognitive Therapy technique of mindfulness meditation practice to improve focus and attention of task oriented behaviors.

Plan:
Client will apply learning from session and attempt adaptation to study behaviors to improve focus on academic work completion. Next session, writer and client will engage in creative activity to allow client to practice adaptation in the therapeutic environment to reinforce still development. Sessions will continue to utilize horsemanship tasks with mindfulness practices to assist client in development of focus and attention during task behaviors.

Other Notes: Client to attend psychiatric evaluation 1/20/2018.

______________________________ _______________

Dr. Carlene H. Taylor, LMHC, LPC, CPCS, NCC — Date
Licensed Clinical Mental Health Counselor

FIG. 9.1. *(Continued)*

REFERENCES

American Psychiatric Association (APA). (2013). *Diagnostic and Statistical Manual of Mental Disorders.* 5th edition. Arlington, VA., American Psychiatric Association.

Baer, R. (2003). Mindfulness training as a clinical intervention: A conceptual and empirical review. *Clinical Psychology: Science & Practice, 10*(2), 125–143. Retrieved from www.wisebrain.org/papers/MindfulnessPsyTx.pdf.

Chronis-Tuscano, A. (2013). Key issues relevant to the efficacy of behavioral treatment for ADHD. *The American Journal of Psychiatry, 170*(7), 799.

Elliot, R. & Greenberg, L. (2007). *The essence of process-experiential: Emotion-focused therapy.* American Journal of Psychotherapy, 61 (3), 241–254.

Green, M., Wong, M., Atkins D., Taylor, J. & Feinleib, M. (1999). *Diagnosis of Attention-Deficit/Hyperactivity Disorder.* Technical Reviews, No. 3. Rockville (MD): Agency for Health Care Policy and Research (US). Retrieved from www.ncbi.nlm.nih.gov/books/NBK44173/.

Kabat-Zinn, J. (1990). Full Catastrophe Living: Using the Wisdom of your Body and Mind to Face Stress, Pain, and Illness. New York: Delacorte.

Polanczyk, G., Willcut, E., Salum, G., Kielig, C., & Rohde, L. (2014). ADHD prevalence estimates across three decades: An updated systemic review and meta-regression analysis. *International Journal of Epidemiology, 43*(2), 434–442.

Sonuga-Barke, E., Brandeis, D., Cortese, S., Daley, D., Ferrin, M., Holtmann, M., … & Sergeant, J. (2013). Nonpharmacological interventions for ADHD: Systemic review and meta-analysis of randomized controlled trials of dietary and psychological treatments. *The American Journal of Psychiatry, 170*(3), 275–289.

Smalley, S. L., Loo, S. K., Hale, T. S., Shrestha, A., McGough, J., Flook, L., & Reise, S. (2009), Mindfulness and attention deficit hyperactivity disorder. *Journal of Clinical Psychology, 65*, 1087–1098.

van de Weijer-Bergsma, E., Formsma, A.R., de Bruin, E. I., et al. (2012). The effects of mindfulness training on behavioral problems and attentional functioning in adolescents with ADHD. *Journal of Child & Family Studies, 21*, 775.

Wong, D., Hall, K., Justice, C. & Wong, L. (2015). *Counseling Individuals Through the Life Spa*n. Thousand Oaks, CA: Sage.

Section 6

AUTISM

10

EQUINE-ASSISTED PLAY THERAPY WITH CLIENTS WITH AUTISM SPECTRUM DISORDER

Tracie Faa-Thompson

AUTISM SPECTRUM DISORDER

According to the *Diagnostic and Statistical Manual of Mental Disorders 5* (APA, 2013), an individual with autism spectrum disorder (ASD) shows deficits under two broad categories:

1. Deficits in social interactions and communication.
2. Restricted or repetitive patterns of behavior and interests.

Tantum (2012, p. xxiv) provides a unique definition of ASD as "a disorder of the unconscious linkage between people, mediated by nonverbal communication." People with ASD struggle with accurately deciphering a myriad of subtle verbal and non-verbal cues of fellow humans.

ASD affects people in many different ways. For some, it is a debilitating condition while others can harness their ASD and utilize their unique qualities. Yet common features among people with ASD tend to be the desire to belong; possible development of an anxiety disorder in their teens and twenties; and experiences of being bullied (Tantum, 2012). Therefore, many people with ASD will benefit from counseling interventions. However, traditional counseling approaches can have limitations for people with ASD because of their tendency to take everything literally. The use of metaphor, which can be very effectively with other populations in equine-assisted therapy (EAT), can be ineffective for teenagers and children with ASD. Even common directions must be specifically concrete. For example, in one EAT session we were working with a group of pre-teens who were setting up an obstacle course. One of the boys with ASD knocked his shin on the plastic pole as he was moving it. It did not look as if he had hurt himself but due to his sensory issues he started hopping around holding and rubbing his trouser leg. Since safety is paramount and we needed to make sure that he was not hurt, my co-director, Jaki, called his name and said, "Pull your trouser leg up," intending for him to roll his trouser leg up so we could see if there was an injury. He immediately grasped a hold of his trouser, lifted his leg in the air, and hopped on one leg. Immediately realizing her mistake, Jaki corrected herself and said "roll up your trouser on your hurt leg so I can see if your leg is scraped."

Animal-assisted therapy (AAT) may be particularly helpful for children and adults with ASD for several reasons. First, a growing number of studies have found that children and adults with ASD are receptive towards animals (VanFleet & Coltea, 2012). Second, people with ASD are not forced into verbal conversation in AAT. Third, in AAT they are not confused by subtle facial expressions of humans. Fourth, they are more apt to understand obvious body movements of animals. Finally, people with ASD tend to enjoy the sensory experiences of touching fur.

ANIMAL-ASSISTED PLAY THERAPY

The International Institute of Animal Assisted Play Therapy was co-founded by Dr. Rise VanFleet and Tracie Faa-Thompson in 2004. Animal-Assisted Play Therapy™ (AAPT) is defined as the integrated involvement of animals in the context of play therapy, in which appropriately trained therapists and animals engage with clients primarily through systematic playful interventions, with the goal of improving clients' developmental and psychosocial health, while simultaneously ensuring the animal's well-being and voluntary engagement. Play and playfulness are essential ingredients of the interactions and the relationship (VanFleet & Faa-Thompson, 2017). It is the therapist's training, skill, and expertise as a play therapist, and their ability to utilize playfulness and affirming humor that helps create the emotional safety clients need to address problem areas.

POSITIVE TRAINING METHODS

At Turn About Pegasus, an equine-assisted program for at-risk youth, we work primarily with horses, although the other animals on the farm might turn up on occasion and invite themselves into a session. All our horses have been trained exclusively with positive reinforcement with ethological methods grounded in science. As a result, they are unafraid to offer lots of behaviors because the worst that will happen is no response from the humans. All our horses are eager to work with clients and bring their own unique selves to the therapeutic interventions. Since horses are sentient beings (e.g., able to perceive or feel things) and not toys, they are trained positively. Through this positive approach, horses offer behaviors and communicate their needs very effectively with their whole selves.

We do not adhere to the pressure–release model, which is popular in many natural horsemanship circles. This approach pushes the horse to the point at which they become scared, resistant, confused, etc., and then allows them to retreat to the last place they were comfortable, before repeating the process. Small steps towards the human's training goal are rewarded by a release of the pressure. This pressure–release model would be questionable if humans were trained in that way. It does not appear to be an effective or ethical method of training since physiology and psychology indicates that a relaxed non-aroused state is needed for learning. Sullo (2009) states that when learners are pushed to the point of fear, they focus on self-preservation rather than the acquisition of new knowledge and the development of new skills. By removing fear, learners take risks and learn more. Thus, a positive approach to training horses is far more effective and ethical.

In AAPT, the therapist invites clients to notice the subtler nuances of the horses' body language, starting with the ears and moving onto other parts of the body. Then clients are encouraged to notice the subtler "language" of the horses such as lip wrinkling, muscle tension, stiffened tail, slight raise of the head, etc. This is particularly helpful for clients with ASD who may often miss social cues of fellow humans. If clients with ASD can learn to "speak horse," then they can transfer this insight to humans.

In order to assist clients in this way, it is important that the therapy team learn the body language of horses, fluently, and then learn the individual nuances of their own individual horses. This requires learning from experts in the field such as ethologists and trainers. It also requires many hours of hands-on experience so therapists are attuned to what the horse is feeling or communicating. Such training will help therapists pick up the subtler body language of not only horses but their human clients as well. Horse and human body language is one of the many core competencies needed by AAPT practitioners (Van Fleet & Faa-Thompson, 2017).

INTERVENTION: WASHING HORSES' TAILS AND FEATHERS

At Turn About Pegasus, four full-day sessions are needed to teach clients about the way horses communicate and what the horses' body language is telling them. By this time, most clients feel more in control of themselves, are comfortable around the rear of the horses, and have let go of their fears that the horses' main aim in life is to kick them. After this is accomplished, we introduce the washing of the horses' tails and feathers (the long thick hairs on the bottom of traditional cobs and draft horses' feet). Clients with ASD tend to have sensory issues and struggle with unfamiliar sensations. In a traditional room-based play therapy session, many clients with ASD would never immerse their hands and elbows in warm soapy water. However, doing so for the horses makes it acceptable.

As in AAPT (VanFleet, 2008), the rewards of washing the horse's tail and feathers are multidimensional for clients with ASD.

- Clients have to work physically, close together as a team to achieve the goal, thereby enhancing their social skills.
- There are lots of sensory opportunities in the lathering of the tails such as soapy bubbles, conditioner, oils, and the difference in texture of the tails. The Arabians have silky tails and the Natives coarser hair. Other sensory stimulations include the feel of sponges, brushes, combs, as well as plastic and metal pourers and buckets; being outside in nature and feeling the grass and the wind; seeing the trees; smelling the farm; and hearing a multitude of birds, small wild mammals, and insects.
- It is fun. The horses are loose and sometimes walk off to a tasty morsel of grass. The clients are left trailing behind the horse desperately trying to keep his tail in the bucket and not slop all the water out of the bucket, laughing all the way.
- This activity teaches frustration tolerance. The physical prompt of the horse's wet, soapy tail motivates clients to persevere despite the frustration. Clients can see the results of their efforts directly in that the horse's tails and feathers are clean, full, and luxuriant. They are always surprised at how much dirt was in the water to begin with and take pride in showing others in other teams how clean they got their own horses' tails.
- It is hard work washing and conditioning tails and then plaiting them. For the horses with feathers, there needs to be a further application of oily mite repellent that has to be painted on with a paintbrush. This is a process that has to be followed in a particular order so clients have to keep focus and concentrate and not get distracted.
- The experience provides the opportunity to take another's viewpoint when horses decide to do their own thing. Horses can only see the experience from their own perspective and are incapable of doing something deliberately to annoy the human. Understanding the horses' viewpoint promotes insight in clients with ASD of how others may feel with them.
- The horses enjoy the sensation of getting their tails and feathers rubbed and stroked. Clients are asked how they know their horse is enjoying the activity. They are asked to observe the horse's whole body (e.g., relaxed body, droopy bottom lip, relaxed nostrils, half-closed eyes, resting back foot etc.). Then they are asked to reflect on what the horse may be feeling, although we never can be sure just like we can never be certain what another human being is thinking or feeling. It can feel much safer to the client with ASD to experiment with attempting to think about what the horse may be feeling than to guess at what a fellow human being is feeling.
- Clients have the opportunity to nurture and care for another creature, which can facilitate empathy. This activity and indeed all the activities with the horses are designed to assist with nurturing empathetic feelings first with the horses and then bridging over to fellow humans. We have never had a client be unkind to the horses in this activity.
- The experience also teaches limits and boundaries because clients often want to wash the whole horse. We do not allow that for the following reasons:
  - Too-frequent washing robs the horses of the natural oils in the skin, which are there for protection.
  - Some horses are not keen on getting washed on their bodies especially near their heads and eyes.
  - Most clients are unused to washing horses and there is a great danger of them accidently getting soap in the horse's eyes, ears, or up their nostrils. If that were to happen, the clients would feel bad and be less likely to want to continue. It would not be an option to ignore the horse's discomfort to save the client's feelings or to hold onto the horse and force them to accept the washing of their bodies.
  - If the weather turns bad and the horses are not dry enough they are in danger of catching a cold or chill.

CASE EXAMPLE

Corey (a pseudonym) was a 15-year-old boy who lived in a specialized children's home for children with autism. As with many children with ASD who have also experienced seriously neglectful family backgrounds, it was difficult to know which of his behavioral traits were due to his attachment difficulties and which were down to his autism as there are many parallels between the two conditions. He also had a diagnosis of ADHD.

When Corey arrived at Turn About Pegasus, he was placed in a group of six teenagers all from different children's homes or foster care placements. The teenagers did not know each other and were meeting for the first time. Corey was the only one with a diagnosis of ASD. The other teens in the group had multiple diagnoses ranging from conduct disorders to anxiety disorders to self-harming and self-abusive behaviors. None of the teenagers were in mainstream education. The group was receiving eight full-day sessions of equine-assisted play therapy and social learning.

At the beginning of his first session, Corey did not want to engage with anyone. He remained unresponsive and did exactly the opposite of what was being asked of him including going to meet the horses. We did not want to push him, no pressure or release, and allowed him to sit where he was comfortable with his care worker. Corey's care staff from the children's home tended to treat him with kid gloves as he often would go from withdrawn to physically lashing out if he was challenged. This was probably due to anxiety rather than anger, but the overt presentation was an angry one. In our program, he was expected to engage to the best of his ability. We always use the five-finger contract (Trotter, Chandler, Goodwin-Bond, & Casey, 2008) so that clients know they will not be asked to do something beyond their capacity. Corey eventually walked through to meet the horses who were eager to meet him. A horse named Buster approached him and turned around to invite him to scratch his bottom. Within minutes Corey was fully engaged and remained engaged throughout his time on the project.

There is a tendency in some areas of AAI towards a form of anthropomorphism by suggesting that the horse knew exactly what the client needed to engage or heal them. Our view at the International Institute for Animal Assisted Play Therapy™ (IIAAPT) is that the animals are being themselves and are not thinking "if I do this or this then I will engage or heal this person." It is the skill of the therapist to provide the therapeutic environment to facilitate the process and not make suggestions about the horses knowing just what the client needed. If the client makes those connections and verbalizes them, then that is acceptable as these reflections are client-led. This is not to suggest that domesticated animals that have lived with humans for thousands of years do not pick up on and respond to people's emotional arousals or states just like any sentient being will pick up on differing emotions. These abilities are both a relationship and survival strategy for humans and animals. This is also one of the reasons why horses are excellent for this work as they are more attuned to human's body language than humans are to them due to horses' superior vision, hearing, and sense of touch and smell (Levison & Mallon, 1997; Melson 2001).

Session four was washing tails and feathers, which occurred on a warm day. Corey chose his favorite horse (Buster, an Arabian) and worked in a team with two other people. His care worker had warned he did not like to get wet and suggested he not do this activity. Yet Corey was up for the challenge and his team worked well, listening to instruction and getting wetter and wetter. The therapy team was watching closely, making facilitative comments. Corey was an exceptional leader and motivator for his team and worked really hard, seemingly not perturbed by the water. All of a sudden, Buster took his tail out of the bucket and with the dexterity of movement unique to Arabians flicked his soap-covered, drenched tail up and down and sideways saturating his team and covering them in bubbles. The girl in the team screamed. Corey was covered in bubbles even in his hair. I looked at Corey and said "Buster must have thought you guys needed to wash your hair too." Corey looked stunned and then burst out laughing as he looked at his drenched team. Then everyone else laughed. He said "I've been in a car wash but never a horse wash." Everyone laughed even louder and Corey was delighted that he had made such a good joke.

Children and adults with ASD are often wrongly characterized as not having a sense of humor or getting jokes. Corey was a joker throughout his time at Pegasus. Although he may not have understood sophisticated metaphorical jokes, he was a master at in-the-moment, slapstick-style humor that Buster inadvertently provided. For example, on another occasion he was walking with Buster who was breathing gently on his neck and he said with a smile on his face and a twinkle in his eye, "Tracie, I have my very own air conditioning."

Since Buster was free and unrestrained, he was being himself when he flicked the water. My therapeutic, gentle, playful but empathetic humorous comments helped facilitate the acceptance of being wet unexpectedly. His care staff were stunned that Corey did not have a behavioral meltdown in that moment due to all his sensory difficulties, his inability to understand or pick up on non-verbal cues, and having to deal with the unexpected. However, Corey understood implicitly that Buster was not getting him wet on purpose but rather just being a horse.

In contrast to Corey's apt understanding, many people in the equine field might have misinterpreted Buster's propensity to not stand quietly and not do exactly as the human wanted as being not very well trained. An alternative perspective is offered by respected horseman Mark Rashid (2016) in his book A Journey to Softness. In response to Rashid's invitation to his pupils to write about their own journey to softness, Michelle Scully discussed how in one of Rashid's videos he demonstrated the differences between softness and lightness. Two horses were shown, one ridden with softness the other with lightness. Michelle stated:

> We see a lot of horses that are highly trained respond almost instantaneously to the smallest ask. What I hadn't noticed before is that sometimes, signs came along with that, such as ear pinning, bit- chewing, tail swishing or tail clamping. I hadn't been in a position to put words to if before, but now it was making sense. Some horses are trained within an inch of their lives, but they are not really digging it. They go through the motions, but their outsides and insides are not in unity.
>
> (Rashid, 2016, pp. 56–57)

Going through the motions yet being disconnected between what is presented on the outside and how they feel on the inside could also be said of many of our clients with ASD. A simple sensory activity like washing tails in an accepting non-pressurized environment can for a while give them the opportunity to feel the connection from within and without.

Corey made excellent progress and continued to be the joker of the group. He also made a great enduring friendship with one of the older girls in the group who was in a group home near him and helped out at local stables. Corey went along to the stables and proved to be a hard worker who had great affinity with the horses. He learned to ride and was always respectful of the horses and concerned in case he may hurt them. A month after our sessions ended, he was reintegrated into mainstream education where he is excelling. He wants to be a veterinarian.

CONCLUSION

Washing tails and feathers conducted in a playful and accepting manner in an outdoor environment, which is relaxing and accepting, can have a multitude of therapeutic benefits for clients and horses alike. Horses that have been trained positively, who are able to work in their familiar natural environment where they have freedom of choice, whether to stay or go, will only enhance the therapeutic experience, often in unexpected ways as seen in this case illustration. Like all our activities in AAPT, this is an activity done with the horses, not to them. It is not about the client exerting control over the horses using certain learned techniques or special equipment. It's about partnership and reciprocity and shared experiences, all bundled up within an atmosphere provided by the human therapeutic team and the horses of acceptance, light-heartedness and fun. It is within this whole package that clients no matter what age or what the presenting issues are can be helped to towards healing.

REFERENCES

American Psychiatric Association (APA). (2013). *Diagnostic and Statistical Manual of Mental Disorders* (DSM-V). 5th edition. Washington, DC: American Psychiatric Association.

Levinson, B. M. & Mallon, G. (1997). *Pet-Orientated Child Psychotherapy*. 2nd edition. Springfield, IL: Charles C Thomas.

Melson, G. (2001). Companion Animals and the Development of Children: Implications of the Biophilia Hypothesis. In A. H. Fine (Ed.), Handbook of Animal Assisted Therapy (pp. 376–382). San Diego, CA: Academic Press.

Rashid, M. (2016). A Journey to Softness: In Search of Feel and Connection with the Horse. North Pomfret, VT: Trafalgar Square Books.

Sullo, B. (2009). The Motivated Student: Unlocking the Enthusiasm for Learning. Alexandria, VA: ASCD.

Tantum, D. (2012). *Autistic Spectrum Disorders Throughout the Life Span*. London: Jessica Kingsley Publishers.

Trotter, K. S., Chandler, C. K., Goodwin-Bond, D. & Casey, L. (2008). A comparative study of the efficacy of group equine assisted counselling with at-risk children and adolescents. *Journal of Creativity in Mental Health, 3*, 254–284.

VanFleet, R. (2008). Play Therapy with Kids & Canines: Benefits for Children's Developmental and Psychosocial Health. Sarasota, FL: Professional Resource Press.

VanFleet, R. & Coltea, C. (2012). Helping children with ASD through Canine-Assisted Play Therapy. In L. Gallo-Lopez & L. Rubin (Eds.), *Play-Based Interventions for Children and Adolescents on the Autism Spectrum* (pp. 193–208). New York: Routledge.

VanFleet, R. & Faa-Thompson, T. (2017). *Animal-Assisted Play Therapy*. Sarasota, FL: Professional Resource Press.

11

Improving Social and Communication Skills for Participants with Autism Spectrum Disorder through Equine-Assisted Psychotherapy

Saan Ecker and Joanne Byrnes

INTRODUCTION

Between 1% and 2% of the population has autism spectrum disorder (ASD) (Christensen, Baio, & Braun, 2012). Reports of diagnosed ASD have grown by 120% between 2000 and 2010, that is, from 1 in 150 to 1 in 68 (Center for Disease Control and Prevention, 2014). It is acknowledged that this extreme growth in rates may be related to expansion of diagnosis criteria or increased awareness, as well as a true increase (American Psychiatric Association (APA), 2013).

Characteristics of individuals with ASD can include: lack of social and communication abilities; aversion to change; low adaptability; difficulties in developing, maintaining, and understanding relationships; deficits in verbal and non-verbal communication; insistence on sameness; restricted and fixed interests; and hyper- or hypo-reactivity to sensory input (APA, 2013). The impact of ASD includes limited social interactions, hindered learning, and limited occupational opportunities. Extreme difficulty with planning, organizing, adapting, and coping with change means that as adults, individuals with ASD may struggle to live independent lives (APA, 2013). Around one-third of young adults with ASD have never been employed and many live in assisted living conditions (Howlin, Goode, Hutton, & Rutter, 2004).

BACKGROUND

Animal-assisted therapy (AAT) is emerging as an option to support individuals with ASD (Mapes & Rosén, 2016). It has been proposed that AAT can assist individuals with ASD to develop sensory and social skills, manage problem behaviors, and improve quality of life (O'Haire, 2013). One rationale for AAT is that social aversion shown by individuals with ASD may be human-specific and not apply to interactions with animals (O'Haire, 2013). Christon et al. (2012, as cited in O'Haire, 2013) found that that 63% of parents of children with ASD reported perceived improvements from AAT. The most frequently reported outcome was increased social interaction. Reduced social isolation and reduced self-absorption are also reported as benefits of AAT for individuals with ASD (O'Haire, 2013).

Research into equine-assisted psychotherapy (EAP) for individuals with ASD has shown promising results although there is a limited evidence basis at this stage. The majority of research into EAP for ASD has been in regard to horseback riding interventions with children (Bass & Llabre, 2009; Fletcher, Grannemann, Richardson, & Trivedi, 2011; Hawkins, Ryan, Cory, & Donaldson, 2014; Memishevikj & Hodzhikj, 2010). Mapes and Rosén (2016) reviewed 12 studies examining the efficacy of EAP for ASD and found that only one study did not show some benefits. Overall, these studies showed that EAP improved physical and social functioning, communication, sensory sensitivity, sensory motivation, self-regulation, adaptive skills, motor skills, and motivation, and led to reductions in severity of ASD symptoms (Mapes & Rosén, 2016).

THEORETICAL APPROACH AND RATIONALE FOR EQUINE-ASSISTED THERAPY

Our therapy training includes Gestalt and Buddhist psychotherapy; family and systemic constellations; psychology as well as various influences of equine-assisted psychotherapy. While we operate from this theoretical background, our methods for working with participants with ASD have been developed through trying different approaches over time and following the lead of our horses. In comparison to evidence-based treatment practices for individuals with ASD, our method is compatible with social interaction and social skills training and the natural teaching aspects of Applied Behavioral Analysis (ABA) models. The rationale for our approach is described more fully in the descriptions of our procedures below.

ETHICAL ISSUES IN ANIMAL-ASSISTED THERAPY PROGRAMS

Horses and Facilities

Our horses are kept in a natural boarding situation with free roam over 100 acres except when they need to have calorie restrictions, at which time they are keep in long "runs" of around 1km round-trip, as per the Paddock Paradise model. They run as a herd and have a dynamic social life within the herd. The mixture of mares, geldings, a stallion, and a one-eyed miniature mare get on very well. They are all high spirited and are not "push button" quiet horses. Some of them are quite bombproof (as well as being spirited) and we tend to use these quieter ones for our ASD clients, in keeping with the limiting of overstimulation that many of our clients appear to prefer.

Horse Handling

Our horses are experienced therapy horses who are used to working with people. Most of them have developed their own "styles" of working with people and each of our 11 horses are very different in what they bring to the therapy sessions. They are handled along natural horsemanship concepts and we work with them to develop their courage and independence. Our horses are very good at "saying" no, which is an essential part of their effect. We coach clients to respect the horse's "no." We believe horses who submit immediately without question are not as valuable in teaching relationship negotiations and also success can be too easily found. That said, our horses have been developed to a high standard of obedience when required as demonstrated by the ability of many the horses to play Parelli's seven games at liberty.

We coach all our clients to read the horses' body language and manage the inclination of most humans to progress and "make" horses do stuff, for the benefit of the horse and also to teach patience, distress tolerance, and a range of other emotional resilience skills. Our sessions emphasize positive social interactions and enjoyable learning for both human and horse. Despite some of our ASD participants having had to leave other (non-animal-assisted) programs because of aggressiveness, we have never had a case of aggressive or abusive behavior. Quite the contrary, these individuals have all developed extremely caring and respectful relationships with their horses.

EQUINE-ASSISTED THERAPY PROGRAM FOR PARTICIPANTS WITH ASD

During our sessions with ASD participants, we work with horses on-ground on halters or at liberty. We focus on interactions and building relationships with the horses. We use metaphors and modeling to relate relationship-building exercises to interactions with people. We also provide a range of learning exercises that allow the development and exploration of new skills using a large variety of props on our farm including a cross-country obstacle course that has jumps, walk-throughs, pedestals, a teeter totter, a labyrinth, round pens, and a sand arena.

Participants

Participants on the autism spectrum attending EAP at Peakgrove are generally Level 2 or 3 severity as described in the DSM-5, requiring very substantial support for deficits in social communication (APA, 2013). Some of our clients are entirely non-verbal, as described in Level 3 and others speak in short, simple sentences (Level 2). In keeping with the higher rate of males with ASD, about two-thirds of our participants are male. Ages of participants with ASD attending Peakgrove range from 6 to 30 years old. Carers, parents, or other family members attend sessions with ASD participants. Having a more extraverted co-participant or a parent or carer work with another horse can help clients overcome imitation.

Goals and Objectives of Our Approach

Our approach for participants with ASD is guided by the following objectives that are related to specific deficits or issues faced by individuals with ASD.

- Emotional regulation
- Building social-emotional reciprocity
- Enhancing verbal and non-verbal communication
- Developing and maintaining relationships
- Experiencing success
- Enhancing mood and motivation
- Breaking inflexibility and rigid thinking patterns.

These goals are discussed below.

Emotional Regulation

The horses play a key role in assisting with emotional regulation, based on the hypothesis that simply being in the presence of horses, under certain conditions, can have a calming effect on the human autonomic nervous system. In conjunction with the Australian University of New England, we conducted a multiple single case research project using our horses at our facility in 2016. The results are pending journal publication but suffice to say this research confirmed the effects of the presence of horses on calming the nervous system of humans.

This research was undertaken with a developmentally normal population; however, based on observations of ASD clients, we believe we can extrapolate this effect to individuals with ASD. Being in the presence of a horse, either at liberty or online has the effect of calming many our clients with ASD who usually have agitated and restless movements. It is worth noting that this is likely to apply to emotionally healthy horses who are not in a stressed state. ASD clients may arrive in an agitated state, walking rapidly in circles. After some time with the horses they will calm and focus and become more "in tune" with their horse. This opportunity to practice regulation of emotional states is important in helping participants cope with everyday stress, and be available for learning and connection with others.

Building Social-Emotional Reciprocity

Social-emotional reciprocity is a difficult concept for many individuals with ASD. A key ingredient in our program for helping participants with ASD develop this reciprocity is the principle of empowerment and autonomy, enabling people to make choices in their own time. We also focus on the empowerment and autonomy of the horse and call this "horse time." Horse time is the time that horses naturally take to move, make decisions, problem-solve and so on. Horses, like people, want to retain their autonomy. Natural horsemanship leader Pat Parelli coaches to wait for the horse to "ask a question." That is, wait until the horse shows some readiness before continuing. We have observed that participants with ASD appear to be tuned into these signs of readiness, or they respect signs of un-readiness to move (e.g., yawning, micro sleeps, looking away).

Particularly for the ASD participants who have strong social introversion or are strongly hyperactive or hypo-reactive to stimulus, we have found that using the same approach of encouraging them do things in their own time to be very effective in growing confidence and in building social and other skills. We coach our participants in this slow and conscious, give and take approach when working with horses.

Observing "Horse Time" Intervention

When negotiating obstacles or tasks, explain or demonstrate the task and then allow participants to take as much time as they want. Look for signs of readiness in both the horse and participant and only encourage when both signal readiness. This timeframe may be outside your comfort zone and they may seem to be waiting for a long time. At a certain point in time the horse may suddenly walk forward without resistance. On closer observation, you can often see that the participant has waited for a sign of readiness from the horse. We believe some of the participants with ASD attending our program have an extremely good ability to read this readiness in horses and we can learn more about reciprocal readiness between horses and humans from them.

We have noted two main benefits from this approach for participants with ASD. One of these benefits is that ASD participants can use the timeframe that they would prefer to operate in, such that they will move forward when there is a shared or reciprocal readiness. They may ask things of the horse in the same way they want to be treated. Another benefit is the change we have noted in the way carers communicate with their ASD charges after witnessing how participants work with the horses. Seeing how effective using "horse time" is in gaining the horse's confidence and willingness, demonstrates the value of this approach to carers.

Carers have learned to look for these signs of readiness in their clients/children. On the basis of this, we run workshops just for carers where carers can practice horse time, waiting for readiness, and exploring 50/50 leadership models with the horses. Exercises where carers and parents can experience reduced levels of control or power and develop strategies to share leadership are the main focus of this workshop. An example is OK Corral's "Appendages" where a group of three or more must stay linked together with only the use of the left and right hand of the group to saddle a horse at liberty, and only the person in the middle can speak.

We have had feedback from carers and parents that time with the horses is one of the few times that ASD participants are able to operate in their own timeframes and provides a space for them to relax without pressure to perform. Horse time means that ASD participants do not have to follow the rigid timelines that they usually have no option but to follow and can, in companionship with their horse, enjoy going at their own pace.

Enhancing Verbal and Non-Verbal Communication

Improvements in speech and non-verbal communication documented in some equine-assisted therapy programs are hypothesized to be as a result of the participant making connections between the commands to the horse and the horse's behavior (Mapes & Rosén, 2016). When the horses responded to the commands, the participants learn that their communication is impacting the horse's behavior (Mapes and Rosén, 2016).

Based on advice from Rupert Issacson (Horse Boy Method), having a range of commands that horses respond to can be empowering for participants with ASD. On the basis of this, we have taught some horses to pick up their legs (Spanish walking style) on the command of pointing to the front legs. All our horses all back up from simple hand signals or the word "back." Horses can comprehend pointing gestures (Maros, Gacsi, & Miklosi, 2008) and most of our horses have learned that pointing means we want them to go in that direction. They are also responsive to following a gaze in a direction.

Hence, ASD participants are able to use these commands to successfully communicate to the horses. This is particularly empowering for non-verbal participants. Individuals with ASD can have difficulty with the concept of pointing, following another's gaze, or showing objects to others (APA, 2013). Finding that these non-verbal and verbal commands can motivate an otherwise resistant horse helps motivate the use of these interactions skills. Getting success using these commands helps expand the range of communication they have with the horses and also with humans. This is similar to social skills training recommended for individuals with ASD. Social skills training may focus on increasing eye contact or inviting a peer for a play date, which contributes to overall social skill development. These skills can be practiced on responsive horses.

For ASD participants that are verbal, we have also noted differences in verbal communication around the horses. In a number of cases, talking has changed from talking about nonsensical matter to talking about the horses, the farm, themselves, and even asking about us. These behaviors suggest stronger social engagement as a result of EAP.

Developing and Maintaining Relationships

In our sessions, we have discovered the benefits of participants diagnosed with ASD working with the same horse at each session over time. This allows the development of a bond between the horse and participant. This bond provides the opportunity to overcome deficits in ability to develop and maintain relationships associated with individuals diagnosed with ASD. The effect of horse and human getting to know each other, and indeed liking each other are clear in the initial meeting of the horse and person at each session. With regular clients who attend at the same time each week, some of our horses turn up at the correct time, appearing as if waiting for the participant who works with them.

The importance of the human–animal bond is of increasing interest in animal-assisted therapy research showing contact with animals can increase relaxation and health as measured by a number of physiological measures including heart rate, blood pressure, and oxytocin levels (Cole, Gawlinski, Steers, & Kotlerman, 2007; Odendaal, 2000; Serpell, 2011; Wells, 2009). However, there is limited information on how horses effect these measures. Lanning, Baier, Ivey-Hatz, Krenek, and Tubbs (2014) suggest that much of the improvements in physical, emotional, and social functioning may be due to the therapeutic effects of the bond between ASD participants and the horse.

We have a strong focus on quality of experience rather than quantity of things they achieve. The emphasis is on helping the participant to stay focused, in relationship with the horse and the therapists and carers. Relationship comes before tasks. In keeping with principles of evidence-based treatment for ASD, we provide positive reinforcement when participants show socially appropriate behaviors with the horse. As therapists, we are also very consciously offering connection with the participants, mostly using the horse as the shared focus rather than a focus explicitly on the participant. This is in keeping with the suggestion by Bass and Llabre (2009) that ASD children in their EAP programs could pay attention to the horse as a shared reference for the child and the instructor/therapist. An example of building an initial relationship using nonverbal social cues is our "Meet, don't move the feet" exercise.

"Meet, Don't Move the Feet' Intervention

Participants are coached in observing their own personal "bubbles" and the horse's "bubble" by asking them to approach the horse in a way that the horse doesn't move away from them. If the horse is about to move due to the pressure of being looked at or advanced upon, participants are coached to stop and move backwards, before the horse moves away. In more advanced sessions they are asked to step back before the horse looks away. Through observing and reading the body language of the horse and approaching and retreating to keep the horse and the participant comfortable and safe, skills are learned about respecting and understanding the personal space of self and others. This also builds confidence in nervous participants. This initial contact with the horse can take several sessions or be quite instant.

Experiencing Success

It can be difficult for individuals with ASD to develop a sense of success in their everyday lives. Repeated small and successful attempts at obstacles and tasks mean that both horse and participant slowly develop confidence and skill to take on more challenging tasks. During exercises with the horses, we gather information about how the participant themselves wants to learn and how they encounter and cope with new things. We can then incorporate that information into their therapy program. We have noticed increasing ability to cope with changes and new things across all of our ASD participants. Another factor in this success is increasing the leadership skills of participants as the horses are "tuning in" to the degree of leadership the participant is showing. Our horses are all quite independent such that if the handler is not concentrating or not giving adequate leadership, even a horse seasoned to an obstacle may refuse to do it. Hence participants need to stay present if they are going to keep the horse focused.

Successes where the horse is motivated rather than pressured require "reading" the horse and noting the horse's level of motivation or interest. Participants receive an abundance of positive reinforcement for demonstrating these skills of reading the emotions of the horse that would be considered socially appropriate behaviors in relation to humans. An example of how we help participants set up for success is discussed below.

Setting Up for Success Intervention

Coach participants to slowly introduce the new obstacle to the horse, using prior preparation and accepting and rewarding small tries (e.g., through allowing the horse to rest). Help the participant understand the horse's performance threshold at any time. For example, at the first try it might be enough for the horse to sniff a new obstacle. Encourage participants to recognize these small tries as successes and see success with the horses to mean that the participant will set up the horse and the horse will do the task themselves (i.e., without force). Importantly, coach that relationship is more important than the task.

Our ASD participants don't generally need to be told not to use force and in most cases, seem to have a natural aversion to forcing the horses. This may come from not being as task-orientated as people from the non ASD population or a good understanding of the need for autonomy in others.

We believe this constant sense of being successful and learning through success is a key ingredient of all learning. Because of its rewarding nature, equine-assisted activities may further stimulate natural development of cognitive concepts (Mapes & Rosén, 2016).

These experiences of success build capacity and confidence for participants with ASD in functioning in a range of real-world situations. Feedback from parents and carers of participants with ASD attending our program suggest that they have "grown tremendously in confidence and have acquired a vast array of life skills through working with the horses" (ASD participant parent feedback).

Enhancing Mood and Motivation

Enhanced mood has been noted in AAT studies and may be related to increases in energy and motivation associated with working with animals (O'Haire, 2013). We have observed with all of our ASD participants increases in eye contact, smiles, and other facial and sign language that indicate positive mood. The overall increase in positive mood, comparing before and after a treatment program and also before and after individual sessions, is quite obvious. This is consistent with studies where animal-assisted therapy resulted in increases in smiling and laughing and positive emotional expression when compared to conventional therapies (Silva, Correia, Lima, Magalhães, & de Sousa, 2011; Martin and Farnum as cited in O'Haire, 2013). Motivation has also increased over time. An example is one adult non-verbal participant with severe ASD who often was reluctant to get out of the car in a range of situations for many years. We addressed this by bringing the pony he works with to the car. This pony is quite a character and would put his head in the car and go to sleep with his chin on the participant's lap or generally interact with him, always causing the participant to laugh at his antics. We never pressured him to get out of the car. This participant now gets out of the car right away.

Breaking Inflexibility and Rigid Thinking Patterns

Offering a wide range of activities can help overcome rigidity and difficulty with novelty that is characteristic of ASD. In combination with the use of consistent patterns with the horses to create confidence, novelty can be introduced to help extend participant's ability to cope with change. In keeping with social interaction skills training approaches for ASD, the sessions with the horses provide a wide range of opportunities, both planned and naturally occurring, allowing a chance to practice skills in both structured and unstructured situations. This is also in keeping with the natural environment teaching aspects in ABA, using what comes up in the environment to enhance learning.

In general, participants with ASD have a particular horse to work with and they are responsible for introducing the horses to the new obstacles as we continue to create them. Horses are also concerned by change and resistant to novelty and we encourage ASD clients to show understanding of the need for very slow introduction to build braveness in the horses. The way they do this can also provide information on how they deal with novelty. We have found consistently that participants increase their ability to cope with novelty over time. Being able to teach the horse to undertake a simple task despite unexpected occurrences that working with a horse brings is empowering for ASD participants in dealing with the unexpected.

CASE EXAMPLE

Mark (a pseudonym) attends EAP sessions with his father Peter (a pseudonym). Mark is in his mid-20s and has been diagnosed with a severe form of ASD. He lives at home with his family. When he first arrived, he had experienced difficulties in group activities such that he had been asked to leave several group programs because of perceived aggressive behavior. His father Peter said that he suffered from some aggressive outbursts. He uses limited speech, with very short sentences but has excellent receptive abilities. During his fortnightly EAP sessions he works specifically with one horse, an experienced older Arabian mare, Bella, who is gentle and kind as well as having a strong spirit. His high receptivity is shown by his strong ability to learn and retain information such as different techniques to lead and move Bella with kindness and skill as well as negotiating different obstacles with Bella.

The activities often involve a long walk with both Mark and Peter leading horses in the forest or large hill paddocks. The walk is interspersed with or followed by a pattern, task or obstacle with the horse. This can include negotiating a "labyrinth puzzle" without stepping off the path or walking Bella over a set of obstacles. Mark has developed a reciprocal relationship with Bella and is always gentle and respectful of her ideas, such that it appears that he uses negotiation rather than pressure to motivate her.

Peter suggests that one of the main benefits of EAP for Mark is the stimulation it provides. For much of the time, Peter reports that Mark is unfocused or absentminded and rarely has the opportunity for such an interactive focus. This interactive focus can be seen in the communication between Mark and Bella when Bella doesn't particularly want to do something, such as leave the herd, and he needs to stay very focused to convince her to go with him. One of the tangible benefits has been an increase in the use of words through giving verbal instructions to the horse. Prior to this, his speech was very limited. It appears that he is rewarded by speaking to Bella through a change in her behavior and is thus motivated to use verbal instructions.

The other notable difference is a reduction in agitated and hyperactive behavior. When he is connected to Bella by the lead rope he will go at her pace, including waiting patiently with relaxation while she rests or grazes. This represents a significant change to his usual behavior. Another benefit that Mark gains from working with Bella is exposure to emotional constructs such as love and respect. Peter says that Mark shows difficulty in understanding such concepts and avoids discussions around them. He shows enormous affection for Bella and will hug her and speak of his affection for her, which is uncharacteristic for him. The bond is obviously a two-way connection and Bella will follow Mark at liberty after he has let her off the halter. The connection between them is very obvious and touching. Finally, an important outcome is that Mark no longer shows aggressive outbursts.

REFERENCES

American Psychiatric Association (APA). (2013). Diagnostic and Statistical Manual of Mental Disorders. 5th edition. Washington, DC: American Psychiatric Association.

Bass, M. M. & Llabre, M. (2009). The effects of equine assisted activities on the social functioning of children with autism. Journal of Autism and Developmental Disorders, 39, 1261–1267.

Center for Disease Control and Prevention. (2014). CDC Estimates 1 in 68 Children Has Been Identified with Autism Spectrum Disorder. Retrieved from www.cdc.gov/media/releases/2014/p0327-autism-spectrum-disorder.html.

Christensen, D., Baio, J., & Braun, K. (2012). Prevalence and Characteristics of Autism Spectrum Disorder Among Children Aged 8 Years. Retrieved from www.cdc.gov/ncbddd/autism/data.html.

Cole, K. M., Gawlinski, A., Steers, N., & Kotlerman, J. (2007). Animal-assisted therapy in patients hospitalized with heart failure. American Journal of Critical Care, 16, 575. Retrieved from http://go.galegroup.com.ezproxy.une.edu.au/ps/i.do?id=GALE%7CA171139138&sid=summon&v=2.1&u=dixson&it=r&p=ITOF&sw=w&asid=11dafa301c45be72a0352793415edf74.

Fletcher, C. L., Grannemann, B. D., Richardson, T. A., & Trivedi, M. H. (2011). Prospective trial of equine-assisted activities in autism spectrum disorder. Alternative Therapies in Health and Medicine, 17(3), 14.

Hawkins, B. L., Ryan, J. B., Cory, A. L., & Donaldson, M. C. (2014). Effects of equine-assisted therapy on gross motor skills of two children with autism spectrum disorder: A single-subject research study. Therapeutic Recreation Journal, 48(2), 135.

Howlin, P., Goode, S., Hutton, J., & Rutter, M. (2004). Adult outcome for children with autism. Journal of Child Psychology and Psychiatry, 45(2), 212–229.

Lanning, B. A., Baier, M. E. M., Ivey-Hatz, J., Krenek, N. & Tubbs, J. (2014). Effects of equine assisted activities on Autism Spectrum Disorder. Journal of Autism and Developmental Disorders, 44, 1897.

Mapes, A. R. & Rosén, L. A. (2016). Equine-assisted therapy for children with autism spectrum disorder: A comprehensive literature review. Review Journal of Autism and Developmental Disorders, 3(4), 377–386.

Maros, K., Gacsi, M., & Miklosi, A. (2008). Comprehension of human pointing gestures in horses (Equus caballus). Animal Cognition, 11, 457–466.

Memishevikj, H. & Hodzhikj, S. (2010). The effects of equine assisted therapy in improving the psychosocial functioning of children with autism. The Journal of Special Education and Rehabilitation, 11(3/4), 57–67.

O'Haire, M. E. (2013). Animal-assisted intervention for autism spectrum disorder: A systematic literature review. Journal of Autism and Developmental Disorders, 43(7), 1606–1622.

Odendaal, J. (2000). Animal-assisted therapy—magic or medicine? Journal of Psychosomatic Research, 49(4), 275–280.

Serpell, G. A. (2011). Animal assisted interventions in historical perspective. In A. H. Fine (Ed.), Handbook on Animal-Assisted Therapy: Foundations and Guidelines for Animal-Assisted Interventions. San Diego, CA: Elsevier Academic Press.

Silva, K., Correia, R., Lima, M., Magalhães, A., & de Sousa, L. (2011). Can dogs prime autistic children for therapy? Evidence from a single case study. The Journal of Alternative and Complementary Medicine, 17(7), 1–5.

Wells, D. L. (2009). The effects of animals on human health and well-being. Journal of Social Issues, 65(3), 523–543.

REFERENCES

Section 7

Oppositional Behavior

12

Equine-Partnered Play Therapy™ for Children with Oppositional Behavior

Hallie Sheade

INTRODUCTION

Oppositional Behavior in Children

As children grow, it is natural for them to test boundaries and work towards becoming independent in order to develop a healthy sense of self as they move towards adulthood. However, some children begin to engage in oppositional behavior that crosses the line from healthy independence-seeking to dysfunctional behavior that interferes with their ability to engage in day-to-day interactions with family, teachers, friends, and other people in their lives. Oftentimes, these children are diagnosed with oppositional defiant disorder (ODD). ODD is one of the most common childhood psychiatric diagnoses and is characterized by defiant or hostile behavior, rebelliousness, being quick to anger, argumentativeness, spiteful behavior, and refusal to follow rules (American Academy of Child and Adolescent Psychiatry, 2009). Most of the child's difficulty is manifested in their interactions with authority figures and can cause impairment at home, school, and with peers. It is important to differentiate true oppositional behavior from responses to stress, crisis, and normal childhood development.

Oppositional behavior often co-occurs with ADHD, anxiety, mood disorders, and learning and language disorders (American Academy of Child and Adolescent Psychiatry, 2009). When treating oppositional behavior, it is important to also treat all co-occurring conditions. Most treatments focus on parent training, social skills, and cognitive processing skills. Of utmost importance is the development of skills related to empathy, problem-solving, self-control, and perspective-taking (Kazdin, 2010; Academy of Child and Adolescent Psychiatry, 2009; Webster-Stratton, 1993). Play therapy is an evidence-based practice that has been found to be beneficial in treating oppositional and aggressive behaviors in young children (Jafari, Mohammadi, Khanbani, Farid, & Chiti, 2011; Meany-Walen, Bratton, & Kottman, 2014; Ray, Blanco, Sullivan, & Holliman, 2009; Ray & McCullough, n.d.).

THEORETICAL FOUNDATION: CHILD-CENTERED PLAY THERAPY

Play is universal among children all around the world. Through play, children explore and investigate their world and their place in the world (Axline, 1969). Play is the natural language of children with toys as their words for communicating experiences, reactions, feelings, sense of self, wishes, wants, and needs (Landreth,

2012). As young children are concrete (as opposed to abstract) and cannot adequately express themselves through just talking, play therapy is an approach based in the language of children (Piaget, 1951; Landreth, 2012).

Equine-Partnered Play Therapy™ (EPPT) is based on the principles on nondirective play therapy and adapted from Child-Centered Play Therapy (CCPT) to be used with children ages three through nine years of age. Inspired by Carl Rogers' person-centered approach, Virginia Axline (1969) developed non-directive play therapy in which the therapist allows the child to lead the play, trusting the child's innate ability to move towards healing. This approach later became called CCPT. Rather than simply a set of techniques, CCPT encompasses a broad philosophy for interacting with children and trusting in their ability to move towards growth and self-direction (Landreth, 2012). Maladjustment is best understood as incongruence between one's self-concept and experience. In CCPT, the therapist's attitudes of unconditional warmth, genuineness, and empathy are crucial in creating a therapeutic relationship in which the child feels free to explore and express him/herself freely and without fear of judgment or expectation (Landreth, 2012).

INTEGRATING EQUINES INTO PLAY THERAPY: EQUINE-PARTNERED PLAY THERAPY™

Children around the world have an innate curiosity and interest in animals (Melson & Fine, 2010). In 1961, Boris Levinson, with his dog Jingles, was among the first child therapists to include animals in the psychotherapy process (Levinson & Mallon, 1997). There are myriad benefits to including equines in the psychotherapy process for young children including facilitation of trust between the child and therapist, increasing child motivation for attending psychotherapy, and creation of a safe, non-threatening therapeutic environment (Chandler, 2017; Levinson & Mallon, 1997). Equines naturally embody the core therapeutic attitudes of being empathic, genuine, and providing unconditional positive regard (Sheade & Box, 2014).

The inclusion of equines in play therapy facilitates the development of emotional regulation, coping skills, social skills, and provides the opportunity for the child to give and receive nurturing (Levinson & Mallon, 1997; Sheade & Box, 2014; VanFleet & Thompson, 2010). As in CCPT, interaction with an equine enables children to process in ways other than talking and allows child and therapist to focus on the process of being in the present moment (Landreth, 2012; Levinson & Mallon, 1997). By integrating equines into play therapy, the therapist has the opportunity to gain valuable information about the child by observation of the child's play and interactions with the equine. Similar to how a child may use toys to indirectly express inner thoughts and feelings, the child may also project onto the equine as a way to express him/herself (Levinson & Mallon, 1997; Sheade, 2017), Finally, the equines respond to the child as a peer, acting authentically and providing immediate feedback to ground the play session in reality (Sheade & Box, 2014).

ETHICAL ISSUES IN EQUINE-PARTNERED PLAY THERAPY™

There are several ethical considerations in the implementation of Equine-Partnered Play Therapy™ (EPPT). This modality should be facilitated by a competent treatment team consisting of a licensed mental health professional (or intern under the supervision of a licensed professional) and a competent equine specialist. As with any psychotherapy intervention, it is important that the mental health professional has received training in play therapy, animal-assisted therapy, and working with young children. The equine specialist should be experienced in working with equines on the ground, reading equine behaviors, managing herd dynamics, and recognizing signs of equine stress and burnout. The equine specialist plays a crucial role by balancing the needs of the child and the equines in maintaining physical safety for all human and equine participants and emotional safety for the equines. It is also important that the equine specialist receive basic training in understanding the nature of play therapy and associated confidentiality considerations (Sheade & Box, 2017).

As the play area will be a much less controlled environment than a traditional office-based play room, it is important to evaluate the space for environmental hazards (e.g., plants, insects, wildlife, weather, etc.). It is also important to evaluate for threats to client privacy and confidentiality and establish facility policies to best protect clients' interests. Clients should participate in a thorough screening process to evaluate for any precautions or contraindications related to health conditions (e.g., allergies, light sensitivity, etc.) and behavioral concerns (e.g., hallucinations, history of animal abuse, etc.). The informed consent should also outline the heightened risk of physical harm associated with interacting with equines (Sheade, 2017).

EMPATHY-BUILDING IN EQUINE-PARTNERED PLAY THERAPY

Goals and Objectives

The goals of EPPT align with the goals of Landreth's (2012) Child-Centered Play Therapy (CCPT). These primary goals are for the child to develop within him/herself self-respect, self-responsibility, self-direction, self-acceptance, self-reliance, and self-control. In addition, goals related to behavioral outcomes include decision-making skills, coping and calming skills, empathy towards others, prosocial behavior, and problem-solving skills (Sheade, 2017). Objectives associated with these goals should be developed in collaboration between the therapist, equine specialist, and child's caregiver as part of a comprehensive treatment plan tailored specifically to meet the child's needs.

Materials Needed

The technique described below was developed for use specifically as part of the EPPT model. Although the technique can be integrated into other modalities, the materials listed below are consistent with application in the EPPT model.

As described in Sheade's (2017) EPPT training manual, the play area is modeled after the playroom developed for CCPT. It is important that the play area be located in a private space separate from other facility activities where the child's play will not be seen or heard by onlookers. The ideal play area size is 10' × 30' for the toy area and 15' × 30' for an open area separate from the toys that the equines can access if desired. Careful consideration should be put in setting up the flooring to ensure maximum comfort for the equines and to protect toys from outdoor elements such as animals, bugs, and weather. Like Landreth's (2012) recommendations, toys should be carefully selected in the categories of Real-Life Toys, Acting-Out Aggressive-Release Toys, and Creative Expression and Emotional Release Toys. In EPPT, "horsey" toys should also be included to enable the child to interact with the horses directly (e.g., brushes) and indirectly (e.g., horse figurines, puppets, etc.).

Miniature equines (horses or donkeys) are recommended in EPPT due to their smaller size in order to appear less threatening to small children and to decrease the risk of physical injury to the child. As equines feel most comfortable in the presence of other equines, it is also recommended to have two miniature equines in order to enable the equines to feel most comfortable and to provide the child with opportunities to observe social dynamics between the equines. In order to enable the child to build a relationship with the equines, the child should work with the same equines each week. The equines selected for participation in EPPT should be thoroughly screened for health and/or behavioral issues that may negatively impact the session or cause harm to the child. Furthermore, the equines should be thoroughly desensitized to all of the toys including all of the ways that a child may play with the various toys (Sheade, 2017).

INSTRUCTIONS

As discussed above, the technique that follows is intended for use in EPPT. However, the technique may also be used in managing oppositional behavior in other forms of equine-assisted counseling. Set up the play area and bring the equines to the play area prior to the start of the session. Should the child begin engaging in behaviors that are causing (or have the potential to cause) undue stress to the equine(s), the therapist can use the following sequence:

1. Verbally reflect the child's behavior and the equine's subsequent behavioral response.
2. If the child continues the behavior, repeat the above and reflect the equine's feeling based on behavioral observation.
3. If the child persists in the behavior, begin using Landreth's (2012), "A-C-T" Limit-Setting method.
   - Acknowledge the child's feelings.
   - Communicate the limit.
   - Target alternatives.
4. If the child continues the behavior, the therapist may restate the limit up to three times contingent on the equine's ability to tolerate the continued inappropriate behavior.
5. Should the child continue the behavior after the limit has been set three times (or if the therapist determines that the equine's well-being is compromised), the therapist may use choice-giving in setting a limit regarding the equine's continued presence in the session.
6. If the child complies with the limit, the equines may stay in the session. If the child does not comply, the equines should promptly be removed for the remainder of the session.

ETHICAL AND MULTICULTURAL ISSUES

In order to maintain a free and permissive environment, limits are set carefully and consistently to protect the well-being of all human and equine participants in the play session, anchor the session in reality, protect the play area and materials, and preserve the therapeutic relationship (Landreth, 2012). When setting a limit, the treatment team must carefully balance the child's needs with the equine's needs in deciding when and how to set the limit in order to convey continued acceptance of the child's feelings, desires, and wishes even if the behavior demonstrated by the child is not acceptable. It is crucial for the equine specialist to be aware of each equine's window of tolerance for various behaviors that a child may demonstrate in session and be able to read the equine's behavior in the moment. Furthermore, it is important that the play area is structured in such a way that the equine may always choose to move away from the child if desired (Sheade, 2017).

It is important that the therapist conduct a thorough intake and informed consent process to discuss the role of the equines in play therapy and to discuss any cultural variables (Sheade, 2017). Like Child-Centered Play Therapy, Equine-Partnered Play Therapy™ is a culturally responsive approach that enables children of diverse backgrounds with opportunities to express themselves beyond talking (Lin & Bratton, 2015). Children of diverse cultural backgrounds will likely have different experiences with and beliefs about animals that may influence their participation and comfort level in the play session (Sheade & Chandler, 2014).

CASE EXAMPLE

Joey is a representation of various child clients who have previously participated in EPPT.

Joey was a seven-year-old African-American male brought to Equine-Partnered Play Therapy™ (EPPT) in order to address concerns related to depression, aggression, and oppositional behavior, and poor social skills. Joey's father was an army veteran who had been deployed overseas several times during Joey's lifetime. In addition to his father's frequent absences, Joey and his mother accompanied his father whenever he transferred from base to base resulting in Joey having to leave old friends behind and make new short-term friendships. Joey's parents were at a loss of how to manage his increasing defiance at home. In addition, Joey's parents reported that Joey was having trouble making friends and often talked about wanting to hurt himself.

The following transcript analysis is about a pseudonym client.

Table 12.1

Transcript Analysis of Case Example

Transcript	*Analysis*
Client goes over to the puppet theater and selects two "scary-looking" puppets. Client proceeds to run towards the miniature horses with the puppets while screaming "Ahhh." The horses move quickly away from the client to the other side of the play area.	Client is trying to find ways to interact with the horses while testing limits and boundaries.
Therapist: I noticed that when you started running towards the horses, the horses moved away.	The therapist is trying to assist the client in connecting his own behaviors with others' responses to his behavior (i.e., the horses moving away).
Client: I know—they're having fun! *Client begins running towards the horses a second time. The horses move away more quickly than the first time.*	Client is aware of the influence of his behaviors on someone else but is unable to recognize the horses' feelings associated with the resulting behaviors.
Therapist: I noticed that when you run towards the horses, they feel scared and so they move away to go somewhere that feels safer.	The therapist has now attached a feeling to the horses' behaviors to assist the client in developing increased empathy and a better understanding of the impact of his behavior on others' feelings.
Client: That's because these are scary puppets! I like scaring people—it's fun! See, the horses are running—they're having fun too! *Client starts to move towards the horses again. Upon seeing client's initial movement, the horses quickly move away again and client attempts to chase them.*	Client is aware that his actions influence others. Client may enjoy the sense of power he feels by being able to scare others and/or influence their behavior in response to him. Furthermore, Client's struggles with empathy are apparent in his difficulty in recognizing that, although he is having fun, the horses are not having fun.
Therapist: I know that you think it's fun to scare the horses, but horses aren't for scaring or chasing. You can choose to pretend to scare the stuffed horse or walking up to the horses slowly to show them the scary puppets.	The therapist first acknowledges the client's feelings, wishes, and wants in order to convey empathy and understanding. Next, the therapist communicates the limit and specifically describes client's behavior (i.e., chasing) and intent (i.e., scaring). The therapist then provides acceptable alternatives that would not cause undue stress on the horses.
Client: Well, I'm having fun! *Client begins running towards the horses again.* *The horses begin to run away from the client.*	Client is testing limits and refuses to comply with the limit.
Therapist: The horses are not for scaring or chasing. If you **choose** to continue scaring or chasing the horses, you **choose** for the horses to leave our play time today.	Due to the client's choice to break the limit and the associated escalation in the horses' fear response (i.e., running away now as opposed to moving away), the therapist has determined that a final choice regarding the horses' participation in session must be stated. The emphasis on the word "choose" conveys the client's sense of personal responsibility for his behaviors and associated subsequent consequences (positive or negative).
Client: Sighs. OK, I won't scare them anymore. I was just trying to have fun. *Client takes a brush and walks quickly towards the horses. The horses move away.* Why don't they like me?	Client has made the choice to comply with the limit. Client is still seeking interaction with the horses but does not fully understand the impact of his behaviors on others' responses to him.
Therapist: I noticed that when you walked quickly towards the horses, they still feel scared and move away.	Therapist is trying to help the client understand the impact of his behavior on the horses' responses of fear even though he is no longer deliberately trying to scare them.
Client: I have an idea! *Client slows down his walk and carefully approaches the horses. The horses allow the client to approach and he begins brushing them.*	Client has been able to integrate the feedback from the horses and therapist and found an empathic, socially appropriate way to interact with them.

EQUINE CONNECTION COUNSELING

EQUINE-PARTNERED PLAY THERAPY™ - SESSION SUMMARY

The following session note example is about a pseudonym client

Date: 1/19/15 **Child/Age:** Joey/7 **Counselor:** Hallie Sheade **Equine Specialist:** Jane Smith

Session #: 4 **Time:** 6:00 **pm (** X **on time;** ___ **late /** 60 **minutes) Horse(s):** Star, Coco

Reason for Counseling/Presenting Concern: Oppositional behavior; depression

Diagnosis (if applicable): n/a

I. Data

Intervention: EPPT **Current Concerns:** Transition to new school

SIGNIFICANT VERBALIZATION: "I'm having fun!" "I like scaring people—it's fun!" "Why don't they like me?"

LIMITS SET:

Protect Child (Physical & Emotional Safety):

Protect Therapist and/or Maintain Therapist Acceptance/Relationship:

Protect Room/Toys:

Structuring:

Reality Testing:

Protect Equines: Limits set several times regarding child running up to horses. Child complied with limit when given final choice regarding horses' continued session participation.

TOYS/PLAY BEHAVIOR:

___nature-related

___sandbox/water/sink

X theater/puppets

___kitchen/cooking/food

___easel/paint/chalkboard

X horse-related

___bop bag/foam bats/etc

X dress up clothes/jewelry/hats/masks/wand

___crafts/clay/markers/etc.

___doll house/doll family/bottle/pacifier/baby

___cash register/money/phone

___camera/flashlight

___medical kit/bandages

___musical instruments

___games/bowling/ring toss/balls/etc.

___vehicles

___animals: domestic/wild/aggressive

___soldiers/guns/knife/sword/handcuffs/rope

___constructive toys/blocks/barricade

___sandtray/miniatures

X live equines

___Other: ___________

DESCRIPTION OF PLAY: *Describe the play behavior, sequence of play and child's affect during play. Also describe interaction with equines.*

The child entered the play area willingly and eagerly as evidenced by walking quickly to the play area from the parking lot. The child greeted the horses verbally and selected several items from the dress up clothes to wear. The child then spent sustained time examining each of the puppets and verbally described each puppet's level of "scariness". The child selected the "monster" puppet and abruptly ran towards the horses. In response to counselor's reflections, the child continued the behavior despite the horses moving away from him. In response to the counselor's limit regarding the horses' continued participation in the session, the child put away the puppets and retrieved brushes. Child experimented with different ways to approach the horses until he was able to walk up the horses and spent the remainder of the session brushing them.

II. ASSESSMENT

PLAY THEMES: *Underline predominant theme(s).*

EXPLORATORY	***RELATIONSHIP***	HELPLESS	
POWER/CONTROL	NURTURING	REPARATION	POWERLESS
DEPENDENCY	GRIEF & LOSS	RESILIENCY	HOPELESS
REVENGE	ABANDONMENT	CHAOS/INSTABILITY	ANXIETY
SAFETY/SECURITY	PROTECTION	PERFECTIONISM	OTHER: ______
MASTERY	SEPARATION	INTEGRATION	

CONCEPTUALIZATION AND PROGRESS

The child demonstrated continued focus on engaging in behaviors to feel powerful and to test boundaries as evidenced by child's efforts to "scare" the horses and initial refusal to comply with limits set. The child demonstrated difficulty in recognizing social cues and perspective-taking as evidenced by child's attribution of the horses as "having fun" when the horses were moving away. The child demonstrated a strong desire to have a relationship with the horses and is working on identifying socially-appropriate ways to interact with the horses and become more empathic as evidenced by child's efforts to approach the horses calmly. Child demonstrated efforts to repair the relationship by engaging in prosocial behaviors to brush the horses after scaring them.

III. PLAN/RECOMMENDATIONS:

To continue Equine-Partnered Play Therapy. Counselor will consult with child's mother during next session.

Play Therapy Next Appointment: Date/Time: 1/26/15/6:00pm

FIG. 12.1. Sample Client Session Note.

EQUINE CONNECTION COUNSELING

EQUINE-PARTNERED PLAY THERAPY™
SESSION SUMMARY

Date: ________ Child/Age:________________Counselor: _______________Equine Specialist: __________

Session #: _______ Time: ______am/pm (___on time;____late /_____minutes) Horse(s):________________

Reason for Counseling/Presenting Concern: ____

Diagnosis (if applicable): ____

I. Data
Intervention: ___________________________________Current Concerns:______________________________
SIGNIFICANT VERBALIZATION:

LIMITS SET:
Protect Child (Physical & Emotional Safety):
Protect Therapist and/or Maintain Therapist Acceptance/Relationship:
Protect Room/Toys:
Structuring:
Reality Testing:
Protect Equines:

TOYS/PLAY BEHAVIOR:

___nature-related
___sandbox/water/sink
___theater/puppets
___kitchen/cooking/food
___easel/paint/chalkboard
___horse-related
___bop bag/foam bats/etc
___dress up clothes/jewelry/hats/masks/wand
___crafts/clay/markers/etc.
___doll house/doll family/bottle/pacifier/baby
___cash register/money/phone
___camera/flashlight
___medical kit/bandages
___musical instruments
___games/bowling/ring toss/balls/etc.
___vehicles
___animals: domestic/wild/aggressive
___soldiers/guns/knife/sword/handcuffs/rope
___constructive toys/blocks/barricade
___sandtray/miniatures
___live equines
___Other: ____________________

DESCRIPTION OF PLAY: *Describe the play behavior, sequence of play and child's affect during play. Also describe interaction with equines.*

II. ASSESSMENT
PLAY THEMES: *Underline predominant theme(s).*

EXPLORATORY
RELATIONSHIP
POWER/CONTROL
DEPENDENCY
REVENGE
SAFETY/SECURITY
MASTERY
HELPLESS
NURTURING
GRIEF & LOSS
ABANDONMENT
PROTECTION
SEPARATION
REPARATION
RESILIENCY
CHAOS/INSTABILITY
PERFECTIONISM
INTEGRATION
POWERLESS
HOPELESS
ANXIETY
OTHER: _________

CONCEPTUALIZATION AND PROGRESS

III. PLAN/RECOMMENDATIONS:

Play Therapy Next Appointment: Date/Time: ____________

____

FIG. 12.2. Blank Template of Client Session Note.

REFERENCES

Axline, V. (1969). *Play Therapy.* Boston, MA: Houghton-Mifflin.

American Academy of Child and Adolescent Psychiatry. (2009). *Oppositional Defiant Disorder: A Guide for Families.* Retrieved from www.aacap.org/App_Themes/AACAP/docs/resource_centers/odd/odd_resource_center_odd_guide.pdf.

Chandler, C. (2017). *Animal Assisted Therapy in Counseling.* 3rd edition. New York: Routledge.

Jafari, N., Mohammadi, M. R., Khanbani, M., Farid, S., & Chiti, P. (2011). Effect of play therapy on behavioral problems of maladjusted preschool children. *Iranian Journal of Psychiatry, 6*, 37–42.

Kazdin, A. (2010). Problem-solving skills training and parent management training for oppositional defiant disorder and conduct disorder. In J. Weisz & A. Kazdin (Eds.), *Evidence-Based Psychotherapies* (2nd edition, pp. 211–226). New York: Guilford.

Landreth, G. L. (2012). *Play Therapy: The Art of the Relationship.* 3rd edition. New York: Routledge.

Levinson, B. M. & Mallon, G. P. (1997). *Pet-Oriented Child Psychotherapy.* 2nd edition. Springfield, IL: Charles C Thomas.

Lin, Y. & Bratton, S. C. (2015). A meta-analytic review of child-centered play therapy approaches. *Journal of Counseling and Development, 93*, 45–58.

Meany-Walen, K. K., Bratton, S. C., & Kottman, T. (2014). Effects of Adlerian play therapy on reducing students' disruptive behaviors. *Journal of Counseling and Development, 92*, 47–56.

Melson, G. F. & Fine, A. H. (2010). Animals in the lives of children. In A. H. Fine (Ed.), *Handbook of Animal Assisted Therapy: Theoretical Foundations and Guidelines for Practice.* (3rd edition, pp. 223–245). San Diego, CA: Academic Press.

Piaget, J. (1951). Play, Dreams, and Imitation in Childhood. New York: Norton.

Ray. D. C., Blanco, P. J., Sullivan, J. M., & Holliman, R. (2009). An exploratory study of child-centered play therapy with aggressive children. *International Journal of Play Therapy, 18*(3), 162–175.

Ray, D. C. & McCullough, R. (n.d.). *Evidence-Based Practice Statement: Play Therapy.* Retrieved from: www.a4pt.org/resource/resmgr/About_APT/APT_Evidence_Based_Statement.pdf.

Sheade, H. E. (2017). *Equine-Partnered Play Therapy: Foundations Training.* Equine Connection Counseling, PLC. Independently published.

Sheade, H. & Box, L. (2014). Playtime with horses: Equine-partnered play therapy. *PATH Intl. Strides, 20*(3), 18–21.

Sheade, H. & Box, L. (2017). EFP ethics and skills for ESMHLs. *PATH Intl. Strides, 23*(2), 22–28.

Sheade, H. & Chandler, C. K. (2014). Diversity considerations in animal assisted counseling. *VISTAS Online.* Retrieved from www.counseling.org/knowledge-center/vistas/by-subject2/vistas-animal-assisted/docs/default-source/vistas/article_76.

VanFleet, R. & Thompson, T. (2010). The case for using animal-assisted play therapy. *British Journal of Play Therapy, 6*, 4–18.

Webster-Stratton, C. (1993). Strategies for helping early school-aged children with oppositional defiant and conduct disorders: The importance of home-school partnerships. *School Psychology Review, 3*, 437–457.

13

Integrating Body-Mind-Attachment Practices into Equine-Facilitated Psychotherapy

A Case Example of Oppositional Defiant Disorder

Leslie McCullough

INTRODUCTION

Out-of-doors, experiential interventions are powerful medicine, and spending time outside bonding with animals provides multiple cognitive, behavioral, and emotional benefits (Melson & Fine, 2015; Trotter, 2012). Even petting a friendly animal is found to release oxytocin, the "feel good" neurotransmitter that offers stress-buffering opportunities for those experiencing anxiety or fear (Chandler, 2012). Children growing up with animals in their lives indicate better emotional regulation and self-control, nurturance, empathy, and caring (Séverine, Booksmythe, Kotrschal, Jennions, Kolm, 2016). Additionally, Parish-Plass (2008) reminds us that in working with children having little reason to trust adults, including animals in therapy sessions can help in enabling a working client–therapist connection (Melson & Fine, 2015, p. 182). More to the point, as our partners in mental health treatment, animal-assisted interventions have proven to be a highly effective alternative or supplement to more traditional means of therapy (Yorke, Adams, & Coady, 2008). This is particularly true when working with clients having attachment, regulatory, and trauma-related issues who are incapable of, or else unwilling to, work in a cognitive/talk-based intervention (Kemp, Signal, Botros, Taylor & Prentice, 2014; Mueller & McCullough, 2017; Trotter, Chandler, Goodwin-Bond & Casey, 2008).

This chapter will define and describe the various faces of oppositional defiant disorder (ODD). Using the lens of attachment theory, the origins of ODD will be addressed, including its influence on and connection to attention-deficit/hyperactivity disorder (ADHD) and conduct disorder (CD). Current best practices will be addressed in terms of efficacy and limitations. Equine-facilitated psychotherapy (EFP) will be defined and described as the equine intervention of choice for oppositional defiant and attending disruptive and impulse control disorders. In EFP practice, the holding environment (or therapeutic milieu if you prefer) of horse, therapist, and therapeutic riding instructor/equine specialist (from here, forward referred to as TRI/ES) serves as a safe space in which a youth experiencing the spectrum of disruptive and impulse control disorders, can feel supported and cared for as she takes the ultimate leap of faith in learning how to belong and trust. Basic practices of reality, Cognitive-Behavioral, dialectical-behavioral, and mind-body-spirit interventions will help illustrate EFP's presentation as a multi-theoretical model (Karol, 2000) in which individual practitioners might utilize their preferred theoretical approaches. Exercises and activities will be suggested as well as explained via case studies.

THE MANY FACES OF ODD AND CURRENT TREATMENT STRATEGIES

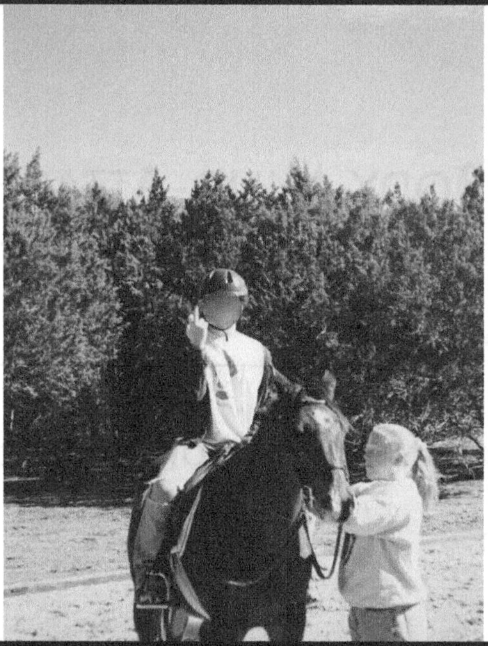

FIG. 13.1.

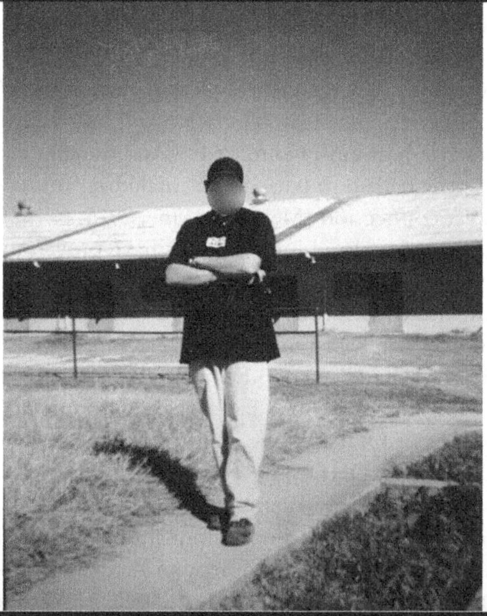

FIG. 13.2.

Many EFP clients present with a diagnosis of ODD, which the *Diagnostic and Statistical Manual, Fifth Edition* (DSM-5) categorizes as an impulse-control disorder, often co-morbid with mood and anxiety syndromes, such as ADHD, CD, and depression (American Psychiatric Association (APA), 2013). Focusing on the disruptive impulse control disorders of ODD, indicators if not diagnoses, typically begin in early childhood (4–5 years) through late childhood and into early adolescence (8–12 years). ODD is the most common clinical disorder diagnosed in children and adolescents, with an occurrence of 6.5% in adolescence (Steiner & Remsing, 2007). Boylan (2014) classified ODD into three subtypes: Cognitive Overload ODD—"irritable/negative affect"; Stimulus Dependent ODD—"headstrong/oppositional"; and the fearful type ODD—"rages and refusals" (Garland, 2001).

Children having ODD typically display negativity towards authority, and exhibit animosity and non-compliance (APA, 2013). Factors contributing to the diagnosis are heavily weighted on the side of familial influences, including physical, neurological, environmental, and traumatic backgrounds. For example:

Genetics: Heritability estimates for the development of ODD exceeds 50% (Eaves et al., 1997). Other genetic associations include ODD with ADHD (Eaves et al., 1997) and depressive symptoms (Rowe et al., 2008).

Parent education/environment: Paternal antisocial personality disorder (APD) and low/poor maternal supervision and discipline appear to invite the development of CD in children, with paternal APD being most significant for the development of ODD (Frick et al., 1992). Low parent education levels and low socio-economic status (SES) can create an unstable home environment, which not only predicts onset, persistence, and severity of childhood mental disorders, but also predicates a substantially elevated life-course of all classes of mental health complications (McLaughlin et al., 2011). Overall, negative family behaviors (harsh parenting, disruptive home environment, etc.) are the greatest contributors to a child's externalizing problems (Jaffee, Moffit, Caspi, & Taylor, 2003).

Traumatic experiences: Research shows that post-traumatic stress disorder (PTSD) is frequently co-morbid with ODD, CD, and ADHD (Steiner, Garcia, & Matthews, 1997). Symptoms of intrusion and hyperarousal can contribute to ADHD's impulsivity and attentional dysregulation or to ODD's aggressive and oppositional behavior.

Neurological: Prolonged stress and anxiety during childhood increase the risk of a child developing anxiety disorders and depression later in life leading to disabling conditions such as phobia, PTSD, and generalized anxiety disorder that persists into adulthood (Qin et al., 2014).

Insecure and disorganized attachment: Research indicates that the mean prevalence of insecure attachment in individuals with CD/ODD is 55.58%; similarly, a mean prevalence of disorganized attachment in individuals with CD/ODD is 30.97% (Theule, Germain, Cheung, Hurl, & Markel, 2016). Specifically, insecure and disorganized attachment styles are more likely to result in individuals having CD/ODD.

Current practices proven to be moderately effective include behavior modification training, medication, and referral to additional treatment approaches. Caregivers and teachers can receive training for "oppositional" or "difficult to manage" preschoolers (Shaw, Dishion, Supplee, Gardner, & Arnds, 2006), and behavioral modification techniques for ODD can help reduce argumentativeness and deliberate attention-seeking behavior. Medication can also be used when an underlying mood, anxiety disorder, or ADHD is driving the behavior (Hood, Elrod, & DeWine, 2015).

Taking a closer look at Boylan's (2014) proposed clinical typology of ODD, we can see why behavioral modification and medication work for only a small portion of children having ODD. By tackling ODD differentially, doors fly open, inviting the development and execution of treatments targeting specific aspects of the varying presentations.

THEORETICAL BACKGROUND

Maslow's (1943) description of the hierarchy of human needs explains human motivation to avoid and/or reduce anxiety by means of satisfying four areas of deficiency involving an individual's need for physiological necessities (food, water), safety and security, social belonging, and self-esteem (Burton, 2012). Youth coming into treatment have likely received fundamental (often limited) physiological attention for nourishment, reasonable clothing, and a bed to sleep in. However, the second tier in Maslow's hierarchy includes the human need for safety, security, and having trust that no harm will befall them, physically, mentally, or emotionally. When children experience the rupture of an attachment, their unmet trust and security needs drive them into states of emotional distress.

They then use maladaptive methods to pursue these needs. EFP seeks to interrupt the devious behavior and remediate feelings of lost trust and security with a safe and secure, unconditional relational-object, the horse.

After creating a safe space, EFP creates opportunities for clients to understand themselves within relationships (social belonging) and develop their ego (esteem) as they learn how to work with the horse as a partner. The goal of therapy is to prepare the way for the client to rise to the fifth level, self-actualization.

Similar to Maslow's hierarchy of needs, Erickson's (1950) representation of psycho-social development via logical, age-specific, birth-to-death, sequential stages have proven an inimitable model across client age, gender, diagnosis, or emotional age, in terms of determining human psycho-social health and dysfunction (McMaken, 2000). Erikson's developmental model not only proffers an orderly, straightforward sequence on how humans master developmental challenges to become strong, well-adjusted adults, but this model also presents the task's explicit opposite. That is, what happens when a child cannot meet the developmental challenge, perhaps getting "stuck," failing to accomplish the age-related task necessary to move forward onto the next stage. Erikson's model begins with trust. Secure attachment offering safety, consistency, and just enough frustration to foster creative alternatives for seeking satisfaction is at the root of "normal" human psycho-social growth.

Keeping Maslow and Erikson in mind, attachment is not bonding (Benoit, 2004). Being neither bidirectional (Tannenbaum, 1995) nor reciprocal (Russow, 2002), attachment develops due to a consistent caregiver's ability to respond to an infant when their "attachment system"—that is, threats to the infant's safety and security (when frightened or hurt, feeling ill; discomfort)—becomes activated. By six months of age, the infant learns to anticipate specific responses from the caregiver and, as a result, develops strategies for dealing with distress when the caregiver is present (Benoit, 2004).

An "organized" attachment therefore describes a child's usual response to predictable parental/caregiver interactions including those that are dismissive or cruel. "Disorganized," on the other hand, defines a child's erratic, ever-changing responses to unpredictable parent/caregiver behavior toward her or in general.

Table 13.1

Types of Attachment and Antecedents

Quality of Caregiving	*Strategy to Deal with Distress*	*Type of Attachment*
Sensitive/Loving	Organized	Secure
Insensitive/Rejecting	Organized	Insecure—Avoidant
Insensitive/Inconsistent	Organized	Insecure—Resistant
Atypical/Atypical	Disorganized	Insecure—Disorganized

Adapted from Benoit (2004).

As a result, the child living with an insecure/disorganized attachment can be experienced as ODD or even CD, due to poorly developed regulatory system and frustration at being unable to form relationships, or cope with stress (Odhayani, Watson, & Watson, 2013), experiences the child is likely unable to verbalize, or is even aware of. A disrupted family environment, social isolation, power disparity, and poor communication can leave the disorganized/insecurely attached, oppositional defiant youth, believing there is no one with whom to confide (Alaggia, 2005). In addition, because of disruptive behavior and emotional dysregulation, the poorly attached and acting out youth is difficult to accommodate in office-based psychotherapy, meaning many do not receive adequate treatment (Kazdin, 2011; Kazdin & Blase, 2011; Mueller & McCullough, 2017).

AN INTRODUCTION TO EFP: A VIABLE SOLUTION

EFP is a specialized form of equine-assisted activities and therapies. It is a method of experiential psychotherapy that addresses mental health challenges by means of a therapist and an equine partnering as co-facilitators in the therapy session (Bachi, Terkel, & Teichman, 2012; McCullough, Risley-Curtiss, & Rorke, 2015). The Professional Association for Therapeutic Horsemanship International (PATH Intl.), an equine professional organization for therapeutic equine activities, defines EFP as, "an interactive process in which a licensed mental health professional working with or as an appropriately credentialed equine professional, partners with suitable equine(s) to address psychotherapy goals set forth by the mental health professional and the client" (PATH Intl., 2017).

Grounded in the natural affinity existing between horses and humans and combined with traditional psychotherapy practices (Bachi et al., 2012), EFP not only offers a more complete psychotherapy experience (Karol, 2007) but also has been shown to significantly decrease arousal symptoms in individuals having experienced abuse-related trauma (Kemp et al., 2014) that manifest as disruptive, impulse-control and conduct disorders (APA, 2013: Mueller & McCullough, 2017).

While many equine therapy programs work with clients who have cognitive or behavioral issues, EFP is distinct in two ways: including a licensed mental health worker in the session, and working with the equine as a partner, not a tool. The Equine Facilitated Mental Health Association describes the horse as a partner in therapy:

> Equines are sentient beings. They are feeling, conscious, perceptive and responsive. With this philosophy, we do not consider the equine a tool to be used. We consider the ethical treatment of equines to include no purposeful scaring, harassing, teasing or threatening physical or emotional abuse. We consider the equine as a partner, a member of the therapeutic team and encourage all members of the team to treat equines with respect.
>
> (PATH Intl., 2018)

Most EFP programs use the Diamond Model (see below), in which the four points illustrate the dynamic relationship between the therapist, client, equine, and TRI/ES. The therapist is a mental health practitioner who uses psychotherapeutic methods to engage with the client. The TRI/ES is a horse professional, and s/he is there to facilitate and observe work with the equine. The signature feature of the Diamond Model is that all four sides are equivalent, meaning energy and input is shared throughout the treatment team and that each member is an equal participant. The peripheral arrows indicate behavior, words, and external/physical energy shared among the team. This energy is fluid and affects every participant, influencing how they each function. Likewise, interior arrows specify internal energy—thoughts, feelings, attentiveness (or not), congruence or incongruence, dissociation, or perhaps anger or sadness—which is felt by all participants and wields great influence among the team. If any one team member becomes overly consumed by his or her own energy, be it internal, external or both, the diamond becomes lop-sided, with the individual exuding the dominant feelings or behavior taking center stage. This could be any member of the team. The goal therefore, is to maintain the "holding environment" wherein physical, emotional and psychic safety is upheld by all participants owning their specific influence.

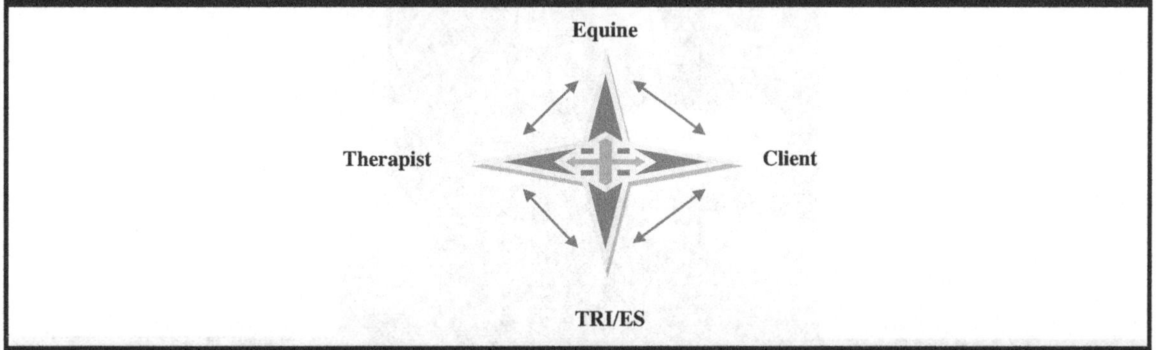

FIG. 13.3. Diamond Model.

The following session descriptions and case studies illustrate the horse–client dyad/relationship and the Diamond Model of EFP. "Therapy" transpires through the dyad's interactions both positive and frustrating, that challenge the client to reevaluate longstanding beliefs about relationships being hurtful and dismissive. Most important, the animal–human bond as "existential theater" (Karol, 2007) provides the setting in which the youth's past tragedies are re-enacted, oftentimes repeatedly, until the client chooses to "flip the script" and allow closeness and trust. The exercises below are designed to facilitate a mutually beneficial and desired, bond between the equine and his human partner.

EFP IN ACTION: A STEP-BY-STEP GUIDE

Step 1: Referral and Assessment

To begin EFP, the client needs to be referred. Youth referred for treatment often come via the usual routes—referrals from parents or other family; foster parents; Child Protective Services or a similar agency; or group homes. After a discussion and assessment, typically in an office setting, if EFP has been determined to be a viable option, a first session is scheduled. What transpires from that point forward, while defined and planned, can assume as many looks as there are clients attending.

Goals are explained, often through a level-system. The "EFP Goals" table describes fundamental goals and activities for a first level. Keep in mind, the activities are individualized according to the clients' treatment plan, which is determined by consensus between client and therapist, parents or guardians, and any protective or juvenile justice agency that might be involved.

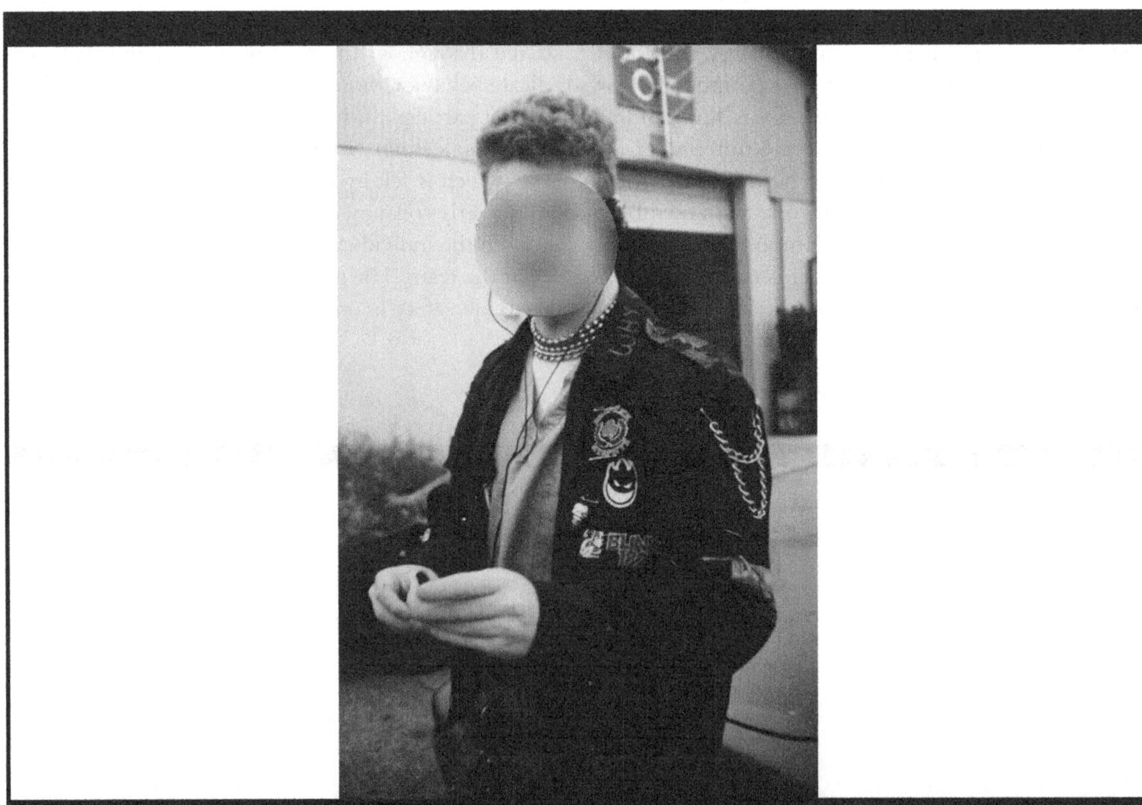

FIG. 13.4.

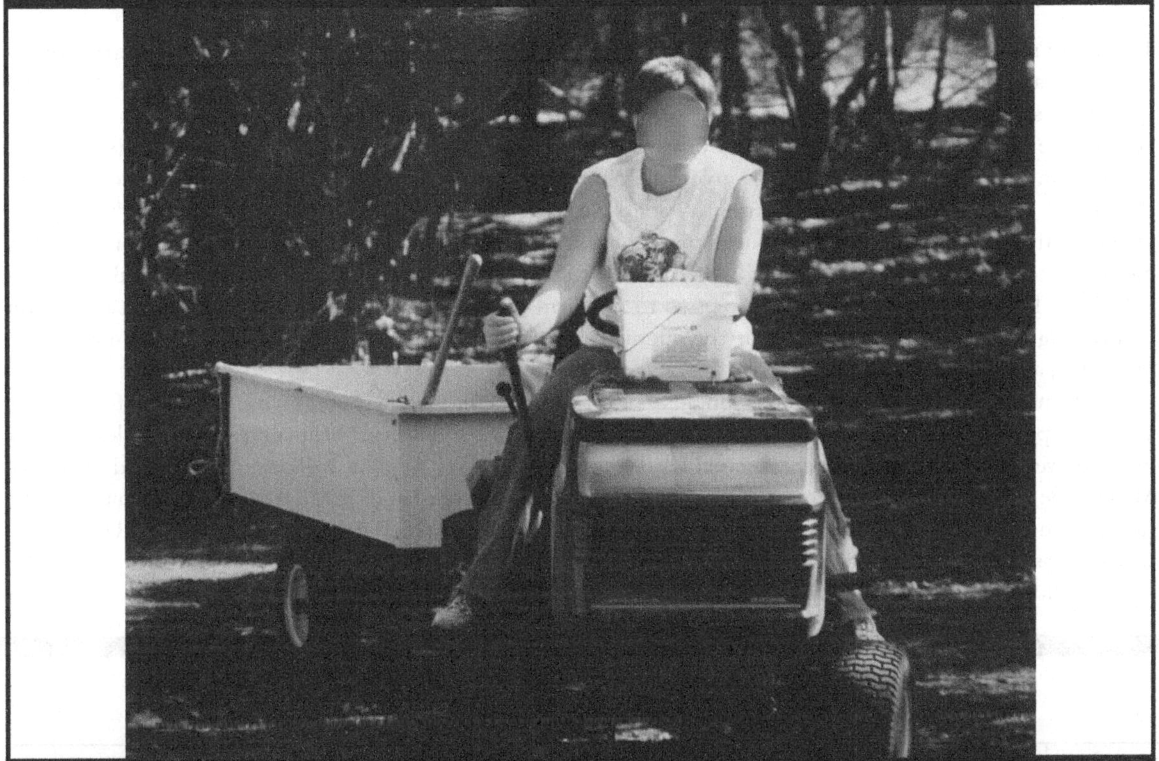

FIG. 13.5.

Table 13.2
EFP Goals

Level 1	1. Horse chooses client (may take up to third session). 2. Client accepts the choice. 3. Client learns to accept the presence of therapist and TRI/ES. • Starts to accept instruction. • Begins to understand that a correction is not ridicule or a challenge. • Can follow TRI/ES instructions part of the time. 4. Becomes comfortable engaging in basic horse care/handling; likes the horse and ground activities. • Leads horse with help. • Leads solo. • Plays lead line games. • Works in the round pen. 5. Rides on lead line, quietly; has basic level of comfort in completing stretches; ride with eyes closed.
Level 2	1. Returns greetings from therapist and TRI/ES. 2. Knows where the halters are kept and can retrieve horse with help. 3. Can give horse space if he is not ready to be caught; can discuss this with TRI/ES: a. without over-reacting; b. in a problem-solving manner; c. with a time-out if horse is reacting to her high arousal; d. practices breathing exercises. 4. Retrieves grooming bucket with few or any direct reminders; can groom horse in reasonably correct sequence. 5. Can find correct equipment for planned activity/helmet if riding; can do this without much help. 6. Can mount horse with limited assistance. 7. Understands how to stop her horse through breathing (no reins) and has experienced success. 8. Can use clip on reins (bit-less halter) to turn right and left without the horse stopping. 9. Can stop in a square box. 10. Rides on the trail (out of arena) while led. 11. Continues to improve ability to follow TRI/ES instructions.

Step 2: The Horse Pick

The client's first session at the barn is about exploring—meeting the staff, seeing where the bathroom is located, learning why certain places are off limits, and being let in on the hiding spots for the chicken's eggs. Unless the client is anxious and wants to stay outside the paddocks, the therapist, client, and TRI/ES go into the fields or paddocks for a full-body meet and greet with the horses. Every horse who is available to work on that day and at that time is given the chance to meet the "new kid" and welcome—or not—to the ranch. The client will be given time to spend with each horse. Depending upon the client's age, language skills, and experiences, awareness may come in squeals of excitement, shock and surprise, being handed a complete equine rebuke, or by being followed by the exact horse the client dismissed earlier as a "loner." It may take another session or two to confirm the match. The horse makes the first invitation by inviting touch. It is not unusual for the client to receive several. By the second or third go-around of meetings, a pairing is confirmed.

The transcript analysis below is an example of a horse pick with Juan (a pseudonym), 14 years of age. He is a juvenile parolee newly released from the state school where he served a one-year sentence for molestation of his three-year-old sister. Juan is at his second EFP session, attempting to make a connection with a draft-cross, Micky. The TRI/ES will communicate any observations to the therapist and step in if necessary to maintain the safety of the horse and the client. The therapist may explain some of the client's behavior to the TRI/ES, and will address the client to discuss the horse's behavior.

The following transcript analysis are about a pseudonym client.

Table 13.3

Transcript Analysis of Case Example: An Example of a Horse Pick

Tri/es	*Therapist*	*Client*	*Analysis*
I'm concerned about Micky's [horse's] behavior, see how he's pinning his ears? I'm going to stay close to keep them both safe.	I see mistrust in them both! Micky looks intrigued, curious, but Juan's fake smile and power-over attitude might get him into trouble.		Juan is self-absorbed, wanting badly for Micky to "choose" him. He'd spoken of his desire to ride a "big" horse. This desire has blinded Juan to the reality that his singularity of mission is interfering with his ability to connect. Juan is unaware that communicating he is less interested in the horse than in what Micky can potentially offer. The TRI/ES stays close for equine support and safety.
	Juan, what do you think Micky is trying to tell you?	I think he likes me! See how he's "licking" my hand?	
	What if I told you that unless you show him more respect you're likely to get bit?	Huh? No way, he's like a big dog!	Self-absorbed and writing his own script, Juan is far less concerned about who and what Micky is than whether or not Micky likes him.
What do you think? Should I intervene, or do you want to let things go on for a while?	Stay close and if you sense Micky getting agitated or into his "dominance mode," just end the interaction. We will process it with him afterwards.		As curious as Micky appears, there is an urgency in his actions toward Juan. And while Juan may likely be "asking to get bit" this is not the point. It is about horse and human safety and opening the possibility for a relationship
I'm sensing Micky tensing even more.	Me too. Do whatever you believe needs to be done.		The TRI/ES has the authority to stop the interaction at any time, which she did.
	Juan, any thoughts on TRI/ES taking Micky away?	I don't know. We were really starting to like each other. Can I meet another horse?	Juan's almost total disregard for his or Micky's safety or even that there was an issue gave me significant insight as to how unaware he was of himself and others. Mostly, that Juan lived in his head with an ongoing narrative about how he wanted things to be. Most concerning was Juan's indiscriminate use of touch. This is especially troublesome in youths who have committed sexual offences.

Step 3: Creating a Holding Space

The primary goal for the therapist and TRI/ES is in creating a safe "holding" environment for the client. A sense of safety is the result of the child's growing experience of certainty, that feeling of OK-ness about the surroundings and those consistent caregivers (horse, TRI/ES, therapist). In EFP practice, the holding environment of horse, therapist, and TRI/ES serves as a safe space in which the client experiencing the spectrum of disruptive and impulse control disorders can feel supported and cared for as the client learns, practices, and acquires skills in self-control, problem-solving, other awareness, and positive interactions. The interactions and their fluidity between the client, equine, therapist, and TRI/ES create a microcosm of a forgiving and loving world, something the client likely does not experience in everyday life. However, as they learn to trust this to be genuine, barriers start to diminish. The once angry, frightened, and skeptical client begins to allow this same experience at home, then school, then anywhere.

Noteworthy, perhaps, its singular contribution to the healing of trauma is that EFP leverages the therapeutic effects of physical touch. Given the deficits in early childhood attachment including emotional touching (Denworth, 2015) coupled with longstanding proscriptions regarding therapists touching their clients (Brooks, 2006), working with horses provides an ideal opportunity for physical touch (Mueller & McCullough, 2017). Inviting touch in the forms of grooming, petting, and riding, the unconditional equine partner offers a safe and sanctioned means by which the client can allow the experience of physical sensation and holding. In the transcript analysis below, we see Kevon (a pseudonym), age eight, who is in his fourth session. He was referred for violent and disruptive disorders in school and diagnosed ODD, bipolar, ADHD. Kevon is grooming Sydney, a 14-year-old Arab, who is not happy with his touch. Again, the TRI/ES communicates any concerns and will step in to maintain safety for the horse and client. Later I conferred with Kevon's psychiatrist on my observations of the session, and he agreed with my assessment of PTSD and likely attachment issues.

The following transcript analysis are about a pseudonym client.

Table 13.4

Transcript Analysis of Case Example: The Power of Touch

Tri/es	*Therapist*	*Client*	*Analysis*
Sydney [horse] sure is yawning and discharging. Is Kevon OK?	I've seen him go over the same area repeatedly, hardly touching Sydney. He is also starting to look checked out. Let me touch base.		The TRI/ES's observations of stress in the horse while getting groomed parallels the client's reluctant and unconscious touch while brushing his horse.
Stays with Sydney. Petting and talking softly to the horse.	Kevon, are you OK? Sydney is telling us there might be something on your mind.	Huh?... *Looks down, shrugs. Plays with the brush bristles.*	From what I'd been observing Kevon is distant, with a glassy-eyed look. Kevon looked as if he were waking from a nap.
Checks in, and reassure Sydney.	Kevon, can I ask you something? *Put my hand out to take the brush and curry comb.*	*Nods. Hands therapist grooming tools.*	I stay engaged and make only as much physical contact as I believed he could handle, as Kevon needed some physicality to come back to present.
Continues to attend to Sydney. When Kevon and I begin to talk, she takes Sydney for a walk to decompress.	Kevon, I noticed that when brushing Sydney, you were barely touching him. In fact, you were so gentle it seemed he could hardly feel you and became worried. Were you thinking about something else when brushing him?	*Nods again. Looks down. This lasts a moment.*	Kevon gradually returns to present as he considers what he was thinking about and whether he wants to tell me. He's been more anxious last week and today and so my gut was saying, "pay attention."

(Continued)

Tri/es	*Therapist*	*Client*	*Analysis*
Continues to walk Sydney.	Can you do a horse breath with me?	*Kevon looks up and gives a tiny smile.*	All clients learn "horse breath"—that big, deep, belly breath in which we snort and "let go" that releases tension. Kevon thought it was silly, but it felt good. All of us doing it together made the practice more fun, less embarrassing.
Walks and checks in with Sydney as she allows him to graze, all the while checking on our status and making eye contact.	OK. Can you tell me where you went just a minute ago? Was it a "lala" land place or were you thinking of something real?	*Shrugs. Breathes and says:* I was worried I would hurt Sydney if I brushed him too hard.	When clients dissociate I "normalize" the experience for them by talking with them about "lala land," explaining how it can both help and hurt us. Kevin's trip today was both.
	Thank you for being so kind and concerned. Sydney was worried that your brushing was so light he could hardly feel it. Horses get nervous about those things. Can you tell me about getting hurt with touch that was too soft or hard?	*Nods. Still looking down. After a pause Kevon started telling me about how his dad would drag him out of bed and beat him with a belt if he wasn't asleep within five minutes of going to bed.*	Having suspected abuse, I wanted to stay on topic but not push too hard or too far. Talking via the horse, speaking for it in terms of the client's issue can be a powerful means of diminishing the fear or threat of punishment. At least with littler kids. It also invites empathy.

Step 4: Processing Emotions

The partnership begun on the day of horse–client mutual selection becomes the foci of attention during therapy. It is to the equine partner that the youth is held most accountable. By means of this relationship between an honest, aware, and unconditional prey animal alongside a mistrusting, emotionally closed and frightened predator, the client begins to see through the eyes of the equine partner. Finding himself on the precipice of having to choose between making a life-changing leap into connectedness or else retreating deeper into the solo comfort of darkness can be a terrifying, vulnerability-making experience. What makes the client's leap even possible is by the time he gets to this point, he is typically no longer incessantly oppositional, or so mad and shut down. And yet, it is also because he no longer wears his protective suit of "badass" everywhere he goes that making the choice to accept attachment is practically a do-or-die decision.

In the next transcript analysis, Kevon is now age 11. After three years, Kevon has learned a lot about self-regulation and has shared his abuse history from both his dad and stepmom. His dad, who has been out of the picture for two years, has come back wanting to see his son. A resurgence of old and mixed feelings has reignited Kevon's previous fury. Unsettled by the boy's agitation, Kevon's horse, Hercules, will not cooperate by lifting his foot for cleaning. The TRI/ES encouraged and helped, but this only made matters worse.

The following transcript analysis are about a pseudonym client.

Table 13.5

Transcript Analysis of Case Example: Processing Anger

Tri/es	*Therapist*	*Client*	*Analysis*
Is standing with arms crossed "glaring" at Kevon, who has the hoof pick in his hand. She is keeping an eye on the horse and looking very serious. She appears ready to spring into action at any second.	Paying close attention to Kevon, I had only just heard about Kevon's dad pushing his grandma to come see him. I look over to my TRI/ES, nod to let her know that things might get heated.	Kevon is clutching a hoof pick. He is grunting and making threatening looks at both horse and assistant. There is a scowl on his face well as a heaviness about him that is new.	There is a sort of stand-off going on. I wonder if it is Marissa (the TRI/ES) or Kevon's horse, Hercules, that has put up the challenge. Likely both. I assess the strength of Kevon's and my relationship with that of his current simmering anger, considering my next move. Under-responding is the only way to go.
She nods her head and backs up but stays close.	Hunkering down to his level. Hey Kev, what's with the ugly face? You look really pissed off!	Looking at the ground, frowning and pounding the hoof pick into the dirt. I am pissed off.	Stating the obvious, being where the client is, using body and verbal language that cannot be misunderstood, helps create a connection that invites comradery and therefore, safety
Attends to Hercules, petting and brushing, talking kindly to the big horse.	Yeah. So, what's going on?	Herc wouldn't pick up his stupid foot and Marissa got all on my ass about how I wasn't being respectful... she's such a bitch!	Letting Kevon vent without judgment including not giving any weight to his derisive descriptions maintains the flow of conversation.
Having exchanged glances acknowledging things were better, she unties Hercules and takes him for a walk.	Yeah. Herc is tough and so is Marissa. But you know that! It's why you like these guys. Guess not today, huh?	Gets quiet, breathes, and stops pounding the hoof pick, but still plays with it.	Being heard and attended to, Kevon's energy decreases. He is reminded of the importance of those individuals on whom he is currently displacing his anger. Following years of horse breath, Kevon instinctively breathes!
Continues to attend to the horse, allowing him to graze as she completes the hoof cleaning job.	Nice to see you settling down. How about you hand me that hoof pick and let's take a walk and figure this out...	Still not making eye contact, Kevon nods, stands up and walks toward the pasture, and his "thinking tree." Kevon apologizes to both Hercules and Marissa.	By maintaining my energy as low as possible and still staying tuned in, Kevon was able to do the same. Our relationship built on three years of honesty, respect, and safety, had everything to do with Kevon feeling safe enough to get still, think, and feel.

Step 5: Reaching a Breakthrough

We tell clients that as prey animals, horses avoid proximity of anyone/thing that is going to hurt or eat them. The youth with ODD who is disrespectful, dismissive, shallow, frightening, and/or frightened, just might want him for lunch! Sooner or later, the youth's highly sensitive, intuitive, boundary-setting, equine partner, "disses" her in a way no human is capable, much less could get away with. Struck speechless by this silent dismissal, the client comes face to face with having to choose. Does she blow off her horse like she has every social worker who brought bad news or foster parent who dared put her in time-out? Or does she accept his honest reproach for what it was, a hard-core reality check? Having been called out as unsafe, and therefore not to be trusted, the client is faced with the awareness that she has become what she fears and hates. Typically, this scene will be replayed until the client is at last able to accept what is right in front of her as truth. It is only then that she can ask her horse for forgiveness, and then accept the partnership.

In the next transcript analysis, Juan is now 15. He had a break in therapy but returned and has been coming for seven months. It is his fourth-to-last session and Juan finally comes clean about the "secret" he has held on to for years, that has prevented him from being real with anyone, including or especially, his horse, Micky.

The following transcript analysis are about a pseudonym client.

Table 13.6

Transcript Analysis of Case Example: Making the Breakthrough

Tri/es	*Therapist*	*Client*	*Analysis*
Listening.	I hear you have something to share with us?	Uh, yeah. But can I just read my letter to you? And Micky?	Juan has delayed writing a letter to his mother, his victimizer, for almost seven months. This is a huge step for him and it is important that he be able to decide who can or cannot be present.
Nods her understanding, knowing Juan will include her when he is ready.	Of course. Look over at TRI/ES.	Sigh of relief. Goes to the field with Joy (TRI/ES) to retrieve Micky.	The relief in finally dealing with his dark past with mom shows in Juan's much lighter mood, his freedom of movement and in how Micky greets him in the field.
Engages in friendly banter with Juan as he grooms and plays with Micky	Sees a very different client and horse.	Hugs his horse in a manner that is more genuine than I have seen to date.	Micky's relaxation with Juan indicates an energy shift from that of cautious curiosity to playful acceptance. He seems to be saying, "Wow!"
Checks on the other horses while I engage with Juan and Micky.	I'm all ears. So is Micky! In fact, I can't remember ever seeing him this attentive.	Yeah. Me too. I'm kinda nervous, this was really hard. But ya, know, you were right, I do feel better, like relieved now that it's out. Juan then proceeds to read us his victimizer letter to his mom.	Juan had convinced himself that his mother's emotional demands on him as a child were normal, that they "made me the man of the house." Confronting his rage and jealousy when she deserted him to his dad to remarry had become internalized as being "jilted by" his primary love-object. Juan is starting to develop abstract and critical thinking skills necessary on a convoluted, emotionally charged experience.
Are you kidding? I've been waiting six months for this to happen! Let's saddle up.	Let's ask TRI/ES. If she says it's OK, then let's do it.	After a good cry, Juan announces: I want to try riding Micky! Is that OK?	Although youth in my program typically begin basic mounted work 4–6 weeks into therapy, Juan's continued self-deception and emotional barriers prevented this from happening. Micky's interest in Juan never wavered and maintained an indisputable connection. As much as anything else attained in therapy, Micky's dogged dedication gave Juan the support and courage needed to complete a difficult journey.

CONCLUSION

In the wake of over-the-top dysregulation and at times, cruel and unyielding behaviors, practitioner awareness that attachment deficits are often driving ODD behaviors will lead to a better understanding of the client. In this broadened scope of awareness, intervention possibilities extend well beyond medication or therapy in an office. Offering therapy in the context of a partnership with equines has proven especially helpful in working with clients who struggle with attachment and security. Horses tell us what the client cannot or will not; they tell us what we cannot hear and do not feel.

REFERENCES

Alaggia, R. (2005). Disclosing the trauma of child sexual abuse: A gender analysis. *Journal of Loss & Trauma, 10*(5), 453–470.

American Psychiatric Association (APA). (2013). *Diagnostic and Statistical Manual of Mental Disorders.* 5th edition. Arlington, VA: American Psychiatric Publishing.

Bachi, K., Terkel, J., & Teichman, M. (2012). Equine-facilitated psychotherapy for at-risk adolescents: The influence on self-image, self-control and trust. *Clinical Child Psychology and Psychiatry, 17*(2), 298–312.

Benoit, D. (2004). Infant–parent attachment: Definition, types, antecedents, measurement and outcome. *Pediatrics & Child Health, 9*(8), 541–545.

Boylan, K. (2014). The many faces of oppositional defiant disorder. *Journal of the Canadian Academy of Child and Adolescent Psychiatry, 23*(1), 8–9.

Brooks, S. M. (2006). Animal-assisted psychotherapy and equine-assisted psychotherapy. In N. Boyd-Webb (Ed.), *Working with Traumatized Youth in Child Welfare* (pp. 196–218). New York: Guilford Press.

Brooks, S. & McCullough, L. M. (2008). The diamond model. In S. Brooks, M. Hogan, L. M. McCullough, & M. Stuart (Eds.), *Equine Specialist Workshop Faculty Manual* (pp. 43–47). Denver, CO: NARHA.

Burton, N. (2012). *Hide and Seek: The Psychology of Self-Deception.* Kent, UK: Acheron Press.

Chandler, C. K. (2012). *Animal Assisted Therapy in Counseling.* 2nd edition. New York: Routledge.

Denworth, L. (2015). The social power of touch. *Scientific American Mind, 26*, 30–39.

Eaves, L. J., Silberg, J. L., Meyer, J. M., Maes, H. H., Simonoff, E., Pickles, A., Rutter, M., Neale, M. C., Reynolds, C. A., Erikson, M. T., Heath, A. C., Loeber, R., Truett, K. R., & Hewitt, J. K. (1997). Genetics and developmental psychopathology: The main effects of genes and environment on behavioral problems in the Virginia Twin Study of Adolescent Behavioral Development. *Journal of Child Psychology and Psychiatry, 38*(8), 965–980.

Erikson, E. H. (1950). *Childhood and Society.* New York: W. W. Norton & Company, Inc.

Frick, P. J., Lahey, B. B., Loeber, R., Stouthamer-Loeber, M., Christ M. A. G., & Hanson, K. (1992). Familial risk factors to oppositional defiant disorder and conduct disorder: Parental psychopathology and maternal parenting. *Journal of Consulting and Clinical Psychology, 60*(1), 49–55.

Garland, E. J. (2001). Rages and refusals: The many faces of adolescent anxiety. *Canadian Family Physician, 41*(5), 1023–1030.

Hood, B. S., Elrod, M. G., & DeWine, D. B. (2015). Treatment of childhood oppositional defiant disorder. *Current Treatment Options in Pediatrics, 1*(2), 155–167.

Jaffee, S. R., Moffitt, T. E., Caspi, A., & Taylor, A. (2003). Life with (or without) father: The benefits of living with two biological parents depend on the father's antisocial behavior. *Child Development, 74*(1), 109–126.

Karol, J. M. (2000). A psychotherapeutic riding program: An existential theater for healing. *Dissertation Abstracts International: Section B. Sciences and Engineering, 60*(11-B), 5776.

Karol, J. M. (2007). Applying a traditional individual psychotherapy model to equine-facilitate psychotherapy (EFP): Theory and method. *Clinical Child Psychology and Psychiatry, 12*(1), 77–90.

Kazdin, A. E. (2011). Evidence-based treatment research: Advances, limitations, and next steps. *American Psychologist, 66*(8), 685–698.

Kazdin, A. E. & Blase, S. L. (2011). Rebooting psychotherapy research and practice to reduce the burden of mental illness. *Perspectives on Psychological Science, 6*(1), 21–37.

Kemp, K., Signal, T., Botros, H., Taylor, N., & Prentice, K. (2014). Equine-facilitated therapy with children and adolescents who have been sexually abused: A program evaluation study. *Journal of Child and Family Studies, 23*(3), 558–566.

Maslow, A. H. (1943). A theory of human motivation. *Psychological Review, 50*(4), 370–396.

McCullough, L., Risley-Curtiss, C., & Rorke, J. (2015). Equine facilitated psychotherapy: A pilot study of effect on posttraumatic stress symptoms in maltreated youth. *Journal of Infant, Child, and Adolescent Psychotherapy, 14*(2), 158–173.

McMaken, M., (2000). *The Relationship between Erikson's Developmental Tasks and children Identified as At-Risk.* Master's thesis. Retrieved from All Graduate Theses and Dissertations. (2630).

McLaughlin, K. A., Breslau, J., Green, J. G., Lakoma, M. D., Sampson, N. A., Zaslavsky, A. M., & Kesslere, R. C. (2011). Childhood socio-economic status and the onset, persistence, and severity of DSM-IV mental disorders in a US national sample. *Social Science and Medicine, 73*(7), 1088–1096.

Melson, G. F. (2000). Companion animals and the development of children: Implications of the biophilia hypothesis. In A. Fine (Ed.), *Handbook on Animal-Assisted Therapy: Theoretical Foundations and Guidelines for Practice* (pp. 376–383). San Diego, CA: Academic.

Melson, G. F. & Fine, A. H. (2015). Animals in the lives of children. In A. Fine (Ed.), *Handbook on Animal-Assisted Interventions* (pp. 179–194). San Diego, CA: Academic.

Mueller, M. K. & McCullough, L. (2017). Effects of equine-facilitated psychotherapy on post-traumatic stress symptoms in youth. *Journal of Child and Family Studies, 26*(4), 1164–1172.

Odhayani, A. A., Watson, W. J., & Watson, L. (2013). Behavioral consequences of child abuse. *Canadian Family Physician, 59*(8), 831–836.

Parish-Plass, N. (2008). Animal-assisted therapy with children suffering from insecure attachment due to abuse and neglect: A method to lower the risk of intergenerational transmission of abuse? *Clinical Child Psychology and Psychiatry 13*(1), 7–30.

Professional Association of Therapeutic Horsemanship International (PATH Intl.). (2010). PATH Intl. Code of ethics. Retrieved from www.pathintl.org/images/pdf/about-narha/documents/PATH-Intl-Code-of-Ethics-05-15.pdf.

Professional Association of Therapeutic Horsemanship International (PATH Intl.). (2015). PATH Intl. FAQ. Retrieved from www.pathintl.org/faq#efp.

Professional Association of Therapeutic Horsemanship International (PATH Intl.). (2017). What is EFP? Retrieved from www.pathintl.org/27-resources/general/193-eaat-definitions.

Professional Association of Therapeutic Horsemanship International (PATH Intl.). (2018). What is the PATH Intl./ EFMHA integration? Retrieved from www.pathintl.org/images/pdf/about-narha/Integration-FAQ-web.pdf.

Qin, S., Young, C. B., Duan, X., Chen, T., Supekar, K., & Menon, V. (2014). Amygdala subregional structure and intrinsic functional connectivity predicts individual differences in anxiety during early childhood. *Biological Psychiatry, 75*(11), 892–900.

Rowe, R., Rijsdijk, F. V., Maughan, B., Eley, T. C., Hosang, G. M., & Eley, T. C. (2008). Heterogeneity in antisocial behaviors and comorbidity with depressed mood: A behavioral genetic approach. *The Journal of Child Psychology and Psychiatry, 49*(5), 526–534.

Russow, L.-M. (2002). Ethical implications of the human–animal bond in the laboratory. *ILAR Journal, 43*(1), 33–37.

Séverine, D., Booksmythe, I., Kotrschal, A., Jennions, M., & Kolm, N. (2016). Artificial selection on male genitalia length alters female brain size. *Proceedings on Biological Sciences, 283*.

Shaw, D. S., Dishion, T. J., Supplee, L., Gardner, F., & Arnds, K. (2006). Randomized trial of a family-centered approach to the prevention of early conduct problems: Two-year effects of the family check-up in early childhood. *Journal of Consulting and Clinical Psychology, 74*(1), 1–9.

Steiner, H., Garcia, I. G., & Matthews, Z. (1997). Posttraumatic stress disorder in incarcerated juvenile delinquents. *Journal of the American Academy of Child & Adolescent Psychiatry, 36*(3), 357–365.

Steiner, H., & Remsing, L. (2007). Practice parameter for the assessment and treatment of children and adolescents with oppositional defiant disorder. *Journal of the American Academy of Child & Adolescent Psychiatry, 46*(1), 126–141.

Tannenbaum, J. (1995). Animals and the law: property, cruelty, rights. *Social Research, 62*(3), 539–607.

Theule, J., Germain, S. M., Cheung, K., Hurl, K. E., & Markel, C. (2016). Conduct disorder/oppositional defiant disorder and attachment: A meta-analysis. *Journal of Developmental and Life-Course Criminology, 2*(2), 232–255.

Trotter, K. S. (2012). *Harnessing the Power of Equine Assisted Counseling: Adding Animal Assisted Therapy to Your Practice.* New York: Routledge.

Trotter, K. S., Chandler, C. K., Goodwin-Bond, D., & Casey, J. (2008). A comparative study of the efficacy of group equine assisted counseling with at-risk children and adolescents. *Journal of Creativity in Mental Health, 3*(3).

Yorke, J., Adams, C., & Coady, N. (2008). Therapeutic value of equine-human bonding in recovery from trauma. *Anthrozoös, 21*(1), 17–30.

Section 8

Eating Disorders

14

The Human–Equine Relational Development (HERD) Approach to Working with Clients Suffering from Bulimia Nervosa

Veronica Lac

INTRODUCTION

Bulimia Nervosa

Bulimia nervosa is one of the most common types of eating disorders, and is an increasing concern within the mental health field. With an estimated prevalence of 1–2% in women, and 0.5% in men (Hudson, Hiripi, Pope, & Kessler, 2007), it is also often underreported and misdiagnosed. Characterized by consuming large quantities of food, followed by compensating for the bingeing, many sufferers are undiagnosed due to being within normal body weight. Symptoms include excessive eating (often in secret), obsession with body weight, feelings of shame around food, self-induced vomiting and/or starvation, excessive exercise, and abuse of laxatives, diuretics, or diet pills (American Psychiatric Association, 2013).

Traditional treatments of bulimia nervosa include the prescribing of antidepressants and the use of Cognitive Behavioral Therapy (National Institute for Mental Health, 2016). While these treatments focus on the symptoms and behaviors of the illness, they may not address the underlying issues that led to its development. More recently, both residential and outpatient eating disorder clinics have begun to introduce more holistic and relational approaches to treatment. The Renfrew Center (2017) and the Prosperity Eating Disorders and Wellness Center (PEDWC) both offer experiential therapies including art, dance/movement, and drama therapies. Additionally, PEDWC also offers mind–body-based instruction through therapeutic yoga, reflexology, and acupuncture.

Bulimia nervosa, as well as the other DSM-5-specified eating disorders are often shaped through relationships in the individual's environment (Morrison, Doss, & Perez, 2009), where these relationships can impact the development and maintenance of body image, weight, and eating concerns. Individuals with eating disorders often hide their eating habits from those around them, further increasing feelings of isolation and lack of support. Taking a relational approach to eating disorder treatment allows for some of these environmental factors to emerge. Additionally, since bulimia nervosa incorporates an aspect of desensitization to the bodily being through overeating, it is important to include a somatic element to the healing process.

THE HUMAN–EQUINE RELATIONAL DEVELOPMENT (HERD) APPROACH

The Human–Equine Relational Development (HERD) approach focuses on an embodied and relational approach to healing, and views the horse as a co-facilitator in the therapeutic process (Lac, 2017). In a nutshell, the principles behind the HERD approach are rooted in existential-humanistic psychology and Gestalt psychotherapy, and are based on the three tenets of what can be referred to as: the Here-and-Now; What and How; and I and Thou (Lac, 2017). The Here-and-Now refers to the ability to remain in the present moment in a fully embodied way. This includes not only awareness of what clients are thinking, but also what they are feeling in their body through all of their senses. It also incorporates what their intuitive feelings in each moment might be. What and How refers to the process by which the practitioner holds a sense of curiosity about what is unfolding in the relationship between the client and the horse(s), without jumping to their own interpretations but simply reflecting back their observations to clients. This phenomenological process allows clients to make meaning of their experiences for themselves (Lac, 2017). I and Thou, refers to the philosophical concept of Martin Buber (1958), who distinguishes between an immersive experience of being with another, versus an objectified relationship. Holding an I-Thou attitude supports the practitioner to be able to become more attuned with the present moment within the relationship, and acknowledges that one cannot avoid making an impact on, or being impacted by, others.

Briefly, the HERD approach to equine-facilitated psychotherapy (EFP) consists of a five-stage model: *Sharing Space*, *Release and Expand*, *Deepening*, *Coming Home to Relationships*, and *Integration* (Lac, 2017). Throughout each session, the practitioner focuses on the client and the horse's process through these stages. *Sharing Space* refers to the beginnings of the process where the practitioner tracks the way that the client and horse start to acknowledge the other's presence. It focuses on breathing and being in the moment. *Release and Expand* refers to the way in which both horses and humans move into/out of relationship in a dance of releasing expectations/constrictions to allow for an expansion of a sense of self, either physically or psychologically. *Deepening* is the stage where authentic connection begins to occur, where clients are able to stay with whatever is unfolding between them and the horse(s). *Coming Home to Relationships* refers to those moments where clients can sink into the relationship and linger for a while, and begin to (re)discover an authentic way of being. Finally, *Integration* allows for clients to take the embodied experience with the horses and translate that into something they can recognize in their everyday lives.

Clients with eating disorders often relate to themselves through a mind–body dichotomy, separating their body sensations, feelings, and processes from their cognitive awareness. The HERD approach works to integrate this mind–body separation through raising the client's somatic awareness. EFP embraces the horse's natural ability to be fully embodied in the present moment. The horse's mode of survival depends on their ability to remain in relationship with the rest of the herd, and have an awareness of their environment. Working with horses in the psychotherapeutic environment allows for clients to experience authentic ways of relating, as horses live in a state of emotional and embodied congruence (Lac, 2017). In the company of humans, horses naturally transfer their ways of being in the herd to humans (Rector, 2005).

Introducing equines into the therapeutic space requires practitioners to be mindful of the ethical considerations of how they partner with their equine co-facilitators. The HERD approach subscribes to the concepts of being a compassionate equestrian in all aspects of relating to horses. As outlined through the 25 principles of the Compassionate Equestrian (Schoen & Gordon, 2015), horses are valued as sentient beings in their own right, and treated with respect, dignity, and compassion when caring for, and working with them. For this reason, within the HERD approach, the horses are mostly at liberty.

CASE EXAMPLE

The following case example outlines the HERD approach, and demonstrates the powerful healing that can occur for clients suffering from bulimia nervosa through an embodied and relational framework within EFP.

Virginia (a pseudonym) was referred for EFP through an outpatient eating disorders clinic by her individual therapist, and had been in and out of residential treatment programs over the past ten years. At 32 years old, she was now in a committed relationship, and was hoping to get married. Virginia wanted to have children, but was aware that she needed to break out of her destructive cycle of bulimia nervosa in order to have a healthy pregnancy. This provided her with a powerful motivation to change her behaviors, but she was still struggling to implement the changes she needed to make. Her bingeing/purging cycle consisted of secret binges in the middle of the night, mostly on weekends, followed by excessive exercise and laxatives. While her weight had not fluctuated too much, and she was within normal weight ranges, her blood work showed high cholesterol and high-risk markers for Type II diabetes. Virginia felt ashamed of her secret binges and reported bouts of depression following her more extreme binge/purge cycles.

In her first session with the horses, Virginia watched the herd grazing in the pasture. My two mares were standing close together eating peacefully. My gelding was by himself in the far corner of the field, dozing in the sunshine.

The following transcript analysis are about a pseudonym client.

Table 14.1

Transcript Analysis of Case Example

Transcript	*Analysis*
Counselor: What's happening for you right now?	Bringing the client into the here-and-now, without prescribing a mode of awareness (i.e., what is happening could be physical, emotional, or cognitive).
Client: I feel sad... I'm looking at that horse over there all by himself. He looks so lonely. It reminds me of how I am when I'm watching other people eat.	Client begins to project feelings onto the horse, and then proceeds to take ownership of her reflections.
Counselor: Where do you feel the loneliness in your body?	Attempt to bring client's awareness into an embodied state.
Client: It's like a numbness in my core. If I focus on it, it gets heavier. Usually when I feel like this, I start thinking about bingeing.	Client begins to articulate the bodily sensation of loneliness that contributes to her mindless eating.
Counselor: I notice you're still watching the gelding on his own.	Phenomenological description of what the client is doing, allowing the client to draw meaning. The client is entering into the *Sharing Space* stage of the HERD model.
Client: Yes. I don't want him to be by himself.	Client's awareness of the need for relationship begins to emerge.
Counselor: How would you like to be with him?	Counselor invites the client to make connection with the horse to facilitate the beginnings of a relationship.
Client: I'd like to go and stand next to him, so he knows he's not on his own.	Client is motivated to make connection with the horse, and in doing so, can begin to reflect on what she may need (support) when feeling on the verge of bingeing. This is the start of the *Release and Expand* stage.

Virginia walked over to the gelding, Arrow. Stopping about ten feet away from him, she looked down at her feet and began to cry. She explained that it had seemed so simple to offer the horse some comfort when she thought he was lonely, but that when she felt isolated, she found it hard to reach out for support. As she spoke, Arrow walked over to her and started sniffing her shoulder. She reached out to pet him on his shoulder. I invited her to move to his side so that she could lean her head and chest on him, and experience being supported in a more embodied way, facilitating the *Deepening* stage of the HERD model. As she lay her head on him, he turned his head towards her, wrapping his neck around her. Virginia continued to cry. I gave them space to experience the moment between them, and watched as she reached her arms around his neck and hugged him tight. After a few moments, Virginia straightened herself up and exhaled deeply. Arrow dropped his head to the ground and began to graze. Virginia continued to pet him on the neck as he grazed. After two or three bites, Arrow took a step forward, lifted his head towards Virginia, and then continued to graze. Virginia adjusted herself and followed him. Again, Arrow moved after a few bites, lifted his head towards Virginia, and she followed and continued to pet him. This dance was repeated several more times. I waited and watched. Virginia was immersed in the experience between her and Arrow, and I wanted to give them time to connect. After a few minutes, I noticed that we were now in close proximity to the two mares who had continued to graze peacefully the whole time we were with Arrow. We were now in the penultimate stage of *Coming Home to Relationships* in the HERD model.

The following transcript analysis are about a pseudonym client.

Table 14.2

Transcript Analysis of Case Example

Transcript	*Analysis*
Counselor: What are you aware of now?	This is an invitation to the client to express their state of being in whatever way they felt able, while staying in the present moment.
Client: *Looking up and around her, she laughed.* I didn't realize we'd traveled so far across the field. I had no idea that we were so close to the other two horses! I think he just needed permission to start eating with the others.	Client is able to return to an awareness of their surroundings while making sense of what they had experienced with the horse.
Counselor: How does this resonate with you?	Counselor begins to integrate the meaning made with the client's way of being-in-the-world.
Client: I need support to be able to eat without feeling ashamed. I need to reach out for that support somehow. I'd like to be able to get to the point where I can eat with others in public without constantly feeling anxious that I'm being judged. Or judging myself.	Client is able to integrate the learning from their embodied experience of being in relationship with the horse, to needing more connection and support in their life. This is the *Integration* stage of the HERD model.

This session was the beginning of Virginia's journey towards reaching out for support from her partner when she felt the urge to binge. Instead of isolating herself and numbing her bodily senses to her need for connection, and feeding the emptiness within her through bingeing, she slowly began to feel the sensations of fullness both physically and psychologically.

CONCLUSION

This chapter outlined the HERD approach to working with bulimia nervosa. A brief case example was presented through the lens of the HERD model, demonstrating the powerful shifts that can occur through a relational and embodied approach to equine-facilitated psychotherapy.

REFERENCES

American Psychiatric Association. (2013). *Diagnostic and Statistical Manual of Mental Disorders.* 5th edition. Washington, DC: American Psychiatric Association.

Buber, M. (1958). *I and Thou.* New York: Scribner.

Hudson J. I., Hiripi, E., Pope, H. G., & Kessler, R. C. (2007). The prevalence and correlates of eating disorders in the National Comorbidity Survey Replication. *Biological Psychiatry, 61*, 348–358.

Lac, V. (2017) Equine-Facilitated Psychotherapy and Learning: The Human–Equine Relational Development (HERD) Approach. San Diego, CA: Academic Press.

Morrison, K. R., Doss, B. D., & Perez, M. (2009). Body image and disordered eating in romantic relationships. *Journal of Social and Clinical Psychology, 28*, 281–306.

National Institute for Mental Health (2016). *Eating Disorders.* Retrieved from www.nimh.nih.gov/health/topics/eating-disorders/index.shtml.

Prosperity Eating Disorders and Wellness Center. (2017). *Equine Facilitated Psychotherapy.* Retrieved from www.centerforhopeofnova.com/EquineTherapy.html.

Rector, B. K. (2005). Adventures in Awareness: Learning with the Help of Horses. Bloomington, IN: AuthorHouse.

Renfrew Center (2017). *The Renfrew Center.* Retrieved from http://renfrewcenter.com/services/experiential-therapy.

Schoen, A.S. & Gordon, S. (2015). The Compassionate Equestrian: 25 Principles to Live By When Caring For and Working With Horses. North Pomfret, Vermont: Trafalgar Square Books.

Section 9
Substance Abuse

15

Equine-Assisted Mental Health Therapy and Alcoholism

Issues in Early Sobriety

Alita Buzel

INTRODUCTION

Alcoholism, also known as alcohol use disorder (AUD) (American Psychiatric Association, 2013), refers to the chronic consumption of alcohol that results in significant problems for the alcoholic and those in contact with them. Alcoholism is said to exist when the following conditions are present: acquiring and drinking alcohol becomes a driving force in the alcoholic's life resulting in failure to fulfill daily responsibilities; the alcoholic experiences significant and escalating health problems; serious legal and emotional consequences result from the poor judgment that characterizes alcohol inebriation; alcohol tolerance escalates with continued use and withdrawal symptoms, sometimes life threatening, might occur when stopping.

Approximately 15 million adults (18+) have been diagnosed with AUD, 9.8 million men and 5.3 million women. In addition, 43% of the US adult population is exposed either to alcoholism or problem drinking in the family. About 66 million of those are children under the age of 18. The cost to society in terms of lost work time, medical costs related to the disease, and the dissolution of families, is staggering (National Survey of Drugs and Statics, 2015).

There are a number of effective interventions in the treatment of alcoholism, but few offer the immediate feedback and hands-on challenges and rewards as equine therapy does. Working with horses addresses many of the issues that alcoholics struggle with, particularly during the early stages of recovery. Some of these, to be further discussed in this chapter, include: dealing with strong emotions such as rage and shame, working on impulse control, developing effective stress responses, repairing frayed relationships, ownership of responsibility, and reframing "control" as a way of managing life.

THE NATURE OF ADDICTION

All addictions, including alcoholism, create a temporary sense of euphoria and/or a release from pain and distress. Once the mood-altering effect of the substance or compulsive behavior wears off, the person is left in a state of withdrawal and discomfort, leading to further addictive behavior (Steinglass, 1987).

What characterizes addicts is the dependence on *something outside of themselves* to create and maintain a sense of inner peace. This results in a state of chronic dependency on that external object, whether that is a line of cocaine, a six-pack of beer, or a sexual encounter with a stranger. Control of access to the addictive outlet becomes a powerful motivator and underlying dynamic.

- Early sobriety, for the sake of this article, extends from approximately three months after cessation of drinking to one year.
- Equine therapy is usually employed as a supplemental treatment option used in conjunction with more traditional interventions from addictions such as 28-day inpatient rehabilitation and Alcoholics Anonymous (AA) meetings.

There are a number of psychological characteristics shared by the majority of people dealing with alcoholism. The following is a list of common emotional issues:

- The overuse of intellectual defenses to explain and justify their addictions, such as denial that there is anything amiss and/or projection of blame onto others for all their problems.
- An inability to tolerate strong, uncomfortable emotions without numbing their discomfort with their addiction reflecting a lack of coping skills and affect tolerance.
- A propensity to become easily frustrated and enraged by everyday stress and/or problematic interpersonal issues.
- A lack of empathy and compassion for oneself as well as others.
- A deep sense of inadequacy, often masked behind a bravado persona.
- A falsely and precariously held belief that they can control everything and everyone in their lives, including the addictive substance.
- Shame cycles that motivate and reinforce the addictive behavior. Promises to oneself and others that they will stop, followed by relapse leading to intolerable levels of shame and self-denigration, which leads to further promises and further relapses.

TREATMENT PLANNING

The following is a review of relevant issues requiring consideration in treatment planning for early sobriety. To begin, ensure that your client is indeed sober. No growth or healing can take place if a person is active in their addiction.

There are usually three different stages in alcoholism recovery, each of which requires differing therapeutic goals and interventions. The first stage is *detoxification and early recovery*, which extends from cessation of drinking until approximately three months of sobriety. This stage might incorporate a hospital stay if it is assessed that the alcoholic needs medical assistance withdrawing from alcohol. Afterward, the recovering alcoholic might attend a 28-day inpatient treatment program and begin daily AA meetings. The second stage, *early sobriety*, usually addresses the first three months to one year after cessation of drinking. During this phase, the alcoholic is optimally attending daily AA meetings and has begun to soberly assess their lives. The third stage is *long-term recovery*, which continues for the rest of the alcoholic's life.

Early sobriety is a critical time of recovery. During this phase, a newly recovering addict will be confronted with overpowering and conflicting emotions without having had the time to master the necessary coping skills or to develop the appropriate support system needed to ensure continued sobriety. The individual will require long-term support, encouragement, and patience. Lowered frustration tolerance, poor affect regulation, increased displays of anger, agitation, and cognitive confusion are to be expected. It is important to keep in mind that the addict's brain is changing rapidly and will do so for up to one year after cessation of drinking (Buzel, 1986).

Equine psychotherapy can begin at any stage of recovery with the goals adjusted to fit the needs of the recovering individual. As there are a multitude of challenges facing an addict, particularly during the first year of sobriety, fluidity in both treatment planning and goal setting is necessary to reflect evolving changes and needs.

INCORPORATING HORSES

Ownership of responsibility, trust, and respect for self and others are basic interpersonal skills that must be developed if sobriety is to be achieved and maintained. In addition, intimate relationships that have been badly bruised by the effects of alcoholism need time to heal. That healing cannot take place until the alcoholic has taken responsibility for his or her behavior. Horses are the perfect therapists to address these issues. They are the litmus test for sincerity and congruity.

The basic goals, at the beginning stage of equine psychotherapy, are to assist the client to self-soothe, recognize and deal with strong emotions, manage complex issues of control/fear/shame, and work on developing a relationship with another sentient creature based on mutual honesty, trust, and respect.

Relationship Benefits

Horses are wonderful teachers of kindness, self-forgiveness, and intimacy. They realize that the herd is only as strong as their weakest member; it is therefore the fragile members that garner extra love and caring (Kohanov, 2001). Horses are also very sensitive to any incongruity between how a person *presents* (e.g., aggressively) and how a person *honestly feels* (e.g., scared and inadequate). Having avoided feeling their own hurt and pain for so many years, alcoholics often have difficulty recognizing and accepting their own vulnerability. In the company of non-judgmental creatures, such as horses, self-acceptance, self-compassion, and self-forgiveness have the opportunity to be safely explored (Hayes, 2015).

Control Issues

Alcoholics believe they have to control everything and everybody. The inability to control the world, in this case the horse, might elicit strong, often primitive, feelings such as: fear/panic, shame/rage, frustration/inadequacy, and blaming/projection of responsibility. Working with the Serenity Prayer, we use the horses to address basic control issues. Accepting what you can control (your own emotions), the inner courage to know what you can't control (the horse), and the wisdom to know the difference (humbleness) gets played out over and over again in the arena with the therapy horse. In other words, you cannot "control" a horse, as you cannot control your addiction. Both are more powerful than you are. However, you can begin to have a relationship with a horse where control is pre-empted by respect, trust, and caring for self and other. Being humble before the power of a thousand-pound horse is not being a wimp. It takes tremendous courage to face something bigger and stronger than you are (Steinglass, 1987).

Emotional Intelligence and Self-Awareness

Up to sobriety, these individuals depended upon alcohol to deaden their uncomfortable feelings, keep emotions at a distance, and basically deny their existence. Learning to first *recognize* and then *tolerate* feelings are some of the major goals during the first year of sobriety. Working with horses gives the alcoholic many opportunities to recognize and face uncomfortable feelings, in addition to exploring core vulnerabilities that connect us to ourselves and others. Masking anxiety and fear behind a bravado demeanor backfires when dealing with a highly sensitive animal such as a horse. Horses become agitated and anxious when confronted by emotional incongruity; their very survival depends on responding to clear messages of danger or safety (Buzel, 2016; Goldman, 1995). Being honest with oneself and accepting human limitations are major goals in early sobriety. Empathy, patience, and even a good sense of humor can develop with the aid of horses.

Cognitive Processing Issues

During the first year of sobriety, the alcoholic's brain is undergoing substantial neurological changes reflected in significant problems in cognitive processing (Buzel, 2016; Eckardt, Parker, Noble, Pautler, & Gottschalk, 1979). Attention, concentration, and memory functions are often negative affected after years of drinking. Working with horses can help address some of these processing issues. The immediacy of every interaction with a horse demands concentration and attention to what is happening, which can be hard to sustain during early sobriety.

However, *not attending to* a huge animal standing directly in front of you is pretty nigh impossible! In addition, the need to remember tasks and sequential instructions when dealing with horses can assist the alcoholic in addressing cognitive processing problems and learn alternative coping mechanisms and strategies (e.g., note taking) that can be generalized to other areas of their lives.

Horses will never judge you, never shame you, and never ask of you what you cannot give. A horse will accept you as the flawed, complex, yet inherently worthwhile person you are. If you try, horses will try. If you respect them, they will, in turn, respect you. This is the ideal milieu for therapeutic healing and change.

GOALS OF EQUINE INTERVENTIONS DURING EARLY SOBRIETY

Exercises and psychoeducation can address:

1. Stress reduction and grounding via mindfulness and deep breathing. Mindfulness, centering, emotional body scans, and deep breathing exercises are explained and taught.
2. Emotional awareness: learning to recognize and label emotions both verbally and somatically.
3. Development of interpersonal awareness: acknowledging your impact on others and increasing empathetic responses.
4. Trust and openness: experiencing the difference between the distancing effect of anger/impatience versus the invitation to closeness that emerges when the client is open and available.
5. Discussion of the above and how it can be incorporated in the client's life.

CASE EXAMPLE AND SAMPLE CASE TRANSCRIPT

Rick (a pseudonym) is a 32-year-old, newly sober alcoholic (five months' sobriety). The counseling unit at his work suggested that Rick get help. He is described as having difficulty at the job with his peers and bosses and rushing through his work resulting in careless errors. Rick is short-tempered, questions orders, blames others for his problems, and seems unaware of the impact of his negative attitude on others. It was reported that he is also having difficulties at home.

Rick grew up in an alcoholic family; his father died an unrecovered alcoholic. He had learning difficulties at school, found making friends challenging, and tended to keep to himself. He started drinking at age 14 and was able to keep it in control until the pressures of job, money, and family all became too much for him, and his drinking increased.

He was sent to detox and a 28-day treatment facility by his place of employment. He has been back at work for about a month and, although he is supposed to be attending daily AA sessions, there is evidence he is avoiding meetings; for example, he failed to turn in his weekly AA attendance sheet to the EAP at work and his employers have noticed a slip in his attitude. When he was offered a supplemental therapeutic intervention to explore therapy with horses, he agreed. Rick was curious about the horses and seemed open to working with them.

It became apparent when Rick entered the barn on his first day of therapy that he was intimidated by the horses' size and obvious strength, a very understandable response. We gave Rick a quick tour of the barn and introduced him to his therapy horse, Miss Lucy, who was quietly standing on cross ties.

As with all equine sessions, we started with a basic centering exercise based around simple deep breathing and moved onto mindfulness by demonstrating "quiet noticing" using all senses; for example, taking in the smell, sound, and appearance of the horses. Rick was amenable to trying, which was a good sign given how strange this must have been for him.

We invited Rick to approach Ms. Lilly and say "hello." He appeared edgy and uncomfortable, looking at the horse nervously. As with all equine therapy work, we take what is happening in the moment and use it to therapeutic advantage. We used his feeling of discomfort to help him learn how to recognize an emotion and label it. In this case, Rick was able to acknowledge that he was nervous, which we assured him was absolutely normal, and he was able to locate the feeling in his body, his stomach. We suggested that he send his breath to his stomach and practice some deep breathing. Reporting that he felt "silly" with this "hippy dippy stuff," he tried it nevertheless and admitted that his stomach felt less tense after a few deep breaths. We returned to this labeling, locating, and breathing into his feelings throughout the session. Most alcoholics deal with a certain level of shame and inadequacy. Typical responses, such as fear, are normalized and all therapeutic movement is acknowledged and supported.

The first equine task assigned to Rick was to groom Miss Lucy. He was shown some basic grooming techniques and encouraged to stay centered and mindful of the moment he was in. Since the horse was on cross ties and "under control," Rick began to relax. He enjoyed the grooming and began to feel a bit more comfortable and competent around his horse.

The first session is usually a "meet and greet" opportunity so we encouraged Rick to spend as much time grooming as he wanted. We invited him to notice how Miss Lucy responded to his touch and ministering, teaching him to recognize horses' relaxation signals. Working on developing empathy, we asked Rick what he thought the horse was feeling. At first, he was taken aback by the notion that this big thing even *had* feelings, but the immediate feedback between his grooming and Miss Lucy's obvious enjoyment (ears front, head down, mouth gobbly) was very empowering. Rick and Miss Lucy were on their way to developing a trusting, healing relationship.

When we felt, Rick had established enough of a beginning connection and was relaxed enough to move onto something a bit more challenging, we asked if he would like to lead Miss Lucy around the arena. We knew this would elicit some anxiety but, as expected with newly recovering alcoholics, Rick approached the task with some bravado, sure that he could easily lead a horse by a rope. When he tried to lead the horse, she shied back, ears flattened to her head, signaling she was not responding to his request. Rick looked upset, then tried to escalate his approach by pulling harder on the lead line resulting in Miss Lucy becoming even more resistant. We asked Rick what he was feeling. "Pissed at the stupid horse!"

Rick was encouraged to try deep breathing and grounding. Suggesting that there might be some feelings underneath his anger, he became quiet. Unable to look at us, he admitted to feeling rejected and "stupid" (a feeling he projected onto the horse). With more gentle questioning, Rick realized he also felt lonely and scared. He was then able to locate these feelings in his body, his heart area and stomach, and began to send his breath into these areas. We suggested he approach Miss Lucy while acknowledging his true feelings. As we expected, the horse approached and nuzzled him. Rick, without our guidance, rested his head on the horse's neck. We left them in this embrace, realizing the power of the moment.

After a few minutes, we asked if Rick wanted to try again to lead Miss Lucy. He nodded, took the lead line, and asked the horse if she would like to come with him for a walk. With a gentleness that had been previously unacknowledged, Rick was able to have someone accompany him because they *wanted* to, not because he forced or scared them into "obeying." The concept of "control" took on a new dimension for Rick that day.

At the end of the session, we debriefed with Rick and asked him what he learned about himself that he could take into his life. He talked about his new-found skill in connecting with others; not by yelling or intimidating, but simply by asking. We suggested that he continue to work on noticing his feelings, both surface, automatic feelings and those hiding underneath. We reviewed the evidence, thanks to Miss Lucy, that nothing bad would happen if he let go of control of his automatic defensive response to life's challenges. When he left himself open, became quietly vulnerable, he invited in caring.

Rick continued to come to therapy at the Barn for the next three months and his progress was excellent. As with all recovering individuals, there were good days and bad, but on the whole, Miss Lucy and Rick did remarkable work.

SUMMARY

Equine-assisted mental health is an effective supplemental treatment intervention during alcoholism recovery. The aims of this type of therapy, depending on the various stages of sobriety, could incorporate: recognition of core feelings, grounding and relaxation techniques, relationship skills, self-forgiveness, and confidence building. Lowered frustration tolerance and impulse control issues should be recognized and addressed as both a result of the brain's detoxification from alcohol as well as overlearned ineffective responses to life's challenges. Patience, support, and reinforcement, during this early stage of recovery, are paramount when working with these clients. Horses exemplify these qualities!

REFERENCES

American Psychiatric Association. (2013). *Diagnostic and Statistical Manual of Mental Disorders.* 5th edition. Washington, DC: American Psychiatric Association.

Buzel, A. H. (1986). Changes in the Cognitive Functioning of Detoxified Alcoholics as Measured by Neuropsychological and Evoked Potential Test Performance.Unpublished doctoral dissertation. New School for Social Research, New York.

Buzel, A. H. (2016). *Beyond Words: The Healing Power of Horses.* Bloomington, IN: AuthorHouse.

Eckardt, M. J, Parker, E. S., Noble, E. P., Pautler, C. P., & Gottschalk, L. A. (1979). Changes in neuropsychological performance during treatment for alcoholism. *Biological Psychiatry, 14*(6), 943–954.

Goldman, D. (1995). *Emotional Intelligence.* New York: Bantam Books.

Hayes, T. (2015). *Riding Home: The Power of Horses to Heal.* New York: St. Martin's Press.

Kohanov, L. (2001). The Tao of Equus: A Woman's Journey of Healing and Transformation. Natato, CA: New World Library.

National Survey of Drugs and Statistics. (2015). *National Survey of Drug Use and Health.* Retrieved from www.datafiles.samhsa.gov/study-series/national-survey-drug-use-and-health-nsduh-nid13517

Steinglass, P. (1987). *The Alcoholic Family.* New York: Basic Books.

16

Triggering Transformations

An Equine-Assisted Approach to the Treatment of Substance Abuse

Shelley Green, Monica Schroeder, Cynthia Penalva, Michael Rolleston, and Valerie Bruce Judd

INTRODUCTION

Equine-assisted psychotherapy (EAP) approaches have been applied to many different clinical concerns, including substance abuse, eating disorders, domestic violence, trauma, PTSD, and physical or sexual abuse (DePrekel, 2012; Karol, 2007; Masini, 2010; Selby & Smith-Osborne, 2013). Clients struggling with the effects of substance abuse, specifically, can benefit from this approach (Kern-Godal, Arnevik, Walderhaug, & Ravndal, 2015), both individually and in group settings. This chapter describes a relational, solution-focused approach to EAP that incorporates attention to mindfulness, allowing clients struggling with substance abuse to work on their individual goals alongside other group participants. The interpersonal exchange that occurs among participants throughout sessions helps them to engage in their own treatment while simultaneously collaborating in the treatment of their peers (Mandrell, 2014). Clinically, the combination of the equine-assisted experiential model and a solution-focused emphasis offers opportunities for heightened awareness and transformation.

DESCRIPTION OF THE PROBLEM

Conventional approaches to treating substance abuse are based on an understanding of addiction as a disease, and typically focus on the clients' presumed deficits, assuming the clients need to be confronted on their "denial" or that they lack the skill or ability to remain sober (McCollum, Trepper, & Smock, 2003). As noted by Dell, Chalmers, Dell, Sauve, and MacKinnon (2008, p. 89):

> Substance abuse programming has generally *not* been holistic in its approach to and understanding of healing, but rather, predominantly disease based. From a health promotion perspective, health is understood to be a state of unity or balance across the physical, mental, social, and spiritual components of an individual's wellbeing, rather than merely the presence or absence of disease.

Clinical approaches that address the addiction without considering the clients' strengths, resources, and resilience miss critical opportunities to engage clients in a collaborative process that can anchor their decision to remain sober.

In contrast, a solution-focused approach to working with substance abuse (Berg & Miller, 1992) highlights clients' strengths and resources, and assumes that clients can build on existing competencies in order to achieve and maintain a commitment to avoid abusing substances (McCollum et al., 2003). As an evidenced-based practice, solution-focused therapy offers an effective, respectful, and collaborative approach to working with clients struggling with addiction (Franklin, Trepper, Gingerich, & McCollum, 2012). Additionally, this model lends itself well to delivery in a group format, making it an ideal choice for this population. Addiction treatment facilities frequently utilize group formats and thus are familiar with and committed to the approach, making collaboration with such facilities more likely to be successful (McCollum et al., 2003).

RATIONALE FOR A SOLUTION-FOCUSED, EQUINE-ASSISTED GROUP MODEL

EAP sessions invite clients to learn about themselves through their reactions to the horse in the context of a therapy group (Masini, 2010). Typical EAP activities elicit discussions regarding the experiences that the participants have in the present moment, as they often require collaboration, communication, and personal reflection. Using more than "a list of interventions," this approach usefully parallels a solution-focused clinical approach—one that adapts to what works for clients, privileging their worldviews, and assuming that they are capable of coming up with their own solutions (Berg & Miller, 1992). Interaction with horses allows the clients to have an array of experiences within the group setting, often through observations and interpretation, which creates the opportunity for vulnerable conversations to emerge (Karol, 2007). Metaphors naturally develop out of these conversations and experiences with the horse, which clients can in turn relate back to their current life situation.

THEORETICAL APPROACH

The clinical work described here has been developed and implemented as a part of a collaboration between the Nova Southeastern University (NSU) Family Therapy Programs and Stable Place, a non-profit organization providing EAP. The work conducted by Stable Place staff—all trained in the NSU model—is consistently informed by a brief systemic approach to therapy (Cade & O'Hanlon, 1993; Flemons, 2002; Flemons & Green, 2007, 2018; Green, 2013, 2014; Watzlawick, Weakland & Fisch, 1974) that privileges our clients' ways of viewing the world and honors their solutions. This non-pathologizing, strength-based approach serves substance abuse clients well by allowing the therapist to meet the clients where they are, and by making sense of their behavior in context (Watzlawick et al., 1974). Without focusing on dysfunction or disorder, the therapist guides the sessions toward strength-based themes and client-led solutions. The horses assist the therapists in shining light on the clients' abilities and strengths in relation to their problem.

The solution-oriented position is informed primarily by curiosity, conveyed through a "nonjudgmental and non-confrontational stance" (Lipchik, 2002). Without minimizing the severity of the problem, "treatment" is based on the understanding that the group process—including observations, meanings, and interpretations—is co-created in collaboration with the client.

Within this theoretical framework, therapists assume that clients want to change; in fact, change is assumed to be occurring at all times and, thus, belief in the clients' ability to change is "built into the model" (McCollum et al., 2003). This offers a particularly optimistic, client-centered context for dealing with the struggles associated with substance abuse.

Incorporating mindfulness practices within this solution-focused approach can be particularly beneficial because of the ability of such practices to promote awareness, present-centeredness, and acceptance for the client in relation to their problem (Germer, 2004). In the treatment of substance abuse, mindfulness practices may help clients avoid relapse by increasing their awareness of negative patterns of thoughts and emotions that could increase the likelihood of relapse triggers (Breslin, Zack, & McMain, 2002).

EAP can also play a key role in the development of mindfulness within clients (DePrekel, 2012). Horses, who are masters of being in the moment, are helpful in demonstrating how to remain calm, cope with triggers, and recover from and let go of anxiety-provoking experiences. In his book *Riding Home*, Tim Hayes discusses how horses' behaviors can relate to the behaviors of those recovering from addiction:

> For horses, the emotional pain from stress is usually expressed physically. Examples would be head shaking, body weaving, pacing, wood chewing, and cribbing, or sucking in air. These are all coping behaviors horses engage in to reduce their anxiety and stress. And just as with addictive behaviors in humans, some of these habitual neurotic patterns can stimulate the horse's brain to release endorphins, the same chemical that provides us emotional soothing. This is identical to the way some humans "self-medicate" their emotional stress and anxiety with compulsive behaviors like exercise, work, sex, or eating, any of which also serve to alter their brain chemistry.
>
> (Hayes, 2015, p. 28)

Hayes goes onto explain that for a prey animal, such as the horse, adjusting to a world created and designed for humans requires the ability to accept, tolerate, forgive, and trust. With this in mind, horses become the ultimate teachers in how to cope with the everyday stresses that could trigger relapse.

DESCRIPTION OF INTERVENTION: TRIGGERS

Through our NSU family therapy partnership with Stable Place, we have worked with a variety of residential treatment centers over the years. Each center we have partnered with brings an array of clients of different ages, genders, ethnicities, and backgrounds that all share a common problem—the struggle to create a life free from their addictions. Despite the differences among the clients, we have found a theme that often brings these individuals together and gives them a common language: the notion of triggers. We began to ask ourselves how we could develop an exercise that could allow our clients to explore how they understand and respond to their own triggers. Through the activity we created, we invite the client to find new ways of responding to triggers constructively and to see their relationship with them in a different light.

This activity begins by having the horses at liberty in the arena while the clients and therapist observe from the outside. The equine specialist enters the arena with a dressage or lunge whip and, with as little effort as possible, demonstrates what happens to the herd when a whip is introduced. When the equine specialist creates movement among the herd in this way, the results can be dramatic; offering clients a clear picture of what triggers the horses' behavior. During the demonstration, the clients are asked to focus on what they notice about the horses' reaction to the whip. This demonstration acts as a catalyst for a conversation about the clients' triggers by exploring what the whip represents (for the horses, and, by extension, how it may metaphorically represent a trigger in the clients' lives).

Following the demonstration, the equine specialist takes the horses in hand and monitors them closely as the clients are invited to go into the arena and meet the horses. The clients are then presented with a crop, a dressage whip, and a lunge whip and are asked to select one. Although our horses are regularly schooled and familiar with training aids, our clients typically are not. Therefore, the clients' selection can provide the therapist with helpful information that can be utilized in a conversation about what trigger the equipment represents for them.

CASE EXAMPLE—LAUREN

Lauren (a pseudonym), age 25, has been in and out of treatment the last few years to address her addiction to alcohol. Lauren began her most recent treatment hoping something would be different this time and yet found it difficult to believe she could avoid relapse. The following excerpt highlights Lauren's experience as well as our team's analysis.

The following transcript analysis are about a pseudonym client.

Table 16.1
Transcript Analysis of Case Example

Transcript	*Analysis*
During the equine specialist demonstration **Therapist:** What are you noticing about the horse's reaction to the crop? **Client:** The horse looks scared. **Therapist:** What do you think he's afraid of? **Client:** He's afraid of how to deal with that whip.	The therapist is beginning to establish the metaphor of the crop being a trigger. The therapist is curious how the client relates to their own triggers, which is informed by what the client is notices in the horse's behavior.
After explaining the activity, the therapist asks the client to select the equipment they will use to approach the horse. Client selects the smallest crop offered. **Therapist:** How did you choose your crop? **Client:** I thought that since the horse was so afraid of the big crop that if he got used to the smallest one first, he wouldn't be as afraid of the bigger ones. **Therapist:** When thinking about your own triggers, how might this relate to your experience? **Client:** I guess for me; I always want to tackle my biggest triggers first. But doing so has landed me back here each time. I'm starting to think that I should try something different.	The therapist is continuing to contextualize the metaphor of the crop with client. The client appeared anxious when selecting a crop and hesitated before selecting the smallest one. The therapist is curious about how this relates to the client's experience of coping with their own triggers.
The therapist invites client to think about their triggers while approaching the horse with the crop. The horse initially responds by walking away from client each time the client approaches. The equine specialist points out to the therapist that the client keeps approaching the horse in the same manner, with their arm stretched out and the crop held high. The client appears to become increasingly frustrated with each attempt. **Therapist:** It seems as though the horse keeps moving each time you approach. What's going on for you? **Client:** I don't know, this happens every time I try to face my triggers. I end up feeling like I'm spinning in circles. **Therapist:** What do you think you would need to do in order to stop spinning? **Client:** That's what I'm trying to figure out.	As previously mentioned, the goal is for the client to introduce the crop to the horse in a way that feels comfortable and allows them to respond constructively rather than reacting out of fear. The therapist notices that each time the client approaches, they become increasingly frustrated. The therapist encourages client to reflect on how they are approaching the horse and how this approach relates to their own recovery process.
Client is invited to try different ways of approaching the horse as a way of exploring what might help them "stop spinning." The therapist observes client take a deep breath prior to showing the horse the crop and moving slowly as they inch closer to the horse. The horse initially takes a few steps away from the client, who continues to move slowly in their approach. The client eventually gets the crop to touch the horse and moves it along the horse's back. The equine specialist notices that the client's intentionality was visibly different during this last attempt. **Therapist:** It looks like you have stopped spinning. What did you do differently this time around? **Client:** I did! I thought to myself that if I was ever going to get out of recovery, I needed to find a way to face my triggers. Whenever I'm faced with my triggers, I become anxious and want to get over them as quickly as possible. I thought that maybe the horse could sense that I couldn't stand being around them so they didn't want to be around it either. **Therapist:** How were you able to get the horse to be around them this time? **Client:** I let the horse see the trigger first, then I slowly approached the horse. I think that by going slow and letting the horse adjust to the trigger as I approached helped with making them feel comfortable. **Therapist:** How do you think moving slowly and letting yourself adjust to your triggers might help you? **Client:** I think that I would be able to learn how to cope and be around them, like the horse did. If I know what's comfortable and allow myself to adjust, I'll be able to face them. I don't have to move fast in my recovery is a process. As long as I remain calm, patient, and keep being persistent, I think this time could be different."	The therapist wanted to invite client to try different behaviors as a way of figuring out what they could alter when facing their own triggers. When the client expressed uncertainty, the therapist encouraged them to use this time as an experiment in order to discover what could work. The client's approach was visibly different from their first attempts. The therapist wanted to reinforce this by exploring what the client believed to be the difference in their behavior and how this could be helpful to them in the future.

Once the clients have selected their "trigger," they are invited to approach the horse with it in a way that feels comfortable. They are also asked to introduce the crop in a way that might elicit a more positive response rather than a reaction that comes out of fear or anxiety, such as the behavior the horse demonstrated at the beginning of the activity. This exercise is intended as a metaphor that can inform and potentially transform the clients' struggles with their own triggers.

As previously mentioned, we believe that holding a non-pathologizing stance serves as a means for the therapist to meet the client where they are at by allowing the client to make sense of their behavior in context. This stance, as well as the use of metaphors, client language, and client-driven solutions, allows the therapist to honor the client's perspective and understanding. The metaphors, solutions, and language that clients generate often relate back to their own personal cultural and life experiences. These elements are incorporated into the sessions by the therapist holding a stance that there are no right or wrong answers in the clients' understanding of what is unfolding with the horses; instead, there are answers that fit and make sense for the clients in their own unique lives.

CASE EXAMPLE—MARK

Mark (pseudonym), age 42, was in treatment for the third time, and attending his fourth equine session at Stable Place. For this activity, Mark chose a lunge whip; he initially expressed a great deal of fear and stood well away for several minutes while he considered how he should approach the horse. Below we describe the unfolding of the session, along with our analysis.

The following transcript analysis are about a pseudonym client.

Table 16.2

Transcript Analysis of Case Example

Transcript	*Analysis*
After some hesitation, client eventually held the whip away from their body, at arm's length, and walked straight at Star (horse). The horse lifted his head and the client beat a hasty retreat. After a few tentative tries that were met by Star with a raised head and a snort, the client slumped his shoulders and walked back to the group, defeated. **Client:** I give up. I can't do this. **Group Members (collectively):** You can do this; why don't you try something different? Maybe there's another way to approach Star. Maybe you can come from a different angle, or hold the whip a different way? **Client:** Nope; not happening.	As mentioned above, we utilize the group process as a supportive—and at times challenging—context in which to promote change. The client was well-connected with his group members and felt that they knew him well. However, his anxiety about approaching Star was shutting down his ability to conceive of doing something different.
Therapist: It seems that Star's reaction to this "trigger" is pretty strong, and that doesn't make this feel safe for you. I'm wondering about the triggers you experience in your life, and how you respond to those. **Client:** It's just all of them—I can't deal with them. My wife, her kids, my in-laws, my sisters... they make me crazy. They are always all over me and I can't take it. I have to escape. It's just too much.	Rather than continue to push client to do something different with Star, the therapist chose to begin making connections between Star's powerful response and the client's reactions to ongoing life difficulties, including the family challenges that he believed created the climate for his relapse.
As the client opened up about the stresses that triggered his relapse, he kept looking over at Star, who stood quietly with his head down. **Client:** Is it OK if I try again now? **Therapist:** Of course, This time he walked to Star's shoulder and stood without moving, the whip at his side. The horse stood motionless. The client gently moved the whip alongside Star, checking to make sure the horse wasn't bothered, then slowly took the end of the string from the lunge whip and touched the horse's wither. Star remained still as the client gently rubbed the string of the whip into his wither and neck. The horse dropped his head and blew. Client carried on rubbing Star with the string, gradually using more and more until he had it bunched in his hand.	The therapist silently observed, alongside the equine specialist, as the client experimented with ways to connect with Star and to allow Star to experience the whip in a different way. Allowing the client to experience a quiet, mindful opportunity to try out new behaviors is central to our commitment to honor the clients' own solutions.
As the client continued experimenting with the horse and the whip, he began talking with the therapist: **Client:** It gets so much easier to control the situation with Star when I just take a little piece of the string at a time. He's cool with it. He hated it before. **Therapist:** Yeah, he seems totally fine now; and you? **Client:** I'm good. I like this. **Therapist:** I wonder what might happen in your family if you were to think about managing one person at a time. Seems like they are pretty overwhelming all together. **Client:** For sure, they are. Laughs quietly. **Therapist:** Who do you think you might be able to start with? **Client:** I think my sister—she actually does listen... sometimes.	The therapist offered the client all the time he needed to explore Star's reactions to his new attempts; only when the client initiated did the conversation begin again. As the therapist observed the client doing something different in the moment and getting a significantly different reaction from Star, she gently began connecting client's experience with the horse to his challenges with his family and with relapse. The conversation generated a much more manageable understanding of how the client could proceed, and how he could create a different relationship with the triggers he had experienced in his family.

REFLECTIONS

These cases reflect our deep commitment to engaging with clients in ways that honor both their struggles and their solutions. We believe interacting with the horses offers powerful opportunities for our clients to try something different, to take risks, to experience change in the moment, and to relate that change back to the struggles of their daily lives. Both Lauren and Mark experienced moments of mindfulness—as Lauren found ways to stop "spinning in circles," and as Mark found ways, bit by bit, to imagine being less overwhelmed by fear, anxiety, and family. We believe that these moments of self-reflection, of experiencing change in the moment, and of imagining the impact of such change in their daily lives, can set the stage for transforming triggers in positive and lasting ways.

The following sample session notes are about a pseudonym client.

Stable Place

Equine Assisted
Individual, Couple, and Family Therapy

Stable Place, Inc.
SESSION CASE NOTES

CLIENT: Group—Substance Abuse **DATE:** 07/01/17

TIME: 2:30pm–4:00pm **DURATION:** 1.5 hrs

THEME OF THE SESSION: Responding to Triggers Constructively/ Not Reacting out of Fear

SESSION PARTICIPANTS:
Stable Place Team: Monica Schroeder M.S., Cynthia Penalva, M.S., Abby & Sheila (ES)
Horses: Casper and Paris

SESSION SUMMARY:

Lauren: Lauren participated fully throughout the activity this week. During the demonstration from the ES, Lauren mentioned that the horses appeared scared and that this seemed similar to how she deals with her own triggers. When asked to select a crop, Lauren had chosen the smallest offered. She mentioned that she thought it would be easier for the horse to become comfortable with the smaller trigger first. When asked if this is how she approaches her own triggers, Lauren said she usually goes for the biggest first and that in doing so, it's caused her to relapse. When asked to approach the horse with her selected trigger, the horse kept walking away from Lauren. Lauren said that this reminded her of her own triggers because she often feels like she's spinning in circles. Lauren was invited to try a new way of approaching the horse, and she was observed to move slowly, remain calm, and eventually made contact with the horse. Lauren said that practicing these behaviors could be helpful for her because it would help her learn to cope and slowly become comfortable with the triggers in her life.

THERAPIST SIGNATURE: Monica Schroeder, M.S. and Cynthia Penalva, M.S.

FIG. 16.1. Session Case Notes.

[Your Logo Here]

SESSION CASE NOTES

CLIENT:

DATE:

TIME:

DURATION:

THEME OF THE SESSION:

SESSION PARTICIPANTS:

Therapist/Equine Specialist:

Horses:

SESSION SUMMARY:

Client Name:

THERAPIST SIGNATURE AND DATE:

FIG. 16.2. Session Case Notes—Blank.

REFERENCES

Berg, I. & Miller, S. (1992). Working with the Problem Drinker: A Solution-Focused Approach. New York: W. W. Norton.

Breslin, F. C., Zack, M., & McMain, S. (2002). An information-processing analysis of mindfulness: Implications for relapse prevention in the treatment of substance abuse. *Clinical Psychology Science and Practice, 9*, 275–299.

Cade, B. & O'Hanlon, W. (1993). *A Brief Guide to Brief Therapy*. New York: W. W. Norton.

Dell, C. A., Chalmers, D., Dell, D., Sauve, E., & MacKinnon, T. (2008). Horse as healer: An examination of equine assisted learning in the healing of first nations youth from solvent abuse. *Pimatisiwin: A Journal of Aboriginal and Indigenous Community Health, 6*(1), 81–106.

DePrekel, M. (2012). Equine facilitated psychotherapy for the treatment of trauma. In K. Trotter (Eds.), *Harnessing the Power of Equine Assisted Counseling: Adding Animal Assisted Therapy to Your Practice* (pp. 59–72). New York: Routledge.

Flemons, D. (2002). Of One Mind: The Logic of Hypnosis, the Practice of Therapy. New York: W. W. Norton.

Flemons, D. & Green, S. (2007). Just between us: A relational approach to sex therapy. In S. Green & D. Flemons (Eds.), *Quickies: The Handbook of Brief Sex Therapy* (revised edition, pp. 126–170). New York: W. W. Norton.

Flemons, D. & Green, S. (2018). Therapeutic quickies: Brief relational therapy for sexual issues. In S. Green & D. Flemons (Eds.), *Quickies: The Handbook of Brief Sex Therapy* (3rd edition). New York: W. W. Norton.

Franklin, C., Trepper, T., Gingerich, W., & McCollum, E. (Eds.) (2012). *Solution-Focused Brief Therapy: A Handbook of Evidence Based Practice*. New York: Oxford University Press.

Germer, C., (2004). What is mindfulness? *Insight Journal*, Fall, 24–29.

Green, S. (2013). Horses and families. In A. Rambo, C. West, A. Schooley, & T. V. Boyd (Eds.), *Family Therapy Review: Contrasting Contemporary Models* (pp. 256–258). New York: Routledge.

Green, S. (2014). Horse sense: Equine assisted single session consultations. In M. Hoyt & M. Talmon (Eds.), *Capture the Moment: Single Session Therapy and Walk-In Service*. Williston, VT: Crown House Publishing.

Hayes, T. (2015). *Riding Home: The Power of Horses to Heal*. New York: St. Martin's Press.

Karol, J. (2007). Applying a traditional individual psychotherapy model to equine-facilitated psychotherapy (EFP): Theory and method. *Clinical Child Psychology and Psychiatry, 12*, 77–90.

Kern-Godal, A., Arnevik, E., Walderhaug, E., & Ravndal, E. (2015). Substance use disorder treatment retention and completion: A prospective study of horse-assisted therapy (HAT) for young adults. *Addiction Science & Clinical Practice, 10*(21).

Lipchik, E. (2002). *Beyond Technique in Solution-Focused Therapy*. New York: Guilford Press.

Mandrell, P. (2014). Introduction to Equine Assisted Psychotherapy: A Comprehensive Overview. 2nd edition. Lubbock, TX: Refuge Services.

Masini, A. (2010). Equine-assisted psychotherapy in clinical practice. *Journal of Psychosocial Nursing and Mental Health Services, 48*(10), 30–34.

McCollum, E., Trepper, T., & Smock, S. (2003). Solution-focused group therapy for substance abuse: Extending competency-based models. *Journal of Family Psychotherapy, 14*(4), 27–42.

Selby, A. & Smith-Osborne, A. (2013). A systematic review of the effectiveness of complementary and adjunct therapies and interventions involving equines. *Health Psychology, 32*(4), 418–432.

Watzlawick, P., Weakland, J. & Fisch, R. (1974). *Change: Principles of Problem Formation and Problem Resolution*. New York: Norton.

17

BEYOND THE COUCH

An Object Relations Approach to EAP Substance Abuse Treatment

Natasha Filippides

INTRODUCTION

This chapter will focus on a psychoanalytic theoretical framework to equine-assisted psychotherapy (EAP) substance abuse treatment. Specifically, an EAP object relations perspective will be applied to treatment of a young adult male with alcohol use disorder (AUD), cannabis use disorder (CUD), and an underlying persistent depressive disorder.

According to the National Institute of Mental Health (2017), in 2014, 20.2 million adults in the US had a substance use disorder and 7.9 million had both a substance use disorder and another mental illness. The Substance Abuse and Mental Health Services Administration (2017) reported that people with mental health disorders are more likely than people without mental health disorders to experience an alcohol or substance use disorder. According to the National Institute on Drug Abuse (2017), alcohol and cannabis are the most commonly used drugs in the US other than nicotine. Substance use disorders can alter and distort desires and priorities, disrupt normal adaptive behaviors, interfere with the ability to have healthy relationships with friends and family, and affect school progress and career success (American Psychiatric Association, 2013).

OBJECT RELATIONS THEORY

At Stand InBalance, an equine interactive program in the Santa Monica mountains of California, a psychoanalytic theory, specifically object relations, is utilized. Object relations theory was born out of Freudian instinct theory. This theory focuses on the significant relationship between the primary caregiver and child; it focuses on nurturance and intimacy (Klein, 1959). Object relations theory purports that human relatedness and contact is the primary force driving human behavior (Klein, 1991). Melanie Klein (1959, 1991) and other object relations theorists begin with this premise, and expand upon the theory by analyzing how an infant's early relationships with his/her primary caregiver, real or fantasized, can create a model for all future interpersonal relationships (Feist & Feist, 2006). The "object" in object relations theory is any person, thing, place, fantasy, memory, or idea infused with "emotional energy." The emotional energy an object can carry ranges from love to hate and often is a mix of both (Hamilton, 1998). An internal object is a mental and emotional image, memory, fantasy, or idea that is connected to a person, thing, or place that has been internalized (Klein, 1959). An external object is an actual person, thing, or place infused with the emotional energy of love and hate (Hamilton, 1998).

According to Klein (1959), an individual's relationships as an adult contain internal psychic representations of one's early childhood objects; for example, the father or the mother. These objects are then introjected into the child's psychic structure and later projected onto the adult individual's intimate relationships. These introjected psychic structures are not actual representations of the primary object, but instead are bits and pieces of one's early childhood experiences (Klein, 1959). How one's internal object relations form is a blueprint for how an individual relates to self, others and the world.

The horses for many clients become a manifestation of internal and/or external objects. One of the most apparent instances where object relations theory becomes evident in the arena is when the client is asked to observe and then interact with the horses and verbalize their reactions. Often clients will comment on what they are noticing in the horses or the horses' interactions with each other. The client may describe her own thoughts, physical, or emotional reactions. The comments made by the client give the therapist a sense of the client's inner world and object relations.

The projective aspect of this therapy helps clients begin to reflect and engage with both the intrapsychic and interpersonal layers of who they are. The horses' non-judgmental, authentic, and attuned nature creates a unique avenue to bypass many ego defenses in order to work on awareness of self and other. The horses can be evocative catalysts for the client to interact with the images and symbols of their internal world. Integrating these aspects occurs through connecting to them externally with the horse and then internalizing what the client has experienced. These profound experiences in the arena can help the client develop a more cohesive sense of self.

RATIONALE FOR EQUINE-ASSISTED PSYCHOTHERAPY

For many individuals, such as the client that will be discussed in the vignette below, substance abuse has served a maladaptive function and unhealthy way of coping. These clients often turn to substances to disconnect from intolerable affect, arising from a multitude of issues from trauma to depression. EAP can help clients address both their substance abuse issues as well as the underlying pathology from which the substance abuse symptoms have arisen. Such clients require an embodied experience merging insight and relational experience, addressing both the intrapsychic and interpersonal dimensions of the individual. Nancy McWilliams (2004, p. 38) wrote:

> Freud learned that there is a difference between intellectual and emotional insight. That is, we can "know" something cognitively and yet not know it at all. To change, we need to appreciate our condition in a way that feels visceral as opposed to cerebral.

Horses are deeply aware of their environment due to their prey animal instincts and are uniquely equipped to "pick up" on the emotional currents in their surroundings. Horses are continually responding to and reflecting the affect they are sensing in the arena. Attending to the client's affect in the experiential sessions with the horses can lead to the work being anchored in emotional insight. Developing insight and making the unconscious conscious, coupled with the profound relational experience with the horse(s) and facilitator(s), lies at the core of EAP's profound ability to effect psychic change (Wolson, 2012).

EAP is an experiential therapy and being open to the experience unfolding is an essential component of how this therapy creates meaningful and lasting change. Often part of the process is to be open to surprise and what emerges in a session, yet safety for the equines, the clients and the facilitators is paramount. The facilitator must take into consideration both the client and horse's physical and emotional safety.

Another aspect of EAP is allowing horses to use their instinctual wisdom and prey animal instincts as feedback in the session. Sometimes incidents such as a foot being stepped on, or a nip may occur as these are basic hazards of being around these large animals that move fast, spook, etc. Safety precautions should be discussed with all clients prior to entering the arena. Clients need to be aware of how horses keep themselves safe, and that they have the right and responsibility to do the same by walking away, asking for support, and using awareness and discernment.

DESCRIPTION OF INTERVENTION: JOIN UP

The goals when utilizing projection of object representations to effect intrapsychic and interpersonal change are to develop confidence, affect regulation, interpersonal skills, a capacity for insight, self and other awareness, and ultimately to develop a healthy integrated sense of self. The materials needed are one horse in a round pen, brushes, a halter, and a lead rope.

The "join up" activity is adapted from the term used to describe exercises developed by natural horseman Monty Roberts. This exercise is used to create an avenue for projection of internal and external object representations. In this exercise the client is required to develop a partnership of connection, safety, and trust through clear effective communication (body language and energy), focus (present in the moment), intention, and calm assertive leadership to have the horse follow him around the arena without ropes or halters. The steps are as follows.

1. Ask the client to choose the horse that the client feels most drawn to that day.
2. Move the horse into the round pen and take the halter and rope off of the horse.
3. Place the horse in the round pen away from the other horses to minimize distraction and have a quite space for the client and horse to focus on each other and their work together.
4. Ask the client to "join up" and connect with the horse so the two can walk together at liberty (without using ropes or halters on the horse's body).
5. Describe that the partnership would consist of the client taking 51% of the partnership and the horse taking the 49% of the partnership.
6. After providing this basic outline of the exercise to the client, observe how the client begins going about the task. Notice the client and horse's body language. Watch how the relationship and dynamics develop in the exercise between the horse and client. Notice shifts, patterns, the unique, and discrepancies.
7. As the facilitator, be aware of countertransference reactions. Use the countertransference as information to inform the session.
8. In a 50-minute session, leave a minimum of 15–25 minutes to process the experience by addressing the following questions and sharing curiosity around relational dynamics and metaphors paralleling life circumstances and relationships for the client.
   - Who or what does the horse represent for the client?
   - Would they give the horse a name? If so what would it be and how did they choose that name?
   - What emotions, feelings, thoughts, or body sensations arose during the experience for the client? Where have they experienced that before in their lives?
   - Help the client use their experience with the horse/s to make a metaphor about themselves and their lives.
   - Help the client integrate the experience affectively by bringing the dynamics with the horse and the parallels they made about their life together in a linking statement.
   - Provide therapist observations, empathic attunement, and affective mirroring.

Multicultural Considerations

When working with clients from different cultures, approaching sessions with an attitude of curiosity for that individual's experience, cultural values, and beliefs is paramount. For this particular exercise and technique the clinician should be attuned to different cultures having different ways of connecting and become curious about what "connection" means to the client.

CASE EXAMPLE AND SAMPLE CASE TRANSCRIPT

The following is a composite case vignette that illuminates the ways in which a client interacts with the projections of internal and external objects with the horses. As the clinician in this vignette, I worked independently with the client as both a mental health professional as well as the equine specialist.

Doug (a pseudonym) is a 24-year-old Caucasian male. He has spent the past three months in a residential treatment center to address his substance abuse issues. Doug currently transitioned out of inpatient treatment and has been residing in a sober living home. He was referred to Stand InBalance as part of his after-care and transition plan to maintain sobriety. Doug's substance abuse issues began in middle school where he tried marijuana and alcohol for the first time. His substance use and abuse escalated in college where he began to drink and use marijuana in excess on a daily basis. Doug's life became unmanageable as he was unable to maintain a job, his interpersonal relationships suffered, and his motivation dwindled. His mother provided an intervention and Doug was sent to treatment. In treatment he began to address the underlying depression that he has been self-medicating for over a decade. Doug's parents divorced when he was ten years old. Doug's father was highly critical of him and Doug felt he could "never do anything right" and that "nothing was ever good enough." Based on Doug's early childhood experiences he was unable to form a strong, integrated self-structure. He has struggled with his identity and has felt a deep sense of shame and inadequacy. His intense feelings of sadness, insecurity, and rejection would often be expressed through an attempt at feeling more powerful and less vulnerable through his substance use.

During a session several weeks into treatment at Stand InBalance, I gave Doug the directive described above for the "join up" activity. Doug chose to connect with the large alpha male horse. Initially Doug walked into the arena with bravado and an inflated confidence. He walked right up to the horse he had chosen. As he began getting to know the 17 hand alpha male horse of the herd, the following exchange occurred.

The following transcript analysis are about a pseudonym client.

Table 17.1

Transcript Analysis of Case Example

Transcript	*Analysis*
Clinician: Would you like to name him?	This provides opportunity for the horse to act as a screen for projection of the client's internal or external object representations.
Client: Yes, I'll call him Pops.	The client naming the horse provides a glimpse into his internal world and interpersonal relationships.
Clinician: How did you come to choose that name?	The clinician begins to help the client develop curiosity to explore the projection onto the horse.
Client: I don't know, just came to me, seems like a good fit for this big guy.	Client demonstrates resistance exploring the projection. Clients defenses are up toward developing a relationship with Pops.
Clinician: How could you invite Pops to connect with you?	The clinician introduces the idea of connection and suggests the idea of inviting the horse into a relationship.
When Pops walks away from the client several times he stated... **Client:** Wow I guess he is a really curious, or maybe he is ADD.	The client is feeling insecure and ashamed about the horse not connecting from the onset. Client externalizes that it is the horse, to defend against feelings of inadequacy and incompetence.

Doug went over to Pops and tried to pet his face. Pops pulled away. He tried to scratch his neck and Pops put his ears back and swished his tale and bobbed his head up and down. The horse was picking up unsafe energy from the incongruence in Doug's external and internal presentations. Doug attempted to get Pops to walk with him by pulling on his head, pushing into his shoulder, and grabbed some mane to try and pull Pops toward him. Pops took a step with Doug and then nipped his shirt sleeve. Doug jumped away from the horse and walked across the arena to me. The following exchange took place.

Table 17.2

Transcript Analysis of Case Example Continued

Transcript	*Analysis*
Client: Screw that horse... what an asshole, he bit my sleeve for no reason. I feel like going back over there and punching him.	The client became angry, from the injury to his ego. He was agitated and beneath his anger deeply hurt, yet unable to connect with the emotions beneath the initial anger.
Clinician: Lets pause a second and talk about what happened. What are you aware of?	Direct the client's attention to their own internal experience. This process of reflection can help the client become aware of his misappraisal of the situation and what was going on beneath the surface that was not being attended to and expressed. (The clinician also called for a pause for safety concerns.)

Transcript	*Analysis*
Client: I don't know why he did that, I am in a great mood and was being friendly with him. You tell me. You are the expert.	The client becomes defensive and is resisting connecting with the underlying feelings. His incongruent affect had felt unsafe to the horse and he struggles with the cues the horse was giving him of putting his ears back, lifting his head, and swishing his tail, which are all signs of setting a boundary.
Clinician: Hmmm, I wonder what the horse was telling you when he was putting his ears back, lifting his head, and swishing his tail? Perhaps he was reflecting a blind spot for you… maybe feelings beneath the surface, deep on the inside?	The clinician used her complementary countertransference to understand the frustration, insecurity, and impotence the client was feeling and unable to express.
Client: I don't know. Maybe he noticed I was frustrated that he wasn't connecting with me. It felt like he was rejecting me when he kept walking away. He did it over and over. I thought I was trying, that I was inviting. It makes me sad. *Tears up and takes a deep breath.* It hurts like when my dad left, or when he was always snapping at me; how I never did anything right in his eyes. How he was big and intimidating… maybe now I know why I named him Pops. I also am super hard on myself. In my head, nothing I do is good enough.	Despite the client's defenses he was able to begin reflecting on how he may have had a role in what occurred between himself and Pops, in other words, developing his observing ego. He began to articulate what was creating the anger and frustration; the painful sadness and shame he felt underneath. He became aware of the horse as representing both his internal critical and rejecting parts as well as his critical and rejecting father. Per conversations with his treatment team, this was the first time the client was able to express these feelings sincerely and authentically.
Clinician: So, like Pops was taking nips at you. so, do you; like your father did, take nips at yourself. I see Pops licking and chewing as you were speaking. I think he was letting you know there were feelings on the inside that you hadn't yet connected to. I wonder now that you know who Pops represents for you, that critical part in you and the pain of the rejection from your past if your connection can develop in a new way.	Pops helped the client metabolize the experience and connect with his affect that had gone unattended for so long. Pops had reflected the incongruence and lack of presence he felt from him earlier in the session. When the client began to speak openly and authentically about his internal world, Pops reflected his congruence by licking, chewing, relaxing his body, and becoming interested in the client. The therapist used a linking statement utilizing the metaphor of "taking nips" to make a parallel between the client's childhood experiences, his relationship to himself, and his dynamics with the horse.
Client: I guess I can try. In the past I would usually be drinking or smoking when I felt any feelings… but I am ready to walk the walk of sobriety… and I am willing to see if this horse can help me with that.	He was able to connect with the ways he had to adapt to survive his childhood and adolescence. At this point the unconscious has become conscious for client. When such patterns become conscious, embodied change can begin to occur.
Clinician: I wonder what it would feel like to clearly communicate what you need to Pops. To picture what it would be like to walk together. To see and feel it from thoughts, to body language to messages. Once you can connect up with something as big as pops, you can connect up with other good things for yourself in life, such as a sober healthy life.	Now that the client is in touch with what he is feeling on the inside, he can then make healthy self-aware choices from that place and learn to communicate his needs clearly and effectively. By practicing this form of self-reflection and using his awareness to inform his choices with the horse in the arena, he can then begin to bridge these skills into his day-to-day life.
After working on the relationship and connection during the second half of the session Doug was able to walk around the arena with Pops. **Clinician:** How did it go?	The clinician checked in with the client after the shift occurred in the session. The clinician left the question open-ended for the client to interpret the shift and the experience that took place for himself.
Client: I can't believe I did it. That felt amazing. I never thought expressing my feelings was useful for anything but intolerable pain and discomfort. I felt the connection. I felt a confidence inside me, and it felt like I was walking taller.	The client had a reparative experience with his horse, beneath the intellectual purely cognitive realm. He had a relational experience grounded in emotional insight. This new experience for the client will aid in his healing process; developing confidence, maintaining sobriety, managing his affective states and helping him continue to develop an integrated sense of self.

Sample Session Progress Note

For this session, a sample session progress note in a narrative format is as follows:

> The client worked on the "join up" activity and named his horse Pops. The client shared feelings of shame and rejection when "Pops" walked away from him and when he nipped at him. The therapist helped the client make a parallel between feelings that arose during the session and circumstances and relationships in his life. The therapist helped the client explore his feelings and learn importance of communicating his needs. The therapist will continue working with the client to develop confidence, self-awareness, and affect regulation toward maintaining his sobriety and life goals.

REFERENCES

American Psychiatric Association. (2013). *Diagnostic and Statistical Manual of Mental Disorders.* 5th edition. Washington, DC: American Psychiatric Association.

Feist, J. & Feist, G. J. (2006). *Theories of Personality.* 6th edition. New York: McGraw-Hill.

Hamilton, N. G. (1998). *Self and Others: Object Relations Theory in Practice.* Northvale, NJ: Jason Aronson.

Klein, M. (1959). Our adult world and its roots in infancy. In M. Klein (Ed.), *Envy and Gratitude and Other Works, 1946–1963* (pp. 247–263). New York: Macmillan.

Klein, M. (1991). The emotional life and ego-development of the infant with special reference to the depressive position. In P. King & R. Steiner (Eds.), *The Freud-Klein Controversies 1941–45* (pp. 752–797). London: Tavistock/Routledge.

McWilliams, N. (2004). *Psychoanalytic Psychotherapy.* New York: Guilford Press.

National Institute of Mental Health. (2017). *Substance Use and Mental Health.* Retrieved from www.nimh.nih.gov/health/topics/substance-use-and-mental-health/index.shtml.

National Institute on Drug Abuse. (2017). *Commonly Abused Drugs Charts.* Retrieved from www.drugabuse.gov/drugs-abuse/commonly-abused-drugs-charts.

Substance Abuse and Mental Health Services Administration. (2017). *Co-occurring Disorders.* Retrieved from www.samhsa.gov/disorders/co-occurring.

Wolson, P. (2012). Working with the relational unconscious: An integration of intrapsychic and relational analysis. *Psychoanalytic Review, 99*(2), 209.

Section 10

SELF-ESTEEM

18

The 7 C's of Well-Being

Corey L. DeMala-Moran

INTRODUCTION

When a client steps into my office for the first time, whether it be a psychotherapy client, equine-therapy client, or someone coming for riding lessons or horse training, I always ask what are they looking to get from our work together. In nine out of ten instances, they are seeking confidence, peace, balance, and healthy, happy relationships. Now the question becomes, how do we help our clients get these things in their lives? Also, what are the tools that make it possible? In 2015, I finally was able to put the finishing touches on a program that I believe helps to answer those questions. It is called the *7 C's of Well-Being*, and it has had a profound effect on many of my clients and upon myself.

The 7 C's of Well-Being came primarily out of my work and training in internal family systems, Eye Movement Desensitization and Reprocessing (EMDR) and Laurell Parnell's Resource Tapping. Then, with the help of Sarah Jenkins's equilateral work (Jenkins & Baker, 2011), as well as training with the Equine-Assisted Growth and Learning Association (Eagala), in Natural Lifemanship (Jobe, Shultz-Jobe, & McFarland, 2016), and a yearlong mentorship with Kathleen Barry Ingram, I was able to add the healing power of horses to the program. This has been truly transformative with respect to my work and my life.

A core component of both the internal family systems (IFS) model and EMDR is that we all have some kind of internal resource/self/center that is both good and necessary in the healing of emotional wounds and negative experience. Schwartz states that, "a major tenet of IFS is that everyone has at the core, at the seat of consciousness, a Self that is different from the parts" (Schwartz, 1995, p. 40). This is the part of us that we want in the driver's seat of our life. For, although all parts have good intentions, it is our true self, the part of us that Schwartz is referring to, which has the greatest capacity for steering our lives in the direction of a life that our clients, and also we, really desire.

The self, in IFS, is believed to have certain qualities and characteristics that help therapists and clients identify when they are in what is called self-leadership, or in other words, the self is in the driver's seat. The 8 C's of Self-Leadership are confidence, calmness, creativity, clarity, curiosity, courage, compassion, and connectedness. The idea being that you can tell that you are leading from your true self when you are experiencing these qualities in any given moment or situation. This framework has been incredibly helpful and is at the foundation of my 7 C's of Well-Being program. As I hope you will see here and will experience with your own clients, in working with my 7 C's, clients are able to develop and increase self-leadership in their lives and relationships.

In addition to the framework of IFS, EMDR, Shapiro and Forrest (1997), and Parnell (2007, 2008), are key components in helping clients to build confidence, peace, balance and healthy, happy relationships. Parnell states, "Within each of us is a hidden potential, a wellspring of untapped natural resources we can use to heal our psychological wounds and help us better navigate challenges we face in our lives" (Parnell, 2008, p. 13). These resources are incredibly important for clients, as they enable them to take the benefit of our work in the barn out into their daily lives.

The 7 C's of Well-Being are compassion, calm, courage, creativity, clarity, congruence, and connection. This program uses a variety of experiences and exercises that help clients tap into the 7 C's they already have, and continue to increase both their inner and outer experiences of each and every C. When clients work through this program and increase their connection to their true selves, their confidence increases. They can find some peace and create balance and the possibility of healthy and happy relationships become a reality. Like the sun in the sky, we cannot always see it, but it is always there, despite the clouds, storms and darkness that may come. The 7 C's of Well-Being help us reconnect with our "inner sun," which lights the way towards the lives we truly desire.

TAPPING IN RESOURCES

Adapted from Laurel Parnell's *Tapping In* (2008).

1. Take a moment to find a quiet, comfortable place and position.
2. If it feels safe to do so, close your eyes and bring your attention inside yourself. If you prefer to keep your eyes open, just allow your eyes to become soft and focus your awareness inside.
3. Bring to mind the resource you would like to work with. It can be an experience you have had, a real person, place or animal, a character from a book or movie, a spiritual figure, or whatever image allows you to have a bodily felt sense of the quality or characteristic you would like to connect with. In this case, find an image that connects you to a bodily felt sense of the C you would like to tap into.
4. Allow the image to become as vivid and detailed as you can be using all of your senses.
5. When you have a felt bodily sense of the C you want, begin to tap right-left (or left-right) on your knees or shoulders (or using whatever method of dual-attention stimuli you choose).

Tap 6–12 times or as long as the image and sensations stay positive. Tapping is a powerful process and although it is not EMDR therapy, the process can activate traumatic memories. If you or your client has a trauma history, keep the sets of tapping short or simply use only the visualization without the tapping. If difficult and/or disturbing images come up, you may want to seek an EMDR or another trauma-focused psychotherapist to help. Tapping is designed to help create supportive resources and experiences, but is not a substitute for psychotherapy.

THE PROGRAM

This program is appropriate for individuals, couples, families, and groups. Although this program can be helpful in an office setting, the addition of horses truly takes the work to an entirely different level. Given that we now know the brain is "experience dependent" and can therefore be changed at any age, the importance and relevance of experiential therapy has never been greater. Nothing beats the experience of connection that one can have with a 1,200-pound animal in a ten-acre field. For clients who struggle with confidence, these experiences with a horse are life- and brain-changing.

However, in doing this work, we must remain client-centered and collaborate consistently with our clients, adapting our treatment plan and goals as needed to ensure safety for all, at all times. Safety, collaboration, and communication are necessary in all therapy, but working with horses increases both the benefits and the risks. We must be mindful that what is an experience of courage for one client may not be for another. For example, for one just walking into the barn (after four sessions) and standing two feet from a horse is an incredible example of tapping into courage. For another client, riding bareback through a field offered a similar experience of courage. Therefore, we much constantly be aware of both what is happening for our clients and for ourselves when working through this program.

Program Goals and Objectives

- Help clients regain access to the resources and strengths that are already within them.
- Create new neural pathways in the brain that increase positive feelings, which provide new choices to old triggers.
- Allow clients to learn to be responsive vs. reactive.
- Build confidence in all aspects of life including home, work, family, and self.
- Assist clients in finding peace and learning to experience and access calmness.
- Create balance in life and at work.
- Learn how to set and keep boundaries, as well as learn to respect the boundaries of others.
- Increase self-awareness and self-regulation.
- Develop grounding/calming skills.
- Create stabilization, which is necessary for trauma treatment and recovery.
- This is not a substitute for trauma therapy!

Materials

This program is highly adaptable and can be implemented with one horse and a small space, or a herd of a dozen on a 100-acre ranch. One of the most important things I have learned on my equine therapy journey is to keep it simple. As a lifelong horsewoman, I am still amazed at how transformative the little things we do every day with horses can be for clients. And frankly, when we approach these everyday little things with mindfulness and intention, we too can be transformed.

The Process

To get started, I will have a discussion with my client or group about the 7 C's, including the definitions of each. Depending on your client, you can provide definitions to clarify or you allow the client to create his or her own. Both work equally well. Trust your gut.

Then you need to get a sense of where they need to start. In essence, what C needs the most attention? You can create a variety of scales to get a measurement for pre/post information. I use a numeric scale of 1–10, with 1 being little to no experience of the C, and 10 being able to tap into that C as much as one needs. I don't use 0 because it is my belief (and one I share with clients) that we all have the 7 C's within us. I believe it is part of our true self that can never be taken away or destroyed. Just this idea alone can be extremely helpful for clients, as it offers them hope.

If you have clients who tend to get stuck in their heads or for whom a number scale may create too much internal self-judgment, I would recommend using a circle, like a wagon wheel. The hub of the wheel is 1 and the end of the wheel is 5. Draw one spoke for each C, and then connect the dots. You can also just get started with whatever C has come up in previous sessions. Once you have decided on a C to work on, you then collaborate with the client to choose an activity or exercise that will provide a positive experience of that particular C.

More often than not, I start by helping clients to find a peaceful or calm place. Once we do that, we tap it in and this allows them to go into the work with the horses already having a resource to use if needed. It may take several sessions to get through it, but trust the process. You can do all of this work outside with the horses or in the barn if it is helpful to do so. I often teach the tapping in of resources outside next to a paddock or in front of the stall of the horse my client has chosen to work with. Now it's time to get to work. All of the above is done in preparation for the work with the horse.

Remember that what is most important is not the elaborate activity you choose, but that you collaborate with your client(s) to find the most appropriate experience for them. Also, as any of us who do this work know, things do not always turn out how we expect them to, nor do they take the time that we think they may. Stay open to what arises and hold the space for your client to get what they need. You will see in my case example that you can never really be sure what will happen, but if you trust the process, results will come.

HELPFUL DEFINITIONS AND KEY COMPONENTS

Courage

- "The ability to do something that you know is difficult or dangerous."
- "Mental or moral strength to venture, persevere, and withstand danger, fear, or difficulty."
- **Key components:** vulnerability, authenticity, resilience, "heart energy," success, and failure.
- **Activity ideas to promote Courage:** haltering/catching a horse in a field, leading, obstacles, and round pen work.

Calm

- "A quiet and peaceful state or condition."
- "A peaceful mental or emotional state."
- **Key components:** mindfulness, consciousness, self-awareness and self-regulation, "back to grazing," neuroscience of calm.
- **Activity ideas to promote Calm:** grooming, haltering/catching and round pen.

Clarity

- "The quality or state of being clear"
- "The quality of being expressed, remembered, understood, etc., in a very exact way"
- **Key components:** understanding and setting intentions and goals, action/motivation, limiting negative beliefs, core values, meaning/purpose.
- **Activity ideas to promote Clarity:** round pen, riding, leading, and obstacles/problem-solving.

Creativity

- "The ability to make new things or think of new ideas."
- "The ability to create."
- **Key components:** imagination, expression, exploration, curiosity, play/fun, beginner's mind, openness, nonjudgmental awareness.
- **Activity ideas to promote Creativity:** round pen, riding/groundwork to music (Rhythmic Riding—Natural Lifemanship: Jobe et al., 2016), painting on horses, artwork and obstacles/problem-solving.

Compassion

- "A feeling of wanting to help someone who is sick, hungry, in trouble, etc."
- "Sympathetic consciousness of others' distress together with a desire to alleviate it."
- **Key components:** self-worth and self-compassion, loving-kindness, forgiveness, empathy, the inner critic.
- **Activity ideas to promote Compassion:** grooming, leading, round pen and liberty work in the field.

Congruence

- "The state of being when what is experienced on the 'inside' matches what is expressed on the 'outside'."
- "A state of internal harmony."
- "The quality or state of agreeing, coinciding, or being congruent."
- **Key components:** self-awareness, communication, understanding emotions, emotion regulation, and false self vs. authentic self.
- **Activity ideas to promote Congruence:** round pen, riding, leading, and grooming.

PROGRAM SESSION OUTLINE EXAMPLE

Session 1

Go over the 7 C's of Well-Being, discussing definitions and rating levels of each C in specific or various aspects of each client's life. Next, observe the herd (or whatever horse(s) you have to use. Ideally, this is done outside in a paddock or arena, although you can make it work in stalls if you have to. Have clients observe the herd looking for examples of some or all of the C's in the horse behaviors. Discuss client's observations and then if they are comfortable, I have clients go in with the horses and spend some time with each horse with the intention to choose a horse to work with for the rest of the program.

Session 2

The client will now go into the paddock/arena/round pen depending on what is available and what the client is comfortable with, and approach, halter, and lead the horse back to the therapist or team. Discussion of this follows and can actually take several sessions, as you will see from the case example at the end of this section.

Session 3

The client will connect with the horses either in a stall or in the paddock. They will then halter the horse and do a grooming session in order to better connect with the horse and themselves. I will often then have clients take the horse for a walk either inside, outside, or both. We are fortunate enough to have a horse-size labyrinth and will have clients explore this space with the horses at this time.

Session 4

In this session, the client will halter/lead the horse to the round pen or arena space. Ideally, this is a smaller space, but you can make it work with whatever you have. We use our round pen most often as it provides a nice sized space for this work. We will often talk about moving a horse and give some demonstrations of how to communicate movement in the round pen. Clients are encouraged to find their own way, as what may work for me, may not work for the client. At this time, I find Natural Lifemanship (Jobe et al., 2016) principles of pressure and connection to be most helpful. The client is asked to move the horse around the round pen in each direction. You can elaborate this by adding different gaits, speeds, directions, etc. You can also work towards getting the horse to stand still, as well as following the client without a lead rope. This all depends on time, space and amount of sessions you have to work with.

SUMMARY

You can use this program as a weekend retreat, a series of daylong workshops, a week intensive, or many individual weekly/monthly sessions. I have worked with it in all of these ways and have had great success. The most important thing is to find the right fit for the client.

I cannot emphasize enough that you must communicate and collaborate with your client in regards to safety and security in all interactions and activities. Remember, for some clients just being in the same vicinity as a horse can be quite terrifying, so use any and all appropriate measures to make sure you are clear about where you client is emotionally and physically. If I have a client with a lot of anxiety or a high arousal level, I will use the 1–10 scale to keep a measure of anxiety/arousal and I will also use grounding skills, as needed, to maintain safety. Having a good understanding of dissociation and resistance on the part of both horses and clients is extremely important. Sarah

Jenkins' work on dissociation and equine therapy is a great resource. Check out www.dragonflyinternationaltherapy.com for more information. Also, I recommend van der Kolk's book, *The Body Keeps the Score.* This book is incredibly helpful in better understanding how trauma and dissociation work and they can be healed (van der Kolk, 2014).

One of the biggest complaints I have heard about equine therapy is that it's all well and good at the barn, but then the client goes home and all bets are off. To help clients better integrate and own the work we do with the horses, I teach my clients (both therapy and riding) how to use Parnell's Resource Tapping exercise (Parnell, 2008). I teach this before we work with the horses and then end each session with it as well. Sometimes we will even do some in the middle of the session. Resource Tapping, not to be confused with EFT or tapping on acupressure points, is a process by which we bring to mind a positive image, allow a bodily felt sense to emerge, and then tap alternating right/left on opposite sides of the body.

Resourcing is a process by which we focus our awareness on a positive experience (in the past or the present), figure, memory, or feeling state for a short amount of time while at the same time maintaining a dual focus on another stimulus such as tapping on your knees or shoulders, hearing sounds or feeling a horse near you. This process allows for the integration of the positive feeling into our nervous system, creating a resource that can be recalled when needed.

Focusing on and tapping into the positive experiences and feelings that the client can have while working with horses, allows them to activate a natural healing system. EMDR founder Francine Shapiro calls this "adaptive information processing." Throughout history humans have used this concept of dual attention stimuli and bilateral stimulation to heal—drumming, dancing, long walks, running, etc. While it is still unclear why this works so well, there are theories that attempt to explain the phenomena, such as the healing properties of rhythm, imagination and visualization.

CASE EXAMPLE

The following is an example of taking a client through the process of The 7 C's of Well-Being. The client is a 38-year-old Caucasian female, currently married with no children. Sue (a pseudonym) is an office manager at a local insurance agency. She came to treatment because of anxiety, an emotional abusive marriage, binge eating, and dissatisfaction with her career. Sue had been in therapy off and on since she was a child and had been in couples therapy with her husband for almost three years. She was fed up with therapy and felt like the horses were her last shot at breaking free from her struggles. Although she had always loved horses, she had no real experience with them and had some anxiety about working with them.

Sue came weekly to work with the horses and the 7 C's and we used the format example from above in six sessions. We had one intake session in my office where we discussed her current symptoms/issues, as well as her history. We then discussed The 7 C's and she used the 1–10 scale to rate how much of each she felt she had in her life, most especially in her marriage and in her work. The results were as follows: Courage 3, Clarity 3, Creativity 3, Calm 2, Compassion 7 (with others, 2 with herself), Congruence 5, and Connection 3 in her marriage and 5 with friends due to the controlling nature of her marriage. She decided that she felt if she had clarity and courage she could better move forward so we started our work with the intention to cultivate clarity and courage.

Next, we moved out to the horses where she did an observation and then took time in the paddock to meet the herd and choose a horse to work with. She chose to work with a horse named Rock. Here is a sample of that discussion.

The following transcript analysis are about a pseudonym client.

Table 18.1

Transcript Analysis of Case Example

Transcript	*Analysis*
Therapist: Have you decided on a horse?	The reasons clients have for choosing to work with a particular horse will almost always give you useful information.
Client: Yes. I want to work with that one with the scar. He and I have a lot in common.	Client is able to talk about how they feel on the inside, and this is a good start and a moment of courage that the therapist can use later.

Transcript	*Analysis*
Therapist: Can you say more about that? **Client:** Yeah. Clearly the horse has been abused and although I don't have scars on the outside, my insides feel pretty much like his outsides look. Plus, he seems kind of skittish and nervous and so do I.	Therapist has a better sense of client's internal experience.
Therapist: How did you get clear on what horse to choose? **Client:** I don't know. I just knew.	Here is an example of a moment of clarity. Now we will explore how the client feels in their body when they have a moment of clarity. Then we can look to find ways to have more, as well as identifying the moments of clarity the client is already having.
Therapist: What do you notice in your body, when you "just know?"	Connecting to the body allows for present moment grounding, as well as more information.
Client: I feel a lightness, especially in my chest.	Once client has the bodily felt sense of an experience of knowing, you could resource this (using Resource Tapping) or use as a marker to resource later.

Sue continued to work with Rock throughout our six sessions together. By building a relationship with Rock, she was able to reconnect to internal resources she did not even know she had. At the end of the six sessions, she rated her 7 C's again and she had an increase in all of them, most especially courage and clarity, both of which she gave a 7, up from 3 at the beginning. This program is flexible and you can use the template as a foundation, building it to fit both client and clinician.

Sample Client SOAP Session Note

Subjective: Client met the herd today and was able to decide to work with horse (Rock). Client reported that they were able to identify a sense of "knowing" and use it to begin to build a relationship with Rock. There was some hesitation in working so closely with the horses, but by the end of this session, client appeared much more comfortable and client stated that her anxiety had decreased.

Objective: Although anxious at first, client appeared to become more grounded as client moved through the session. Client still is apprehensive about the possibility of building trust with a horse, but seems to have a connection with this horse and his lack of trust (due to his past abuse) actually appears to help client feel more at ease.

Assessment: Client appears to be able to stay grounded and with some sense of self-energy. Client and counselor discuss several parts of her that were apprehensive, but all were able to give client space in order to connect with the horse. The progress of clients work is good and client is showing improvement in her ability to stay present.

Plan: Continue therapy. Next session client will do grooming and possibly take horse for a walk. Client and counselor and will continue to look for moments of courage and clarity, as well as the other C's. Client will resource these moments, building up a positive experiences and new neural pathways.

REFERENCES

Jenkins, S. & Baker, J. (2011). The Equine-Assisted EMDR Manual: A Guide to the Integration of Eye Movement Desensitization Reprocessing and Equine-Assisted Therapy. Tempe, AZ: Dragonfly International Therapy.

Jobe, T., Shultz-Jobe, B., & McFarland, L. (2016). *Fundamentals of Natural Lifemanship: Trauma-Focused Equine Assisted Psychotherapy (TF-EAP TM)*. Liberty Hill: TX Natural Lifemanship.

Parnell, L. (2007) *A Therapist's Guide to EMDR*: Tools and Techniques for Successful Treatment. New York: W.W. Norton & Company, Inc.

Parnell, L. (2008). Tapping In: A Step-by-Step Guide to Activating Your Healing Resources through Bilateral Stimulation. Boulder, CO: Sounds True.

Schwartz, R. C. (1995) *Internal Family Systems Therapy*. New York: Guilford Press.

Shapiro, F. & Forrest, M. S. (1997) *EMDR Eye Movement Desensitization & Reprocessing*. New York: Basic Books.

van der Kolk, B. A. (2014). *The Body Keeps the Score*. New York: Penguin.

19

Stepping into the Arena with Your Inner Ally

Sara B. Willerson and Vanessa M. Sanford

INTRODUCTION

What has become known as "The Man in the Arena Speech" is a section from President Theodore Roosevelt's 1910 speech at the Sorbonne University in Paris, France entitled *Citizenship in a Republic*. Roosevelt's speech inspired the title and focus of well-known author and researcher Brené Brown's bestselling book, *Daring Greatly* (Brown, 2012a).

This quote and Brown's Daring Way™ curriculum subsequently brought the authors of this chapter together. Vanessa M. Sanford and Sara B. Willerson were colleagues and occasional program collaborators. Sanford completed the Daring Way Certified Facilitator training and returned home with an immediate email to Willerson about the power of this program and how they had to co-create something between this curriculum and Willerson's equine-facilitated psychotherapy practice. After watching Brown's TED Talk, The Power of Vulnerability (Brown, 2012b) and reading Roosevelt's speech, Willerson knew the horses were absolutely walking the talk of this program, which centers around the concepts of vulnerability, self-worth, shame resilience, and wholehearted living.

When partnering with horses, whether it is equine-facilitated psychotherapy or learning, the arena *is* the nature-based therapy office. Brown states, "Vulnerability is the core, the heart, the center, of meaningful human experiences" (Brown, 2012a, p. 12). When we step into the arena with a horse, they are asking, inviting, and supporting us into that open heart centered space of who we are. This practice of vulnerability, being and owning the heart of who we are, may open up all sorts of questions around our self-worth and shame-based messages from the outside. In *Walking the Way of The Horse*, author Leif Hallberg cites equine facilitated programming elder Barbara Rector's wisdom reminder that "horses facilitate awareness of our own instinctual nature and its influence on our thoughts, behaviors and feelings" (Hallberg, 2008, p. 115). Through relationship with a horse, we have a four-legged ally holding space for us to step into the core of our being, connect with our strength within, and expand into the present moment of our world.

OPENING THE GATE TO THE INNER ALLY

Two roads diverged in the woods—or pasture—both leading to self-worth. One path depends on Western culture's focus of external performance and praise while betting on empty promises of a destination full of high self-esteem without a backup plan. Another path opens to horses, nature, self-compassion, and a deeper knowledge of how brains are wired for story, gently guiding a practice of curiosity instead of a destination. Brené Brown, discusses one of the most important seats in the arena self-compassion. She refers to the research of Kristin Neff (2011), when learning what to let go of and what to cultivate in order to live a wholehearted life. In Brown's "10 Guideposts for Wholehearted Living," she weaves in the three components of Neff's definition of self-compassion: self-kindness, common humanity, and mindfulness (Brown, 2010).

These components of self-compassion are Spiritual Sherpas, the diplomatic guides offering guidance to shame resilience, self-trust, acceptance, and self-worth. This work challenges old belief systems of using armor to protect and self-esteem as the measure to self-worth. The quest is to transition to new patterns of partnership with an inner ally (self-compassion), and permission to remove the armor. Neff (2011) explains that the fundamentals of self-compassion can be understood through identifying our actions in response to a loved one suffering, and turning that desire inward. Brown (2010) asserts that self-kindness is treating yourself like a friend; actively self-soothing and acknowledging how imperfect it is to be human.

The opposite of self-kindness is self-judgment. Neff (2011) claims that self-judgment turns a moment of suffering into a storyline that defines us by the suffering. Sometimes we can find ourselves saying things like, "I'm such a failure," "I suck," "I'm not good enough," "What's wrong with me?" The idea is to catch the inner dialogue and then practice self-kindness. For example, "I am really mad right now and messed up and made a bad choice."

The next element of self-compassion is common humanity, the recognition we are not alone. The opposite of common humanity is isolation. The instant reaction of "should-ing" all over yourself with thoughts of "I should have or could have done this better" creates a sense of isolation and abnormality. To feel alone in our suffering and have the inner dialogue, "no one would understand" breeds isolation. The challenge is to become aware of this initial and typical story and then practice common humanity by saying, "I am not alone, others struggle too" (Neff, 2011). This narrow lens can omit the compassionate self-awareness that we are not alone and to be human is to be imperfect. Brown explains "When we fail or make mistakes, that doesn't separate us from others, that is precisely what unites us to others" (2017). In Western culture, there is a learned expectation, "This is not supposed to happen to me." Having an awareness of common humanity can widen the lens and allow us to remember, *we* instead of *me*.

The third component of Neff's research is mindfulness or "courageous presence." With multiple definitions of mindfulness, Neff describes it as "the ability to pay attention to what is happening in the present moment, as it is happening" (Neff, 2011, p. 84). The power of mindfulness, according to Neff, is breaking down the counterpart to mindfulness—over-identification. When we are able to look kindly at our struggle and remember we are not alone, we are less likely to get hijacked by our story and know it is a moment of struggle instead of the struggle defining us. Move from an old way of saying "This is painful and it will never go away" to the new mindful expression of "This is a painful moment." Brené Brown says, "The most dangerous stories we make up are the narratives that diminish our inherent worthiness. We must reclaim the trust about our lovability, divinity, and creativity" (Brown, 2015, p.82).

THE BRIDGE TO SELF-WORTH

Self-esteem is a commonly used phrase to measure how good or bad we feel about ourselves. "At its core, self-esteem is an evaluation of our worthiness, judgment that we are good, valuable people" (Neff, 2011, p.138). Whether the path is self-esteem (external) or self-compassion (internal kindness), the intention is to create a bridge to self-worth. This clarification is important to unpack, especially when opening the gate to self-trust, self-love, self-awareness, and self-acceptance.

Self-esteem campaigns a perception that to feel well, things must go well. The hope is to cut away from an external value system based on performance and praise, known as self-esteem, and migrate into an internal value system based on courageous acceptance, called self-compassion. This brave acknowledgement is based in kindness, knowing we are not alone, and being present with our negative emotions. The war between self-esteem and the individual wanting to feel above average can fester rivalry, competition, and judgment. These ruthless traits can create lack of follow-through, fear of failure, and dependence. Through a peaceful treaty with ourselves, self-compassion can cultivate cooperation and contribution, establish a stronger focus on effort, joy in the process, acceptance and self-sufficiency (Dweck, 2006).

The need for high self-esteem encourages us to ignore, distort, or hide personal shortcomings, and collectively misses the ability to clearly and accurately see ourselves. Self-esteem is contingent on the latest failure or success, and fluctuates depending on our ever-changing circumstances (Neff, 2011). Sculpting an inner ally (self-compassion) instead of allowing the inner enemy (shame) to corrode our self-worth means having to step into an arena and brave a new relationship with our true self.

Self-compassion is one of the most crucial seats to be aware of when stepping into the arena and the understanding of how different it is from self-esteem. This new relationship requires vulnerability and removing the armor used for protection. What is armor? Armor is a hiding place from pain. It is a shield that protects, but also creates a barrier to authenticity and wholehearted living. Examples of armor we may carry include people-pleasing, acting cool, avoidance, constant change, busyness, and social media. Having support and leadership from a harmonious herd role models what an inner ally looks and feels like.

THE THEORETICAL ARENA FOOTING

Attunement through horses partnered with Brené Brown's Daring Way™ curriculum, is easily supported by Choice Theory, Experiential Theory, and Humanistic Theory. Choice Theory explains that human behavior is based on internal motivation (Glasser, 1999). Learning how to connect to an inner ally of self-compassion rather than external sources can lead to what Brené Brown says, "You either walk inside your story and own it or you stand outside your story and hustle for your worthiness" (Brown, 2015, p. 45). The narrative is so powerful and can either pull us towards vulnerability and wholehearted living with self-worth or lean us back into armor overusage and shame.

Experiential Theory is the process of learning through experience (Kolb, 2015). Having the opportunity to learn concepts on vulnerability, shame resilience, courage, and self-worth followed by practice with horses allows meaningful integration. Meaningful integration to feel what it is like to take off the armor and stand surrounded by compassion and empathy embodied in a massive four-legged being. Brown believes, "We move what we're learning from our heads to our hearts through our hands" (Brown, 2015, pp. 6–7).

Humanistic theory is based on the understanding that the person is a whole being (Rogers, 1995). One of the focuses incorporated into this partnership is remembering that our bodies do not simply carry our thoughts from place to place. This can be referred to as neck-down work. Neck-down means we connect all of ourselves (mentally, physically, emotionally, and spiritually) instead of just focusing on the armor we feel burdened to carry. Brown states that this wholehearted, "neck-down" way of living means "Owning our story and loving ourselves through that process is the bravest thing we will ever do" (Brown, 2010, p. ix).

This ensemble of the Daring Way curriculum, partnership with horses, and theoretical perspective sets the alliance for Brown's credo that self-compassion, more than self-esteem, leads to self-worth. The harmonious chorus of these three theories link internal motivation, active learning with all parts of self, and wholehearted embodiment of an inner ally.

A PARTNERSHIP OF ETHICS

In *Horse Sense and the Human Heart*, McCormick and McCormick (1997, p. xxix) reflect that when partnering with horses:

> we discovered a force—an unseen but ever-present energy that bathes the spirit and requires that we be completely present and true to our own nature. A horse's ability to connect with people is uncanny. Its size and presence somehow force us to become physically, mentally and spiritually more aware and more human.

The McCormicks' writings are a beautiful and powerful reminder of the importance of knowing and understanding horses when we are partnering with them in a therapeutic setting. Without this relational knowledge of our four-legged facilitators, we may miss their cues and communication around their needs and well-being. It is paramount that as professionals we do our own personal healing/development work, participate in ongoing equine behavioral learning/ training opportunities and membership communities and, most importantly, ensure that we truly know and understand each of the equine members on the treatment team. When we as facilitators have a deep understanding and relationship with these sentient beings, we know and are attuned with their desires, mood, interests, healing gifts, and when, most importantly, they need and/or ask for a break. Equine facilitated healing work is intense for all parties involved, horse and human, and as the main facilitator, the horse's entire being *must* be cared for physically, emotionally, mentally, and spiritually.

THE STEPPING INTO THE ARENA WITH YOUR INNER ALLY—INTERVENTION

Supplies needed:

White board or flip chart and multicolored pens to write with

- Round-pen or enclosed space
- Horse at liberty (no tack) in an enclosed space
- Chairs outside enclosed space for group members to sit and observe (labeled metaphorically or literally with the words empathy and compassion)
- Rocks with inspirational words in a container of some sort
- Thank-you carrots.

This activity is a reflective experience for participants to begin integrating The Daring Way concepts of vulnerability, defensive armor, and the cultivation of self-worth. The exercise occurs at the end of the first day and has been used with people aged 12 and older. Participants have already created connections with the herd of horses they are partnering with throughout the program and have been introduced to core concepts of vulnerability, armoring up (ways that we may protect/shield ourselves from being in an open-hearted space), and cultivating self- compassion with ourselves and others as tools to bring into the arena space.

Prior to stepping into the experiential partnership space with a horse, group members participate in a discussion and identification process of their own "armor" that shows up when contemplating being in the vulnerable space of the wholehearted arena. This discussion is accompanied by a symbol of a shield drawn on a whiteboard (flip chart paper or even a large piece of butcher paper can be used) with participants naming their armor and these parts being listed on the symbolic shield. The combination of mental, verbal, and visual processing is a reminder that there is no shame in "armoring up." Armor, at times, has held an important role and was created, most likely, from a need for protection, problem-solving, and possibly survival. There is honor in expressing gratitude for the armor and recognizing when it is helpful and when it gets in the way of being wholehearted.

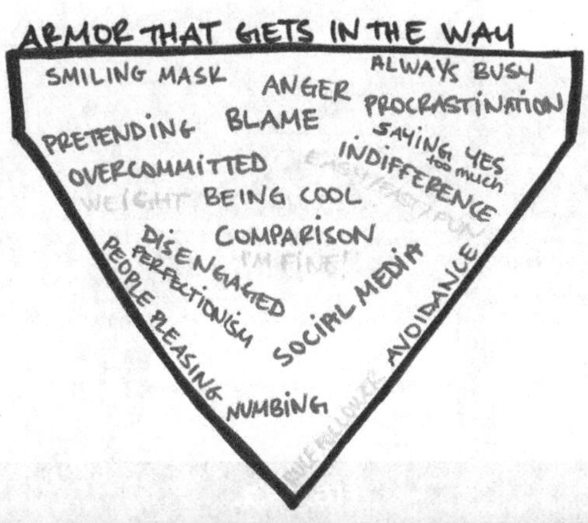

FIG. 19.1.

The Stepping Into the Arena With Your Inner Ally activity is designed for each participant to partner with the horse of her/his choice in a round pen space (or the horse may have chosen the participant). If the horse and/or person prefer a larger space to connect and explore, a larger arena is also an option to move the experience into, as is the open pasture. This is a ground-based activity that does not require tools or tack.

At this point in the retreat weekend, participants are beginning to have a sense of a theme or even a message their horse partner(s) is starting to share with them. One participant in a past program noted, "Maybe what I am supposed to be focusing on is joy instead of grief." Another stated, "I am tired of opting out of my vulnerability... I am learning to be vulnerable because I can opt out of it... I have to give myself permission to be vulnerable."

Prior to entering the round pen, the participant is guided by the facilitator to take some deep breaths, get grounded, and notice the current sensations in their body. The facilitator supports the participant in noticing how their body is holding or even responding to this newly emerging theme or equine wisdom message. The participant is also encouraged to notice if there is any defensive armor showing up as they step more deeply into partnership with their vulnerability and true self. How might that armor be supporting or blocking this new theme, story, or message? Once the participant is attuned to their internal process, they step into the round pen with their four-legged ally. Participants do have the option of having the facilitator join them in the round pen with their horse if desired.

While the participant is in the round pen, the other participants are seated in chairs a respectful distance from the round pen but close enough to observe the interaction. It is what Eponaquest co-founder Kathleen Barry Ingram (2017) refers to as "the sacred space of possibility." When one of us is in the arena, marred with dirt and sweat, while erring and striving valiantly, those who are seated in the stands hold the seats of empathy and compassion as allies and sources of support. Having these chairs allows for armor to soften and offers space for self-compassion.

Once in the round pen, horse and human step into a space of unlimited potential and awareness. The importance of knowing each horse, their personality, healing gifts and ways they communicate is incredibly important in this relationship space. It is from this place that participants can step into a spirit of exploration with themselves and with their horse ally as guide. It is through their interactions with each other, hearing what each is saying and doing, that a heart centered space of vulnerability and self-compassion is created.

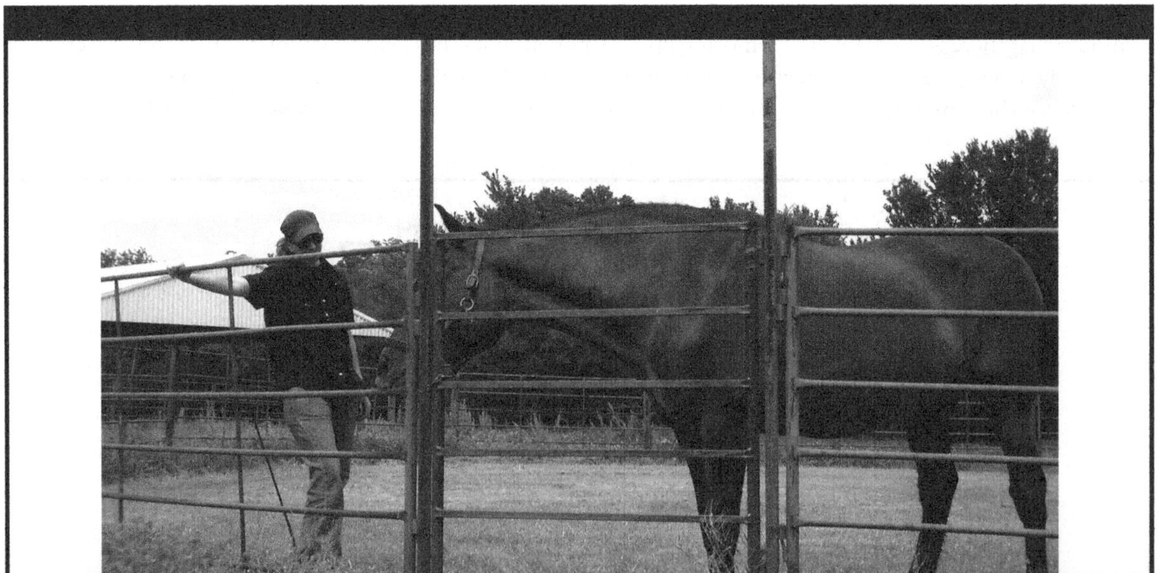

FIG. 19.2.

Once the participant feels they have received the message from their horse and experienced the embodied practice of vulnerability and self-compassion, they take a moment to thank their four-legged partner and give the gift of a carrot. Upon exiting the relationship space, participants are invited to reach into a bag of word-themed rocks (believe, strength, dream, create, faith, nurture, inspire, etc.) with the guidance that their horse partner is giving them one more gift from this vulnerable connection space of self-worth. The group member reaches into the bag without seeing the rock they are choosing, going by intuitive feel. Each time the participant is surprised at how aligned and accurate this "blindly" chosen rock is. This additional token is *always* aligned with the equine-guided work they completed moments previously. Stepping into the arena of self-kindness and openness to receiving are additional components of self-compassion.

The participant shares their experience with their human herd and all take turns offering observations from the seats of empathy and compassion. This is the adhesive to connect with the Inner Ally and practice the three aspects of self-compassion in a supportive community setting. Through this reflection process, all are connected with the Inner Ally through the collaborative message of "Me too!" The magical moments of having all senses wide open and knowing in our bones what an Inner Ally looks, feels and sounds like, is the gift of this activity.

CASE EXAMPLE—REAL-TIME PARTNERING WITH A FOUR-LEGGED ALLY

A past participant gave permission for her experience to be shared in this book. Natalie (a pseudonym) is employed as a law enforcement officer where vulnerability is a safety hazard when holding the perimeter and ensuring safety for others. From the beginning of the program weekend, she was acutely aware of the paradox between her professional role and this invitation to step into vulnerable connection with her inner ally. She quickly identified with Domino, the lead mare in the herd, whose role it is to keep an eye on the perimeter and all members in her herd safe. Natalie was able to voice her desire of leaving the armor of her professional role outside of the arena and allow Domino to hold this sense of responsibility instead. Natalie chose to partner with Magno, a massive 17h draft gelding who is the protector in the herd. When she stepped into the round pen, Natalie initially remained by the gate. The colossal gelding she had chosen as her partner attempted to move her away from her perimeter hold by grazing around her feet and gently asking her to move. Natalie expressed her struggle with releasing her hold on the mental concept of vulnerability into the embodied practice of the inner ally. At that moment, Domino stepped into the periphery of her vision and Natalie interpreted this as the mare letting her know, "I got this perimeter. Trust me." At that moment, Magno stepped between her and the gate and clearly asked her to trust him as well. Natalie chuckled and was well aware of what her equine ally was saying to her. She took several deep breaths and released her hold on the fence and stepped toward him, putting her hand on his sizeable shoulder. As she held this space of vulnerable connection, her gentle giant leaned in toward her, as a beautiful confirmation of trusting her experience and allowing the old armor and belief systems to wait outside. Charles Feltman says "Trust is defined as choosing to risk making something you value vulnerable to another person's actions" (Feltman, 2009, p. 7). Natalie and her massive ally stayed together, quietly connected, to honor this release from perimeter holder to acceptance of the inner ally.

Each member of the horses' Heart & Soul® herd has their own unique way of supporting their human participant in this space. At times, the participant may need some assistance in understanding what is happening between themselves and their four-legged partner. In this integrative experience, there are elemental aspects of horse language that can be challenging for our human, logic-based language. The way to speak a common language is through the practice of compassion. Some questions to be considered in creating a common tongue include the following.

Transcript	Analysis
Counselor escorts client into the round pen with their horse, Magno, and closes the gate. Counselor takes a step back from the round pen and watches.	Counselor quietly observes initial interaction between client and her horse. This allows space for client and horse to explore each other at liberty.
Counselor: What is happening between the two of you?	After a while, client starts looking around as if she is unsure. Counselor asks supportive question to encourage connection between client and horse.
Client: I don't know.	The counselor is gently guiding the client in returning to a connection space with her horse.
Counselor: What are you noticing about Magno right now?	Client is now looking back at her horse partner and counselor is helping client begin to see the horse step into the role of the Inner Ally.
Client: Well, he is standing there by the gate eating.	Counselor quietly pauses to allow client space to consider this observation.
Counselor: What are you feeling in your body right now? **Client**: *Puts her hand on her belly.* I feel something in my gut. *Magno turns his head and looks right at her belly.* **Client:** *Smiling.* Oh! I get it! That is what he saying to me!	This question begins to help the client lean into self-compassion through awareness of sensations in her body. Client becomes aware of her horse validating her internal experience.
Counselor: *Pauses and reminds client to take a deep breath.* What is he bringing your attention to right now? *Magno takes several side steps moving client further away from the gate and client then puts one hand on the fence.* **Counselor:** Just take some deep breaths and be with your horse in this moment.	Counselor is gently supporting client in stepping into self-compassion and moving towards an understanding of her personal armor. Counselor is aware that the horse is actively stepping into the role of Inner Ally with client. Counselor is encouraging client to take a breath to embody this interaction
Counselor: What do you think Magno is doing with you right now?	Counselor supporting translation between horse and human language.
Client: *While laughing.* He is telling me to trust him and he's got this.	Client has allowed the horse to truly step into the role of the Inner Ally with her.
Client releases hand from the fence and places it on the shoulder of the horse and takes a deep breath and smiles.	Client is embodying her connection with her Inner Ally.
Counselor: What armor is showing up at this time?	Counselor continues to assist client in deepening her awareness of this integration.
Client: My role has always been to protect the perimeter. It is hard to trust another to take over that role.	Client is able to identify the real-time application of this work.

FIG. 19.3. Transcript Analysis of Case Example.

The facilitator can use these simple questions to actively assist the presence of the Inner Ally. These curious inquiries support the participant in stepping into vulnerability and identifying, honoring, and at times, shifting any armor that may be presenting as a result of this internal paradigm shift toward the Inner Ally. This is the courageous presence of self-compassion.

REFERENCES

Brown, B. (2010). The Gifts of Imperfection: Let Go of Who You Think You're Supposed to Be and Embrace Who You Are. Center City, MN: Hazelden.

Brown, B. (2012a). Daring Greatly: How the Courage to be Vulnerable Transforms the Way We Live, Love, Parent, and Lead. New York: Gotham Books.

Brown, B. (2012b). *Brené Brown: The Power of Vulnerability*. Retrieved from www.ted.com/talks/brene_brown_on_vulnerability.

Brown, B. (2015). *Rising Strong*. 1st edition. New York: Spiegel & Grau.

Brown, B. (2017). *Self-Compassion and Heartfelt Apologies with Kristin Neff and Harriet Lerner.* Retrieved from www.courageworks.com/classes/self-compassion-with-kristin-neff-brene-brown.

Dweck, C. S. (2006). *Mindset: The New Psychology of Success.* New York: Random House.

Feltman, C. (2009). The Thin Book of Trust: An Essential Primer for Building Trust at Work. Bend, OR: Thin Book Publishing Co.

Glasser, W. (1999). *Choice Theory: A New Psychology of Personal Freedom.* 1st HarperPerennial edition. New York: HarperPerennial.

Hallberg, L. (2008). Walking the Way of the Horse: Exploring the Power of the Horse–Human Relationship. Bloomington, IN: i-Universe.

Ingram, K. B. (2017). *Sacred Place of Possibility.* Retrieved from www.sacredplaceofpossibility.com.

Kolb, D. A. (2015). Experiential Learning: Experience as the Source of Learning and Development. Upper Saddle River, NJ: Pearson Education.

McCormick, A. & McCormick, M. (1997). Horse Sense and the Human Heart: What Horses Can Teach Us About Trust, Bonding, Creativity and Spirituality. Deerfield Beach, FL: Health Communications, Inc.

Neff, K. (2011). Self-Compassion: The Proven Power of Being Kind to Yourself. New York. HarperCollins.

Rogers, C. R. I. (1995). On Becoming a Person: A Therapist's View of Psychotherapy. Boston: Houghton Mifflin.

Roosevelt, T. (1910). *Citizenship in a Republic.* Paris, France: Speech delivered at the Sorbonne.

Section 11

Social Skills and Communication

20

Social Skills and Communication

The Path of Life through Mindfulness and Experience

Rob Pliskin

INTRODUCTION

In 2015, suicide was the third leading cause of death in the United States for children aged 10–14 and third leading cause for youth and young adults aged 15–24. In 2014, New Zealand's youth suicide rate for teenagers aged 15–19, was twice that of the US. Some antecedent conditions to youth suicide include family dislocation and violence, sexual abuse, poverty, bullying, often compounded by youth depression, anxiety, and other mental disorders. In the face of these conditions, youth can end up feeling empty and hopeless. Much of their behavior becomes maladaptive and problematic, with appropriate social skills undeveloped or shut down and communications "trapped" inside (Illmer, 2017; NIMH, 2017a, 2017b). How can equine-assisted psychotherapy (EAP) horses and teams help clients in this situation?

Kolb's Experiential Learning Theory describes one powerful way clients can learn to bring well-being and positive change into their world. It is this author's view that we have sayings such as "experience is the best teacher" for good reason. According to Kolb, "Learning is the process whereby knowledge is created through the transformation of experience" (McLeod, 2013).

Table 20.1

Kolb's Experiential Learning Cycle

1. **Concrete Experience:** A new experience or situation is encountered, or reinterpretation of existing experience.
2. **Reflective Observation of the New Experience**: Of particular importance are any inconsistencies between experience and understanding.
3. **Abstract Conceptualization**: Reflection gives rise to a new idea, or a modification of an existing abstract concept.
4. **Active Experimentation**: The learner applies them to the world around them to see what results.

Source: MCLEOD (2013).

It is evident that the cycle is a strong theoretical foundation for understanding the power of EAP as an experiential approach.

An example of one approach that dovetails with Kolb's work is mindfulness. Mindfulness practice introduces new behavior in the experimentation phase of the cycle, which assists the client in bringing positive change into the client's own here and now, which then can support continuing change for the client in further iterations of experience (Ozen, Gibbons, & Bédard, 2016). As an example, Ozen et al. (2016) found mindfulness-based stress reduction helped participants with traumatic brain injury significantly reduce depression and enhance quality of life in a 12-week group. After one year, 70% of group participants were reached for follow-up and had maintained clinically significant improvements. Brown, Ryan, and Creswell (2007) set the theoretical stage for mindfulness in EAP:

> as a receptive attention to and awareness of present events and experience. First and foremost, mindfulness concerns a clear awareness of one's inner and outer worlds, including thoughts, emotions, sensations, actions, or surroundings as they exist at any given moment.

Models of equine-assisted programming including EAP can reduce the impact of anxiety, depression, and other risk factors for client welfare, including suicide risk. In a comparison of equine-assisted counseling to classroom-based counseling for students at risk for academic and/or social failure, Trotter, Chandler, Goodwin-Bond, and Casey (2008) showed statistically significant reductions in negative behaviors and significant increases in positive behaviors of participants after 12 weekly counseling sessions. In another example Signal, Kemp, Botros, Taylor, and Prentice (2014) found that an equine-facilitated program in Queensland, Australia, was effective for children and adolescents who had been sexually abused. Importantly, this effectiveness extended across gender, age, and indigenous/non-indigenous status of the participants. These results are two examples among many.

EAP grounded in Kolb's Cycle puts faith in the client's ability to garner the inner resources to learn and change during the facilitated experience, and to discover, embrace, and apply them outside the arena (Eagala, 2017). This is the purpose of the Path of Life.

Ethical standards of practice bring together the ethics of mental health, counselling, and coaching for clients as well as the ethics of partnering with equines into one ethical stream. Evans and Grey (2012) explore animal-assisted therapy (AAT) with the lens of ecology in social work. Thus, looking beyond the corral, what is the client's relationship with animals? Should the animals in clients' lives be protected? Is the facilitator morally obliged to report animal abuse in which the client states being involved? When looking towards the equines in a program, what needs to be done to insure their welfare and well-being? Can an intervention for the client in a session also be beneficial for the equine(s)?

Walker, Aimers, and Perry (2015) join Evans and Grey (2012) to consider the role of social work educators in making these issues relevant in social work training. Given the role of animals in the world of some clients, AAT can help the client further build ethical strength into the clients' whole experience.

Finally, the Equine-Assisted Growth and Learning Association (Eagala), builds equine wellness and welfare into its Code of Ethics through its Ethics Committee (Eagala, 2017). This author is currently engaged in a project with the explicit role of extending information and educating members on issues of equine welfare and wellness and the continuing application of its principles and practice. Equine welfare and wellness will continue to be a component of outreach and training, including continuing education for certification. With 4,500 Eagala members in 50 countries, the reach of this initiative is truly global. It demonstrates the growth of equine-assisted programs worldwide and the importance of making the ethical consideration of equine welfare and wellness central to this work.

DESCRIPTION OF INTERVENTION: THE PATH OF LIFE

Goals

1. Increase awareness of personal strengths and self-efficacy to support self-expression.
2. Learn verbal and non-verbal social skills and communication with others to meet needs and wants.

3. Learn and practice mindfulness techniques to integrate into daily experience.
4. Use mindfulness techniques to practice affect regulation and express feelings.

Objectives

With guidance clients will:

5. Practice awareness to stay personally safe, helping keep group members and horses safe.
6. Practice using a numerical scale of subjective experience to communicate and regulate affect.
7. Safely participate in the steps of a group experience with equines.
8. Give and receive feedback during and after the experience.

Materials Needed

- Arena or similar space in which 1–2 groups of clients and several horses can move about safely.
- Assorted props such as poles, swim noodles, cones, plastic barrels, etc.
- Halters, lead ropes of various lengths, or optional baling twine, yarn, ribbon, etc.

Step by Step—Pre-teaching

The first three pre-teaching steps integrate mindfulness practice directly into the experience. They can be taught prior to or during the session and adapted by clients outside the sessions in daily life.

1. Pre-teach: Safety Pledge, from Adventures in Awareness (2017).
    - "This is a safety pledge we take to keep ourselves safe and help keep everyone and the horses safe when we go in the arena. I will say it so you can hear it, and then we will all say it together."
    - "I [say your name] pledge to keep myself safe so I can help keep the group safe and the horses safe."
    - "OK, does everyone agree?" Get a yes from all who participate.
    - "OK, I will say the pledge now a few words at a time. You repeat after me and say your name instead of mine."
    - Repeat the pledge in short phrases with the clients repeating after you until the group completes the pledge.
    - Tell clients now the can do what they need to do to keep themselves safe. Remind and encourage them to be mindful to help others and the horses.
    - Refer to the pledge as an intervention if necessary during the experience to help clients be mindful.
2. Pre-teach: 360-Degree (Situational) Awareness
    - "Did you know that horses can see around them almost 360 degrees? Like, in a full circle, except just behind their tail." It helps them know what is going on around them at all times." Demonstrate. Have clients demonstrate.
    - Demonstrate peripheral vision, with arms straight out to sides where you can look straight ahead and still see your fingers moving in your peripheral vision out of both eyes.
    - Have clients practice this. Call it "soft eyes."
    - Tell them to be looking with "soft eyes" at what they are doing but still be aware of other things happening around them during sessions.
    - Check with clients during sessions to reinforce the use of "their 360." Use it as a preventative intervention when necessary.
3. Pre-teach: 0–10 subjective scale of experience (e.g., Crandall, Lammers, Senders, Savedra, & Braun, 2007).
    - "This is an easy way to express your feelings, or anything that is going on for you. For example, you might be very happy on your birthday. How happy? Or you might be anxious or afraid. How afraid? It's easy to tell someone when you pick a number from 0 to 10 with 0 meaning "not at all" and 10 meaning "extreme, very much, a volcano erupting!"
    - Move from example situations to, for example, fear of horses, others, etc., eliciting client responses.
    - Tell clients you will check in with them from time to time and this makes it easy and quick.
    - Use the scale as a mindfulness intervention throughout the session.
    - Tell clients they can use the scale as a "360" for how they are doing "inside," checking in with themselves.

THE PATH OF LIFE DESCRIPTION

The Path of Life is a group experience of the Equine Pathfinders Foundation at Dune Lakes Lodge, Helensville, New Zealand. It is often chosen during Kids Camp, a week-long residential camp for school-aged children and youth of mixed ages, genders, ethnicities, and cultural backgrounds. It is easily adapted for individual, couple, and family sessions. Tell clients:

1. Imagine what is ahead of them in their lives. This is their Path of Life. It may be something they want to do when they grow up or a character trait they want to develop, anything.
2. Consider what might be possible challenges or obstacles along their Path.
3. They will build a Path of Life together, including its obstacles and challenges, using any of the props available. Then they will choose a horse to lead down the path.
4. Everyone gets a turn leading the horse down "their" path.
5. The leader will have help from the rest of the group.
6. Each person will have a role. Their role will change each time it is someone else's turn.
7. Clients then create the Path and choose a horse. Intervene as necessary during this step using the mindfulness practices and subjective scale as a base to maintain flow.
8. Support clients to help them become mindful of flow, maintaining it, or re-establishing it. For example, ask:
   - What do you need to do to keep going? To make it better?
   - On a scale of 0–10, what is your [fear, frustration, anger] number right now?
9. Show clients their roles for leading the horse on the Path. A basic list of roles for a four-person group is:
   - One leader
   - One left-side walker
   - One right-side walker
   - One driving (leading) from behind.
10. Describe the order of go, or rotation. Example:
11. Clockwise around horse, after one turn on the Path:
    - Leader moves to right-side walker
    - Right-side walker moves to driving from behind
    - Driver moves to left-side walker
    - Left-side walker moves to leader.
12. Interventions and debriefs.

At any time, any client may ask to stop the process with the word "Stop" in the interest of the safety of the group or a horse, or their own physical or emotional safety. After each turn of the Path, clients can share feedback on what worked for them to help others. Sample questions to ask at any time including a final debrief after all turns on the Path:

- What was the best part of this experience? What was the hardest part?
- What worked the best to get through the obstacles?
- What did you learn about yourself? What did you learn about being in a group?
- How was it different at the end from how it was at the beginning?
- How can you behave as a good group member?

MULTICULTURAL AND ETHICAL GUIDELINES FOR CLIENTS

At Intake

Request that clients and/or their parents list or discuss any issues of a multicultural nature. Make adjustments. Ethical standards of practice regarding multicultural issues should already be a working part of any professional facilitation and its policies and procedures.

In session:

- Add volunteers that increase diversity of staff.
- Make speaking in the group about personal experience optional.

- Allow for privately speaking.
- A hand gesture or other "stop sign" can support privacy with no explanation needed.
- Leave open the opportunity for 1:1 guidance and assistance during session with trusted staff.
- Provide a least restrictive environment in a way that supports every individual's participation without being labeled. For example, the Path of Life takes place in a "Kids Camp" week in which some campers are referred by the New Zealand Ministry of Vulnerable Children or are otherwise involved in Ministry services. All personal information about attendees is kept confidential.
- Sessions themselves offer training and practice in resolving interpersonal issues. Learned mindfulness and other practices can be implemented in the here and now when multicultural and other issues arise.

MULTICULTURAL ETHICAL GUIDELINES FOR EQUINES

It is this author's view that equines live in their own culture. From this culture, we can learn how to keep and manage horses for their own benefit. This is an ethical responsibility that needs to be embodied in policies and procedures for the safety and well-being of all equines on a daily basis. Managing horses and involving them in session work from this lens not only benefits them, it can mitigate the possibility of harm to clients (Evans & Gray, 2012; Walker et al., 2015).

Before Session

- Attend to basic horse-keeping needs; check for condition, injury, and soundness.
- Select horses that are fit emotionally and experienced for the session plan.
- Aggressive biting or kicking equines should not be involved in any session.
- Plan session to allow for number of horses, proximity, available space, and number and make-up of clients.

During Session

- At least one staff member observes horses and makes interventions regarding their physical and emotional safety and the safety of clients.
- At least one staff member monitors behavior of clients in the interest of injury or abuse of equines or clients in the session.

After Session

- Equine care regarding cool down, grooming, watering, feeding, and turnout, with check of condition and soundness.

CASE EXAMPLES

This Path of Life session is a group experience facilitated in the Eagala model, which requires clean language without interpretation, with guided interventions for physical and emotional safety as well as learning by the group members during periods of debriefing. Client responses shown are a compilation. Quoted in-session and post-session responses are from the two actual clients below who took fictional names.

Kylie (a pseudonym) was brought up by her grandparents from infancy. An intelligent 15-year-old female in a championship school dance group who rated her social skills, confidence, and comfort with peers at 2 on a 0–10 scale. She became upset in groups easily and as a result was bullied in school, becoming school avoidant. She just "didn't fit in socially."

Fia (a pseudonym) is an intelligent 16-year-old female who sings and writes songs. She rated her comfort level around people at "negative 5… Shutting the world out was my general strategy in life." Her default was to become "stubborn" and "stroppy" even though she knew its effect on others, and became constantly anxious in this cycle. Consequences included school removal. Fia became a cutter.

Madeline (a pseudonym), despite being intelligent and caring was "burdened with stress from home," not comfortable at school, struggling to make friends. "I truly believed I would not go anywhere in life." She is in the care of her grandmother and has been hospitalized for previous periods of suicidality.

CONCLUSION

The Path of Life connects clients' internal resources and experience with their external experience moving forward in the here and now as positive change. Embodied in mindfulness, it teaches clients to respond in ways that enhance current experience rather than being stuck in ways that used to impair it.

The following transcript analysis are about a pseudonym clients.

Table 20.2

Transcript Analysis of Case Example

Transcript	*Analysis*
Facilitators: We are going to [facilitators describe the steps of the experience and its meaning]. Your first job is to come up with a name. Take a couple of minutes to decide together...What name did you choose?	Assess clients' and horses' participation and group dynamic. Answer clients' questions about the steps. Choosing the name allows for increased personal interest in the session. Facilitate the discussion if necessary.
Clients: The Path of Life! Yeah, the Path of Life! Yeah.	Clients appear to express varying levels of engagement evidenced by their verbal and non-verbal communication.
Facilitators: OK great! Let's review the safety pledge. Name one thing you are going to do to be safe. How will you help others and the horses be safe?	Interventions for physical and emotional safety. Naming mindfulness practices for a client if necessary; group mindfulness practice such as breathing together for five deep, long breaths to calm group process.
Clients: *One client repeats the pledge from memory.* I am going to use my 360! I am going to stay calm.	Clients expressing answers to group, this is further opportunity to assess individuals and group process, as well as to focus clients for the experience.
Facilitators: OK then, let's do it, you have ten minutes to create the Path.	Time structure allows best use of the time scheduled for the session, and helps clients practice focus when there is a time limit for their activity.
Facilitators similarly guide clients through steps of choosing a horse, bringing them to the Path, and finding their roles for the first turn. **Facilitators:** How is the horse doing folks? What is the horse telling us?	The horse is fidgety, ears flicking, head up, Children are excited, verbal, and moving quickly. Group intervention is needed. This begins the intervention and begins to focus the group.
Clients: He is getting nervous. We are all crowding around him yelling.	Clients are bringing their awareness into focus, becoming mindful of their impact.
Facilitator: What can you do to change things for him? And yourselves?	Leading the clients into their own mindfulness intervention.

Transcript	*Analysis*
Clients: We can just slow down and breathe.	Clients have found the intervention and are guided to it by facilitators, practicing their own intervention. They become calmer. The session continues with the first go through the Path, as practice.
Facilitator: How was that? Each role, tell how it was and how you think it might be better.	This is individual critique but in group context so it serves group goal as well as support for individual expression.
Client, Kylie: If you say "follow my voice" instead of telling me to go left or go right, it will be a lot easier, and less confusing.	Client feels safe and confident enough after completing the first turn to give individual feedback to the group.
Facilitators manage successive turns on the Path, clients generating their own feedback to each other about the roles.	Minimal intervention is made as clients claim more ownership of the experience. Readiness to intervene for physical or emotional safety is maintained.
Client, Fia: *Leaves group to stand in corner at the rail facing outside the arena, scowling.* It's too crazy and confusing, I can't handle it.	Client is expressing social anxiety and choosing default response, but not completely abandoning situation.
Facilitator: What is your anxious number now? I am so glad you stayed in the arena. What can you do to lower it and stay present?	Facilitator supports client expression of anxiety and choice to remain physically present, and to assume responsibility for lowering anxiety and staying emotionally present.
Client, Fia: My number is off the charts. Thank you, I do want to stay. *Makes brief eye contact, is breathing deeper.* I can take a "time out" and walk back to my spot doing my breathing. I know it's empty now and the group needs me.	Client is becoming emotionally present with support from the facilitator and exercising choice to engage in a mindfulness technique as a self-care intervention in the here and now. Client expresses awareness of group connection.
Facilitator calls group into circle for debrief and closure.	Opens opportunity for clients to give their experience as an individual and a group member a voice.
Client, Kylie: It felt good to be more confident and help and lead others. Learning to respect and trust myself and everyone and to cooperate, like how we had to communicate better to build the Path and go through it. I realized I know more than I thought I did, and I could help others with what I learn. It felt better at the end including everyone and figuring out how to make it work. And then being able to put the right kind of energy into it.	Client expresses her gains in self-confidence and resultant gains in social skills and communications.
Client, Fia: I went from confused to calm. We'd done something, we achieved something, and I was part of it. I felt more connected to everybody. Every time we started I'd be nervous and every time I'd come out feeling better about myself and more centered in my own space. I had to respond instead of automatically overthinking it. That really helped me more than anything. Hey, it doesn't have to be terrifying. I can even be a leader and help with things.	Client expresses enhanced personal centeredness and social comfort, resulting in greater connection to the group and contribution to its achievement.
Client, Madeline: I gained more confidence in myself; like I can do more than I thought I could; I became a stronger person; learned how to behave around horses and feel better around new people; I feel like a better person; yeah, learned how to deal with difficult situations in life; look, I am smiling more and more!	Client expresses increased self-efficacy, social comfort, improved mood, confidence with and learning how to handle difficult social situations.

The following sample group session note are about a pseudonym clients.

EAP GROUP SESSION NOTE FOR: Kids Camp A, K, M, Ak, D, M, M2, F
Date: 16/2/17 **Time:** afternoon **Weather:** fine, warm, slightbreeze
Staff: RP, RWJ
Outside Staff: Volunteers N, A
Horses/Equines: Bailey, Sienna, Texas
EXPERIENCE: The Path of Life. 1) Create Path; 2) Name Path; 3) Choose horse; 4) Take Roles; 5) TakeTurns through the Path Forward

Clients	*Horse(s)*
Beginning Clients milling, circled up somewhat listless (heat?) Wake up nicely when describing session. A, K, M pipe up on how to keep safe. F- attending? Less active as others go at it to build path.	Horses quiet in shade at east end of arena. Notice when Cts start creating Path, Bailey moves further away but with T and S.
Middle Clients esp M2, D, Ak, loud, quick, somewhat off task esp as horse and roles are chosen, everyone else excited but focused, raising voices. Intervention for calm—A and M suggest breathing "we just need to slow down and breathe." First round goes ok. F walks away from group rigidly. Says she can't handle the confusion. Private intervention—walking, moving, breathing, being aware of anxiety number to bring it down. Rejoins group after two minutes or so. Group is highly engaged for The Desert. Sharing planning and gamesmanship. Focused, aware of environment and each other, positive, light.	Horses stir, ears flicking, bodies turn towards group. B and T hang back,S is chosen . S starts swishing tail, moving feet, flicking tail as group moves around her, head goes up, eyes widen. S calms down when given space and quiet. S follows quietly on slack lead rope except for a couple of starts and a stop. T and B step away from the rail and take a few steps around with S from time to time, smell props, etc.
End Lots of group focus, calmer, quieter, smiles in finishing around of the path	Horses are calm and quiet as they leave the

Assessment: Good feedback from debrief. M2 seems low energy. F appears more relaxed and connected. See individual notes

Plan: Continue regular camp schedule. Group is performing. Check in with M2 on energy, F on anxiety.

By: ***Date:***

FIG. 20.1. Sample Group Session Note.

EAP GROUP SESSION NOTE FOR:

Date: **Time:** **Weather:**

Staff:

Outside Staff:

Horses/Equines

EXPERIENCE:

Clients	*Horse(s)*
Beginning	
Middle	
End	

Assessment:

Plan:

By: ***Date:***

FIG. 20.2. Blank Group Session Note.

REFERENCES

Adventures in Awareness. (2017). *Resources, Purpose Statement.* Retrieved from www.adventuresinawareness.net/purpose.ht.

Brown, K. W., Ryan, R. M., & Creswell, J. D. (2007). Mindfulness: Theoretical foundations and evidence for its salutary effects. *Psychological Inquiry 18*(4), 211–237.

Crandall, M., Lammers, C., Senders, C., Savedra, M., & Braun, J.V. (2007). Initial validation of a numeric zero to ten scale to measure children's state anxiety. *Anesthesia and Analgesia 105*(5), 1250–1253.

Eagala. (2017). Retrieved from www.eagala.org.

Evans, N. & Gray, C. (2012). The practice and ethics of animal-assisted therapy with children and young people: Is it enough that we don't eat our co-workers? *British Journal of Social Work 42*(4), 600–617.

Illmer, A. (2017). What's behind New Zealand's shocking youth suicide rate? Retrieved from www.bbc.com/news/world-asia-40284130.

McLeod, S. A. (2013). *Kolb—Learning Styles.* Retrieved from www.simplypsychology.org/learning-kolb.html.

NIMH. (2017a). *NIMH Answers Questions About Suicide.* Retrieved from www.nimh.nih.gov/health/publications/nimh-answers-questions-about-suicide/index.shtml.

NIMH. (2017b). *Suicide.* Retrieved from www.nimh.nih.gov/health/statistics/suicide/index.shtml.

Ozen, L. J., Gibbons, C. & Bédard, M. (2016). Mindfulness-based cognitive therapy improves depression symptoms after traumatic brain Injury. In S. J. Eisendrath (Ed.), *Mindfulness-Based Cognitive Therapy: Innovative Applications* (pp.31–45). New York: Springer.

Signal, T. D., Kemp, K., Botros, H., Taylor, N. & Prentice. K. (2013). Equine facilitated therapy with children and adolescents who have been sexually abused: A program evaluation study. *Journal of Child and Family Studies, 23*(3), 558–566.

Trotter, K. S., Chandler, C. K., Goodwin-Bond, D., & Casey, J. (2008). A comparative study of the efficacy of group equine assisted counseling with at-risk children and adolescents (abstract). *Journal of Creativity in Mental Health, 3*(3), 254–284.

Walker, P., Aimers, J., & Perry, C. (2015). Animals and social work: An emerging field of practice for Aotearoa New Zealand. *Aotearoa New Zealand Social Work Review 27*(1), 24–35.

21

Teaching Social Skills and Communication to Adolescents through Equine Interventions

Phyllis Erdman and Sue Jacobson

INTRODUCTION: THEORETICAL APPROACH

Social and emotional competence is increasingly being recognized as an effective way to build resilience in adolescents and is gaining support in practice, policy, and research. In fact, many states have now drafted or implemented social and emotional learning goals in their educational standards as a way to promote social and emotional competence in children (LeBuffe, Ross, Fleming, & Naglieri, 2013). In the National Association of School Psychologists (NASP) Model for Comprehensive and Integrated School Psychological Services (2010), one of the core competencies for school psychologists is providing effective services to help children and youth succeed academically, socially, behaviorally, and emotionally. School psychologists are also expected to understand and identify risk and protective factors, and promote overall wellness in students (www.nasponline.org/standards-and-certification/nasp-practice-model/about-the-nasp-practice-model).

Research shows that students in well-implemented social emotional learning programs showed positive outcomes compared to students in control groups in a wide range of domains (Durlak, Weissberg, Dymnicki, Taylor, & Schellinger, 2011). We also know that good communication accompanied by skills in problem-solving, taking responsibility, and decision-making all contribute to positive interrelationships. Additionally, children's ability to express emotions, ask for help when needed, and maintaining an optimistic view of life experiences all contribute to enhanced self-concept, which in turn serves as a protective measure to increase resiliency and can buffer children from adverse experiences (Rak & Patterson, 1996).

RATIONALE FOR USING EQUINE-ASSISTED INTERVENTIONS

Research has shown that equine-assisted interventions have a positive impact on children's adjustment in various socio-emotional, cognitive, and behavioral domains (Bowers & MacDonald, 2001); positive behaviors (Chandler, 2005; Pendry, Roeter, Smith, Jacobson, & Erdman, 2013); behavioral and mood disorders (Mann & Williams, 2002); self-esteem (Brown & Alexander, 1991; Gatty, 2001); feelings of social acceptance and peer popularity (MacDonald and Cappo, 2003); interpersonal communication (MacDonald, 2004); anger (Kaiser, Spence, Lavergne & Vanden Bosch, 2004); and social competence, specifically self-awareness, self-management, personal responsibility, decision-making, goal-directed behavior, and relations skills (Pendry & Roeter, 2013). When compared to more traditional, classroom-based counseling activities, equine-assisted interventions are more strongly associated with lower levels of internalizing and externalizing behavioral problems in young children (Trotter, Chandler, Goodwin-Bond & Casey, 2008). Bachi, Terkel, and Teichman (2012) looked at the impact of an equine-facilitated psychotherapy program on self-control, self-image, trust, and general life satisfaction in an Israeli school that included a stable. They found that there was trend in improvement in these areas.

Lentini and Knox (2009) suggest that animal-assisted programs, particularly equine-facilitated psychotherapy (EFP) programs, are effective at decreasing anger, depression, dissociation, and aggression as well as increasing self-esteem, self-confidence, attention-span, and social interaction. Hence, evidence exists for incorporating equine interventions into programs designed to help children build social emotional skills, thus leading toward overall improved social competence.

CASE EXAMPLE

Jerry (a pseudonym) was a 13-year-old eighth grader, who was referred to our EFP program by the school counselor for behavioral issues, primarily acting out in class and refusing to follow directions. He had been living with his grandparents for the past year, following the recent drug-related death of his mother. His parents divorced when he was four and his mother had been his custodian parent. However, he stayed with various relatives off and on following the divorce due to his mother's continued drug-related problems and inability to care for him. He had very little contact with his father, and saw him about once a year during brief visits. Both Jerry and his grandfather, Joe, were interviewed prior to starting the program to inquire about what they wanted to obtain by Jerry's participation in EFP, and then again following completion of the program. Joe was getting very frustrated with Jerry's lack of follow-through and continuous problems at school, and he was feeling resentful that he had such a huge responsibility at this point in his life; however, he loved his grandson very much. It was clear that Jerry was sensing the burden that his grandparents were feeling. We selected Jerry for the program thinking that the exposure to our program and to the horses would help him understand how his behaviors and communication style were affecting others, and to take more responsibility in making choices about his behaviors. Below is the assessment and plan for this session. This was our third session with Joe and Jerry out of a total of nine.

The following assessment/session plan are about a pseudonym client.

PATH to Success

Client Assessment/Session plan

Participant's Name: Joe and Jerry

School personnel's description of child's behaviors during the school day:
Doesn't pay attention in class; disruptive; doesn't follow directions

Parent's description of child's behaviors at home:
He is lazy; doesn't do what he is asks; is rude.

Significant health issues, including any required medication. None

Please check any past/present/impending circumstances in the family:
(Check all that apply)

X divorce	X frequent relocations	physical/sexual abuse
remarriage	eating disorders	attempted/completed suicide
X legal problems	psychiatric disorder	debilitating/terminal illness
X alcohol/drug abuse	X financial crisis	other ____________

Has this child ever attempted suicide or harmed her/himself in any way?
X No Yes (explain)

Is there any reason to believe this child is currently thinking about suicide or harming her/himself in any way
X No Yes (explain)

Has this child ever harmed anyone else, or had thoughts, or made threats about harming anyone else?
X No Yes (explain)

Has this child ever harmed an animal, or had thoughts, or made threats about harming an animal?
X No Yes (explain)

Is this child currently being treated by a mental health provider?
No X Yes (explain) Meets regularly with school counselor; also, sees outside counselor

What are three things that parents would like to see change.

1. More respect shown to us
2. Do his schoolwork and not have to be asked all of the time
3. Get better grades

Planned Intervention for this session:
We decided it was best to have Joe and Jerry work together in the program, since many of their problems stemmed from their own relationship. We wanted Joe and Jerry to work together with the horses to help improve their relationship and communication; to help build teamwork; to help each understand the other one better.

Post Session Summary
Joe and Jerry paid attention to each other and worked toward a common goal—moving the horse. They also seemed to understand that responding to a gentle request was easier and more helpful than yelling or nagging at the horse. They were able to connect this to their own interactions, as well as with others.

FIG. 21.1. Client Assessment/Session Plan.

The following is a sample of the initial meeting with Joe and Jerry as co-participants.
The following transcript analysis are about a pseudonym client.

Table 21.1
Transcript Analysis of Case Example

Transcript	*Analysis*
Initial interview with client Jerry	
Counselor: What do you hope to gain from participation in this program other than how to ride a horse? **Client:** To be nicer to people.	Counselor wanted to understand what client hoped to gain from the program other than learning how to ride.
Counselor: Tell me more about that **Client:** People are always getting on my case and it makes me mad. I get frustrated and do not want to do anything they ask me to do. And then they just keep getting madder at me.	Client is aware, at one level, how others perceive him, but is unable to articulate his underlying feelings and frustration.
Counselor: What do you know about horses? **Client:** They're big and they can get what they want from people who ride them... because of their size and how strong they are.	Client sees power over his actions as something good, but probably seems powerless in his own life. Learning how horses communicate what they want and how humans can communicate to horses will help him gain control over his behaviors in a positive way.
Counselor: How about if you learned how to communicate with a horse (e.g., how to move a 1,200 pound horse with just your finger)? **Client:** Pretty cool. I'd like to see how that works.	We trying to help the client understand that pushing and throwing your size around is not the way to get what you want, and that there are easier more socially acceptable ways to ask for what you want.
Initial interview with client Joe	
Counselor: What do you hope Jerry gains from the program? **Client:** He needs someone to show him the right and wrong way. I try to do that, but I feel like I keep saying the same things over and over... like I'm really nagging.	His grandad is frustrated because he knows what he wants Jerry to do, but does not know how to get him to do it. Having both participate will help them gain an understanding of their behaviors toward each other.

DESCRIPTION OF INTERVENTION AND SESSION GOAL

The goal of this session was to help Joe and Jerry learn more effective and respectful communication techniques. This would not only help in their interpersonal relationship, but also help Jerry learn how to communicate with others more clearly and respectfully, which should improve his social relationships. The objective was to learn to communicate with the horse using four levels of firmness in cuing the horse to move its hindquarters a step or two to the side. Materials needed are a halter, lead rope, and grooming kit.

At this point in the program, Jerry and Joe were comfortable working with the horse and had started to form a bond with the horse. With the horse haltered and tied, they spent a few minutes grooming the horse together. The horse activities always start with grooming, which helps the participants become comfortable and helps toward building a relationship with the horse. After grooming, Joe and Jerry were asked to bring the horse to the center of the arena. The equine specialist told them they were going to try to get the horse to move its back feet a step or two sideways without moving the front feet. Jerry and Joe were asked how they might do this and how the horse might perceive their technique. Is it fair, rude, polite, understood, confusing, nagging, etc.? The equine specialist explained the concept of using levels of firmness to communicate starting with a very light cue and increasing incrementally until the horse gives the desired response. These can be thought of as "suggest, ask, tell and insist." The equine specialist also stressed that as soon as the horse gives the desired response the pressure should be stopped. Using their fingers (rather than a flat palm), Jerry and Joe would each get the horse to move its hindquarters by going through the following phases: press the hair (suggest), press the skin (ask), press the muscle (tell), and press the bone (insist). Questions were then asked to Jerry and Joe: Which phase caused the horse to move? Did it take more or less pressure than you thought to get the horse to move? Now try it again. This time did the horse move sooner or later than last time? Why do you think this is? Did the horse seem to be paying attention to you? How does this relate to how you might communicate with each other/another person?

At the conclusion of the nine-week program, we interviewed Jerry and Joe again. Fortunately, we were beginning to see evidence that they were connecting the lessons they learned in the equine program to their interactions with others.

Table 21.2

Transcript Analysis of Case Example Continued

Transcript	*Analysis*
Post interview with clients	
Counselor: What did you each learn from participation in the program? **Client, Jerry:** How to work together. Also, how to be more respectful. I think Grandpa learned how to be calmer too when he talks to me now **Client, Joe:** I realized I nag a lot. Like when you taught us to move the horse, and use the four phases, you started out so gently, but then added more pressure if they didn't move. That makes sense.	Both clients learned respect by interacting with such a large animal, yet not forcing the horse to do things. Grooming also helped them connect emotionally to the horse, and to each other.
Counselor: Tell me more about you think it changed the way you interact with your grandpa or with others. **Client, Jerry:** I think I follow directions more. I realize I frustrate people, so it seems like if I cooperate more, they treat me better. **Client, Joe:** He didn't get to go to a friend's house because he didn't clean his room, but he knew that and accepted it. He took more ownership for his behaviors	Jerry learned about taking responsibility for his behaviors, and that he has choices. He also realized changing his behaviors allows others to change their reactions to him in more positive ways. Joe learned that he could stop nagging so much and let Jerry learn the consequences of his behaviors.

PATH to Success
Client Assessment/Session Plan

Participant's Name:

School personnel's description of child's behaviors during the school day:

Parent's description of child's behaviors at home:

Significant health issues, including any required medication.

Please check any past/present/impending circumstances in the family:
(check all that apply)

divorce	frequent relocations	physical/sexual abuse
remarriage	eating disorders	attempted/completed suicide
legal problems	psychiatric disorder	debilitating/terminal illness
alcohol/drug abuse	financial crisis	other ___________________

Has this child ever attempted suicide or harmed her/himself in any way?
No Yes (explain)

Is there any reason to believe this child is currently thinking about suicide or harming her/himself in any way?
No Yes (explain)

Has this child ever harmed anyone else, or had thoughts, or made threats about harming anyone else?
No Yes (explain)

Has this child ever harmed an animal, or had thoughts, or made threats about harming an animal?
No Yes (explain)

Is this child currently being treated by a mental health provider?
No Yes (explain)

What are three things that parents would like to see change.
1.
2
3.

Planned intervention for this session

Post Session Summary

FIG. 21.2. Client Assessment/Session Plan—Blank.

REFERENCES

Bachi, K., Terkel, J. & Teichman, M. (2012). Equine-facilitated psychotherapy for at-risk adolescents: The influence on self-image, self-control and trust. *Clinical Child Psychology and Psychiatry, 17*(2), 298–312.

Bowers, M. J. & MacDonald, P. M. (2001). The effectiveness of equine-facilitated psychotherapy with at-risk adolescents: A pilot study. *Journal of Psychology and Behavioral Sciences, 15*, 62–76.

Brown, L. & Alexander, J. (1991). *Self Esteem Index Examiner's Manual.* Austin, TX: Pro-Ed.

Chandler, C. (2005). *Animal Assisted Therapy in Counseling.* New York: Routledge.

Durlak, J. A., Weissberg, R. P., Dymnicki, A. B., Taylor, R. D., & Schellinger, K. B. (2011). The impact of enhancing students' social and emotional learning: A meta-analysis of school-based universal interventions. *Child Development, 82*, 405–432.

Gatty, C. M. (2001). Psychosocial impact of therapeutic riding: A pilot study. *Equine-Facilitated Mental Health Association, 5*(2), 8.

Kaiser, L., Spence, L. J., Lavergne, A. G., & Vanden Bosch, K. L. (2004). Can a week of therapeutic riding make a difference? A pilot study. *Anthrozoos, 17*, 63–72.

LeBuffe, P. A., Ross, K. M., Fleming, J. L., & Naglieri, J. A. (2013). The Devereux Suite: Assessing and promoting resilience in children ages 1 month to 14 years. In S. Prince-Embury and D. H. Saklofske (Eds), *Resilience in Children, Adolescents, and Adults: Translating Research into Practice* (pp. 45–59). New York: Springer Science.

Lentini, J. A. & Knox, M. (2009). A qualitative and quantitative review of equine facilitate psychotherapy (EFP) with children and adolescents. *The Open Complementary Medicine Journal, 1*, 51–57.

MacDonald, P. M. (2004). *The Effects of Equine-Facilitated Therapy With At-Risk Adolescents: A Summary of Empirical Research Across Multiple Centers and Programs.* The Center for the Interaction of Animals and Society (CIAS). Philadelphia: University of Pennsylvania School of Veterinary Medicine. Retrieved from www2.vet.upenn.edu/research/center/cias/pdf/CIAS_AAI_white_paper.pdf.

MacDonald, P. M. & Cappo, J. (2003). Equine-facilitated therapy with "at-risk" youth: Does it work? *Strides, 9*, 30–31.

Mann, D. & Williams, D. (2002). *Equine Assisted Family Therapy for High-Risk Youth: Defining a Model of Treatment and Measuring Effectiveness.* Unpublished manuscript.

National Association of School Psychologists (NASP). (2010). Model for Comprehensive and Integrated School Psychological Services. Retrieved from www.nasponline.org/standards-and-certification.

Pendry, P. & Roeter, S. (2013). Experimental trial demonstrates positive effects of equine facilitated learning on child social competence. *Human-Animal Interaction Bulletin, 1*(1), 1–19.

Pendry, P., Roeter, S. M., Smith, A. N., Jacobson, S., & Erdman, P. (2013). Trajectories of positive and negative behavior during participation in equine facilitated growth and learning program for horse-novice youth. *Journal of Extension, 51*(1), 1R1B5.

Rak, C. F. & Patterson, L. E. (1996). Promoting resilience in at-risk children. *Journal of Counseling and Development, 74*(4), 368–373.

Trotter, K. S., Chandler, C. K., Goodwin-Bond, D., & Casey, J. (2008). A comparative study of the efficacy of group equine assisted counseling with at-risk children and adolescents. *Journal of Creativity in Mental Health, 3*, 254–284.

22

EQUINE-ASSISTED SOCIAL EDUCATION AS A CO-INTERVENTION TO PREVENT DROPOUT BY IMPROVING SOCIAL SKILLS AND ENGAGEMENT IN LEARNING

Ritva Mickelsson

INTRODUCTION

The purpose of this chapter is to give an example of how a school-based program involving horses worked together with mental health professionals to engage pupils in assigned mental health care sessions and to decrease dropout. By using equine-assisted social education, the goal was to improve social skills, motivation, and learning.

Growing interest toward horses in human mental and social rehabilitation around the world, as well as meeting social, emotional, psychological, and mental health needs of young persons are underlined in the social schemas of many Western countries. In Finland, equine-assisted activities have been recognized as a method of care, education, and rehabilitation for pupils with various special needs. Some of these young people are the ones who dropped out from school. While a variety of adolescence programs have been established to support education and motivation, there have been persistent complications in reaching young people's continuous attention and actively and constructively getting them to participate in these programs (Slesnick, Meyers, & Meade, 2000; Stanton, Cole, & Galbraith, 2004) or the context of the school environment has not been suitable for the programs to meet their targets (Ringeisen, Henderson, & Hoagwood, 2003).

Dropping out of school and not achieving a diploma of basic education are factors that contribute to decreased success and well-being in life. Unemployment is more likely to be evident without a high school diploma. The cost of dropouts for a society consists of lower tax contributions, higher reliance on welfare and, in some cases, even higher rates of crime. In my earlier career, as a special education teacher, school dropouts were one group of pupils that I worked with. Each pupil had a story, making it easy to understand why learning and going to school were not part of their daily routines. I taught many of these pupils in their home, public library, or any other suitable place that would foster learning. I realized that a large part of these pupils' problems stemmed from difficulties in communication.

I wanted to improve communication and build trust, and it was also essential to improve their social skills and motivation towards learning. Good communication embraces willingness and was also bidirectional (Schüler, 2000). Because, I had experienced the value of equines building a bridge between a teacher and a pupil, I felt strongly that equine-assisted activities would be appropriate for these school dropouts I worked with. I found that once equine-assisted activities were introduced, communication and interaction between pupils and adults became more equal, natural, and open when horses were around. These were the times of real, spontaneous conversations, facing each other in a different way, with growing respect.

In 2002, the University of Eastern Finland created an equine-assisted activities program for professionals working in the fields of education, health, or social services. The program was called Equine-Assisted Social Education, and its purpose was to support the social growth and welfare of at-risk children, adolescents, and adults, through working in groups with horses. The equine-assisted activities provided a method for people who had various problems; for instance, social and psychic problems or difficulties integrating with communities or taking part in a group. It also provided children with a possibility to promote their own shared peer activities, to be empowered, and to experience nature. Another purpose of this program was to improve social skills and enhance self-esteem. The stable area, with its strict structure, provided a safe environment to participate in activities. The horse mirrored the feelings of clients and approached them, no matter what their background or capabilities.

BRIEF DESCRIPTION OF THE ISSUE/PROBLEM

School dropout is a health, economic, and social justice issue. Although the status dropout rate (representing the percentage of 16- to 24-year-olds not enrolled in school, and not having earned a high school diploma or similar certificate) had decreased during the past 15 years being 10.9% in 2000 and 5.9% in 2015 (National Center for Education Statistics, 2018), every dropout pupil was at risk. According to Freudenberg and Ruglis (2007) good education not only forecasted educational achievement but also predicted good health by enabling better income, guiding to health information, and helping to acquire social support, for example. Research suggested that health has direct and indirect effects on dropout rates, while mental illness and emotional disturbance were also significant reasons to quit school.

There have been numerous interventions to prevent dropout, and promising results were gained in programs engaging pupils in their schools and connecting them to caring adults. Other activities supporting pupils included opportunities for out-of-school programs and academic content that had relevance to the pupils. The sense of community was also related to the positive outcomes for pupils embracing advanced social skills, achievement, and motivation. The level of fulfillment of basic psychological needs (sense of belonging, autonomy, and competence) defined the degree of engagement with school (Battistich, Solomon, Watson, & Schaps, 1997), or increased the sense of well-being (Ryan & Deci, 2000, 2002).

When the situations of pupils and dropout interventions were complicated, it was inevitable to organize a multi-professional cooperational approach. A need for new methods and individual procedures aiming to open new activities and possibilities for the pupils, as well as supporting and motivating them to attend weekly sessions at psychiatric care, were also established.

DESCRIPTION OF INTERVENTION—EQUINE-ASSISTED SOCIAL EDUCATION

The objective of this program was to improve well-being and daily routines of two dropout middle school pupils. The purpose was to work in cooperation with mental health services (psychiatric health care for adolescents), engaging pupils to attend weekly sessions and meeting with their mental health professionals. Another purpose was to teach the learning tasks defined in curriculum to pass that school grade (Kjäldman, 2005).

Theoretical Approach

This intervention program was designed to support both social and life skill competence, as well as improving engagement in learning. The social emotional learning interventions guided pupils to join and become a member of the group. Interventions that involved empirical approaches with hands-on activities had more positive impact than those interventions with conversation or academic teaching and learning (January,

Casey, & Paulson, 2011). By the capability theory of Amartya Sen, education and capability were closely related (Saito, 2003). According to Sen's theory, the basis of adolescents' well-being in society were the following ideas:

1. Everyone possesses capabilities.
2. It is essential how these capabilities are practiced and how much freedom and possibilities for actions is given.
3. An own "voice" and values are the source of motivation (Palola, Hannikainen-Ingman, & Karjalainen, 2012).

In addition, experiencing positive things had an impact on human emotional health increasing ability to meet emotional difficulties. Active membership in social networks and feeling the group identity enabled to enhance health outcomes (Music, 2011).

We live and experience life through our "map" formed during the history of our life events. This map determines the meaning of words and experiences, largely at a subconscious level. Connection comes into being when meeting a person on his/her own map. If this connection is not real, the meaning of communication and signals is not correctly understood (Leitola, 2001). In this program, the shared map of the pupil and the teacher was built using equine-assisted activities. Motivating pupils to learn and engaging them with their tasks was easier when communication was clear, and messages were understandable. Equine activities generated pleasant experiences together with the teacher, and favorable outcomes in learning were possibly a result of positive changes and development of the pupils. Also, the behavior and concentration of the pupils were better in the stable environment.

RATIONAL FOR UTILIZING EQUINE-ASSISTED INTERACTIONS

Equine-assisted social education offered a tool for motivation, since the pupils were interested in animals. Because they both had skipped school for several months, a new source of motivation was needed. Despite the best efforts of the schools, the girls refused to continue in mainstream classes. Therefore, teaching and learning were also placed in the stable environment and in the kitchen of the house, where there were two dogs welcoming the pupils to "stable school" and who were present at the time of learning. Soon it was noticed that both pupils wanted to be around horses, so much so they were even willing to take public transportation to reach the stable and attend learning sessions. Maybe that helped them to also accept the idea of travelling by bus to attend weekly sessions in mental health care.

When I started working with these pupils, the fall term was already over, and they had missed almost half of the school year. I knew I needed to create a confidential relationship and get to know them well in order to succeed in the task I had taken on with them. My duty as a teacher was to inform the schools how learning was proceeding, and if the pupils were attending as we had planned. I was informed if the pupils were skipping their mental health meetings. In such a case, the pupils were offered only school subjects and learning, not equine activities. That happened only once. When it was understood that mental health services and equine-assisted activities were "one package", that they could not skip one and still participate in the other, participation in mental health weekly meetings became a routine.

Horses helped me to get to know the pupils quickly. That would not have been possible inside the school building in such a small time. Horses put us at the same level, which would not have been the case at school, where teacher has a strong role as "the boss" for the pupil. Being around the horses with the pupils and taking care of the horses, I had a chance to discuss and hear a lot of things, thoughts, and hopes that the pupil had at that time. This information helped me to plan their route through the comprehensive education and to the next level of education.

Ethical Issues in Animal-Assisted Therapy Programs

Involving animals in intervention programs sets certain ethical concerns for the counselor. The animals had to have appropriate protection, so that they were not pushed toward their physiological or psychological limits. In addition, the staff and clients were to minimize all possible risks and inconvenience for both the people and the animals. Counselors should know the animals and their methods of communication, and choose suitable animals for the program (Beck, 2000).

The pupils were reminded that equine-assisted interventions were voluntary. It was fine just to watch or take part in chosen activities, if that was what they wanted to do. There are always other ethical issues when working with special needs pupils. Some of the pupils could feel they were labelled, instead being part of mainstream pupils.

GUIDELINES IN IMPLEMENTING WITH CONSIDERATION OF MULTICULTURAL ISSUES AND ETHICS

The intervention program included equine-assisted social education as support for comprehensive education. The keywords of the method were *cooperation, function* (activities), and *experiences*. Activities included daily routines at the stable environment (mounted or not mounted, grooming, driving, feeding, watching the behavior of the horses in herd, maintaining the places, etc.). During these activities, horses were natural and practical "bridges" to create and develop human–equine bond, as well as human–human bond, based on faith and respect. With the assistance of horses, pupils confronted their own inner limits, and the horses helped them to overcome such limitations.

In this case, horse-handling was part of education, meaning it was free of charge for the pupils. Being with horses was enjoyable for the pupils, and it was a pleasure to see those pupils happy and feeling good, but at the same time I had to keep in mind that this intervention would be completed in the end of spring term. Equine-assisted activities and horseback-riding lessons were expensive in Finland due to the high cost of maintaining horses, especially in our area by the capital city. Equine activities and riding are considered luxury sport. Stable-owners could receive more positive social attention to their line of business by including equine-facilitated social rehabilitation among other activities at their stables. This would require educated counsellors and suitable horses for this kind of special work. Not all stables were able to welcome "at risk" pupils to participate in stable routines. There was much prejudice toward and misunderstanding of special pupils due the lack of trained personnel at the stables. To avoid such problems, the personnel and stable-owners needed to be guided into the therapeutic agenda and to be made aware of the benefits of this method, both to the special pupils and to their own stables as self-contained societies.

HOW TO IMPLEMENT THIS INTERVENTION

Treatment Goals

Two of the goals were to improve self-image and self-esteem. Teachers' and peers' roles for shaping pupils' self-image were essential when considering being compared to others both academically—considering capability and talent—or socially. Convenient experiences with horses let the pupils feel that they were successful, as horses did not criticize or point out the mistakes that had been made. As Korpinen (1990) noted in her research, the best things a teacher could offer the pupils were empathy, frankness, and unconditional positive approval. The quality of interaction was valuable with horses, since they were interested in the pupils, and taking care of horses was an enjoyable duty.

There ar six important factors to improve positive self-image when working with adolescents and offering equine activities:

4. Let the pupil feel that you are supporting them. Be there to help the pupil to begin the task. Let them try it by themselves first, being near and ready to help in needed.
5. Let the pupil feel they are responsible. Give them meaningful and significant tasks. Let them feel that they are an important part of the entity.
6. Let the pupil feel capable. Give them tasks that they can manage and thereby gain a sense of success.
7. Teach the pupil to set realistic goals. Plan equine activities and stable routines together. All the activities should involve objectives to be learned.
8. Help the pupil assess themselves realistically. Have a discussion with them after activities. Talk with them about the goals and tasks and how they felt they accomplished them. Let them think about various other ways to meet the goals.
9. Encourage the pupil for giving realistic self-praise. Teach them to find something positive and to be thankful for every day.
10. Start with equine activities, but transfer these ideas into daily routine.

Step-by-Step Description

1. **Planning:** When planning the session, have contact with mental health care professional (information of participation in weekly sessions, etc.), parents (information regarding how homework was done, if the pupil needed help, if there was progress in given projects, etc.), and school counselor (information and material for learning tasks, etc.). Decide which subjects to study at that session; plan and make study material.
2. **Arrival:** Meet and welcome the pupil at the door with dogs; have some snacks and a discussion about tasks that were done, daily routines to be accomplished, etc.
3. **Teaching and learning:** Go through homework and projects, give new homework.
4. **Getting ready to go out to the stable:** Plan what to do today; have conversation regarding who else would probably be there and how to face and greet them.
5. **Going to the stable:** Meet other people and have small talk with them.
6. **Choosing the horse to work with:** Discuss why the pupil made that decision.
7. **Grooming the horse:** Discuss the chosen topic (themes connected into this program quite often deal with self-confidence, decision-making, and self-support in addition to seeing positive opportunities in one's life).
8. **Riding or driving:** Attach school subjects in stable environment (mathematics, physics, ethics, chemistry, language, etc.).
9. **Ending equine session:** Take care of the horse and let him on pasture; have conversation about what went well, what felt good/would like to have more, what was uncomfortable and not wanted again, etc.
10. **Ending the session:** Remind about the next time and homework/other tasks.

The method of "solution-centered approach" was implemented during the intervention program. That meant there were multiple solutions for the problems. The concrete and realistic goals were created and settled with the pupil (Kemppinen, 1997). Equine-assisted social education was well-suited to this approach, while the focus was on personal resources. These strengths were helping adolescents' healthy growth and development. While it would have been challenging to become inspired about given goals, the adolescent's own hopes were the starting point when forming goals to be achieved during the process (Furman & Ahola, 1999).

Table 22.1

Furman's (1999) Six Steps for Development

Step 1	Finding an Interesting Goal • transferring your "faults" into goals • adding other goals • choosing a goal • predicting the benefits of chosen goal
Step 2	Mapping Your Resources • recognizing your strengths • noticing support and help from others • noticing new strengths • experiencing "disadvantages" as resources
Step 3	Defining Abilities and Know-How • recognizing abilities and skills • recalling former successes • assessing previous progress
Step 4	Setting a Project • reification of the goal • perceiving the change as a step-by-step process • giving an influential name or symbol to the goal
Step 5	Investing in Change • investing in achieving the goal • publishing the goal • asking support from others
Step 6	Confirming the Improvement • noticing gained improvement • constructive attitude toward setbacks

To increase motivation toward learning, the tasks and goals were created by the pupils themselves (Furman & Ahola, 1999). In the process of learning, the emphasis should be in situational learning, in which knowledge and skills were used in daily life. The more useful and pleasant the school is experienced as by the pupil, the more motivated and engaged in learning he will be (Kemppinen, 1997). In addition to developing oneself, the whole environment is developing during the process. Everyone who was interacting with the person in the program had an own share of this mental development (Furman & Ahola, 1999).

CASE EXAMPLE

Brief Description of Clients and Case History

There were two special education pupils in this program, both were girls with a history of dropping out. They were appointed to "private teaching lessons," which meant they were given school tasks to be studied at home and met with their teacher twice a week for three hours, altogether six hours a week.

Anna (a pseudonym) was a 16-year-old female. She repeated the ninth grade in middle school, which is the last grade of compulsory education in Finland. She had severe learning problems and was diagnosed in middle school as not being able to reach the goals of the normal curriculum. She had an individualized learning plan for all school subjects and was also released to study Swedish. Anna lived in an apartment house, so the stable environment by the national park with fresh air and exercise brought her vitality. She was diagnosed with depression and school phobia, and in the beginning of the fall term she had decided not to attend classes in her own school any more. She was assigned to have mental health services once a week but was not motivated to participate in the sessions. Anna also had weekly occupational therapy and her own support person from child care center. Despite loving animals, she was afraid of big animals like horses. Anna was overweight, her motoric capability was low, and she got out of breath after a short time walking. She did not want to mount a horse or work with big horses, but she liked the Shetland pony gelding, and chose to drive him.

Betty (a pseudonym) was in the eighth grade. Even though she was only 14 years of age, she looked older. She had enjoyed horseback-riding as a hobby when she was younger. She started to work with a Fjord mare, but that horse was not "challenging enough" for Betty. On the second time, she chose a Finnhorse gelding, which was faster and also better trained for dressage. There were understandable reasons for Betty to choose that Finnhorse, since she had been riding a lot with these national breed horses. She also "saw" something familiar in that gelding, since she had been taking care of the "half-brother" of that horse before.

Both Anna and Betty had "burnt their bridges" regarding schools and friends, making it impossible to organize teaching in their own schools.

ASSESSING THE PROGRAM

The goal of the program was to cooperate with mental health professionals as well as engage dropout pupils in learning. During the program, pupils became engaged in learning and planning for the future. They both had positive attitudes toward animals even before the intervention started. It was observed that the longer the intervention lasted, the stronger the engagement in learning, which could have been the product of the emotional reward that comes from working with horses. The role of the parents was also significant—their positive attitude and trust made it possible to succeed.

Equine interventions "demand" that pupils be trustful and responsible. They had to make decisions, and got daily routines with tasks to be reached every day. Both girls caught up and received their certificates for that school year. Feedback from parents, schools, and mental health professionals was positive and encouraging. Parents were relieved that the difficult situation of their child was being cleared up. Equine-assisted activities were well recognized by the mental health services, when Anna described with details all the situations and activities that were done at the stable. The therapist said later that equine-assisted activities were playing a significant part in her rehabilitation and increased functionality (Kjäldman, 2005).

Client: ____
Teacher/Counselor: ____________________________________

	In the beginning of the intervention	**In the end of the intervention**
What are the things, the client is capable of ?		
What are the clients character strengths (1-5)? https://www.viacharacter.org/www/		
What kind of other competence does the client have?		
What are the special interests of the client?		
What kind of situations were comfortable/easy for the client?		
What kind of situations were difficult for the client?		
In what areas/activities are difficult for the client?		
What kind of problems does the client have? How did these problems show up? Who observed the problems and in what kind of situations?		
When did, these problems begin?		
Have there been eras, when these problems did not exist?		

FIG. 22.1. Blank Client Session Note.

REFERENCES

Battistich, V., Solomon, D., Watson, M., & Schaps, E. (1997). Caring school communities. *Educational Psychologist, 32*(3), 137–151.

Beck, A. M. (2000). The use of animals to benefit humans: Animal-assisted therapy. In A. H. Fine (Ed.), *Handbook on Animal-Assisted Therapy: Theoretical Foundations and Guidelines for Practice* (pp. 21–40). San Diego: Academic Press.

Freudenberg, N. & Ruglis, J. (2007). Reframing school dropout as a public health issue. *Preventing Chronic Disease 4*(4).

Furman, B. & Ahola, T. (1999). *Solution-Oriented Self-Development.* Helsinki: Hakapaino.

January, A. M., Casey, R. J., & Paulson, D. (2011). A meta-analysis of classroom.Wide interventions to build social skills: Do they work? *School Psycology Review, 40*(2), 242–256.

Kemppinen, P. (1997). *Adolescent as a Prisoner By His/Her Own Self. Part I.* Vantaa: Kannustusvalmennus Oy.

Kjäldman, R. (2005). When I dropped out from school, I got up and mounted a horse. In S. Okulov & K. Koukkari (Eds.), *When Riding Pedagogy Turned Into Equine Assisted Social Education: The Basis and Implementation of Equine Assisted Social Education as Experienced in In-Service Training.* Kuopio: University of Kuopio.

Korpinen, E. (1990). Sense of selfhood experienced by comprehensive school pupils. *Research 34.* Research Center of Behavioral Sciences, publications A. University of Jyväskylä.

Leitola, K. (2001). *NLP for Learning.* Helsinki: Tammi.

Music, G. (2011). *Nurturing Natures.* Hove and New York: Psychology Press.

National Center for Education Statistics. (2018). Retrieved from https://nces.ed.gov/fastfacts/display.asp?id=16.

Palola, E., Hannikainen-Ingman, K., & Karjalainen, V. (2012). *Young Dropouts as Clients in Social Services: Case Study in Helsinki.* Helsinki: National Institute for Health and Welfare in Finland.

Ringeisen, H., Henderson, K., & Hoagwood, K. (2003). Context matters: School and the "research to practice gap" in children's mental health. *School Psychology Review, 32*(2), 153–168.

Ryan, R. M. & Deci, E. L. (2000). Self-determination theory and the facilitation of intrinsic motivation, social development, and well-Being. *American Psychologist, 55*(1), 68–78.

Ryan, R. M. & Deci, E. L. (2001). On happiness and human potentials: A review of research on hedonic and eucaimonic well-being. *Annual Review of Psychology, 52*, 141–166.

Ryan, R. M. & Deci, E. L. (2002). Overview of self-determination theory: An organismic dialectical perspective. In E. L. Deci & R. M. Ryan (Eds.), *Handbook of Self-Determination Research* (2nd edition, pp. 3–33). New York: University of Rochester Press.

Saito, M. (2003). Amartya Sen's capability approach to education: A critical exploration. *Journal of Philosophy of Education, 37*(1).

Schüler, T. (2000). Communication with horses: Mounted work and riding. *Kuratorium für Therapeutisches Reiten e.V.*

Slesnick, N., Meyers, R. J., & Meade, M. (2000). Bleak and hopeless no more: Engagement of reluctant substance-abusing runaway youth and their families. *Journal of Substance Abuse Treatment, 19*, 215–222.

Stanton, B., Cole, M., & Galbraith, J. (2004). Randomized trial of a parent intervention. *Archives of Pediatrics & Adolescent Medicine, 158*(10), 947–955.

Section 12

COUPLES AND FAMILY

23

Couples in Balance

Realigning Roles

Vallarie E. Coleman

INTRODUCTION

While many couples struggle with relationship challenges, having a partner with post-traumatic stress injury/disorder (PTSD) can exponentially increase marital difficulties (Khaylis, Polunsy, Erbes, Gewirtz, & Rath, 2011). In general, PTSD affects roughly 10% of women and 4% of men during their lifetime and about eight million adults will have PTSD in a given year (National Center for PTSD, 2016). According to the US Department of Veterans Affairs, for those in the military the rates are even higher—roughly 11–20% of veterans who served in Iraq or Afghanistan and as many as 30% of Vietnam veterans have PTSD (National Center for PTSD, 2016).

Research has found that avoidance and numbing symptoms of PTSD have the strongest correlation to interpersonal difficulties (Pietrzak, Goldstein, Malley, Rivers, & Southwick, 2010; Rodrigues, 2014; Weissman et al., 2017). This can take the form of detachment; diminished areas of interest; avoidance of activities, places, and social interaction; avoidance of thoughts, feelings, and conversations; and restricted affect, such as loss of joy or loving feelings. Not only do the symptoms associated with PTSD negatively impact the survivor, they also create emotional and interpersonal difficulty for significant others, often resulting in high levels of relationship discord and distress (Khaylis et al., 2011; Price & Stevens, 2017). Family violence, caregiver burden, compromised parenting, sexual problems, and aggression are common (Price & Stevens, 2017). Furthermore, relationship conflict has been found to exacerbate PTSD symptoms and negatively impact the survivor's recovery (Khaylis et al., 2011; National Center for PTSD, 2016; Taft et al., 2009).

Couples therapy is a complex undertaking that requires clinicians to attend to multiple levels of interactional and intrapsychic dynamics (Johnson, 2003). Attachment theory combined with an object-relations perspective provides a useful lens for understanding and treating couples. Attachment theory (Bowlby, 1988) postulates that "seeking and maintaining contact with significant others is an innate, primary motivating principle in human beings across the lifespan" (Johnson, 2003, p. 5). When loved ones, such as a spouse, are physically and emotionally available it provides a sense of love and security that helps individuals mitigate "undesirable emotional states" (Mikulincer & Shaver, 2007, p. 190). When an attachment figure is inattentive and non-responsive then emotional distress and dysregulation persist, leading to intense affective states such as anger, fear, and sadness (Rheem, Woolley, & Weissman, 2011). From an object-relations perspective, early internalized experiences of self and others are mental representations that are consciously and unconsciously played out in our adult relationships—particularly with romantic partners (Johnson, 2003). Understanding the ways in which these relational templates contribute to choice of partner and the resulting relational dynamics is an important factor in creating change. However, therapeutic change does not just result from insight; rather it is a "consequence of experiences that change procedural [implicit] memory" (Fonagy, 2001, p. 164).

RATIONALE FOR EQUINE-ASSISTED COUPLES THERAPY

As an experiential form of therapy, equine-assisted psychotherapy (EAP) is an effective mode of couples treatment that can serve as an adjunct to in-office sessions or stand on its own as a form of therapy. For couples struggling to overcome the impact of PTSD, EAP can be especially impactful due to the natural prey instincts of equines (e.g., horses or donkeys) and their fight-or-flight nature. A persuasive paradox for healing is how horses can be both "relaxed and ready" at the same time (Gunter, 2007, p. 20). Equines must maintain vigilance for survival while being able to graze, drink, and rest in the safety of the herd. These herd dynamics serve as a powerful model for trauma survivors who struggle to overcome hypervigilance and increase healthy dependence and improve communication with their significant others. The equines are invaluable co-therapists that provide non-judgmental, direct feedback though their non-verbal posture, proximity, and body movements. This is particularly effective with couples as they find that the equines quickly and clearly give them feedback about the adverse impact of their discord versus the favorable results of their congruent and collaborative interactions. When this feedback is harnessed by the therapist for reflection and interpretation it is often readily accepted.

There are any number of effective EAP exercises that can help couples to overcome the impact of PTSD and rebalance their relationship. Initial exercises should focus on building rapport between the couple, the therapist, and the equines. In the initial phase of treatment, the therapist gains an understanding of the clients' individual attachment styles and the impact of early experiences, and helps the partners to recognize and understand feedback from the equines. The couple participates in exercises that help deepen their awareness of negative relationship patterns and utilize skills that create positive connection with each other. The following exercise, Navigating a Day with PTSD, is one that can be implemented in the early to mid-phase of treatment.

DESCRIPTION OF INTERVENTION: NAVIGATING A DAY WITH PTSD

The goal of Navigating a Day with PTSD is for the couple to "let go" of negative interaction patterns and come together as a team to overcome challenges in their day-to-day relationship. The couple must effectively communicate and balance roles in order to move the horse/donkey through the obstacles without being pulled into unproductive, undesirable interactions and emotional states. Alternatively, this exercise can also be used as a relational assessment tool.

The materials needed are:

- one or more equines in an arena/paddock
- nine trot/ground poles
- one barrel
- one flag pole
- two rail razers
- six cones
- one halter
- a 12-foot lead rope and a 5.5–6-foot lead rope
- duct tape to write on
- a 3 × 5 index card
- a binder clip
- a sharpie.

Depending on the size of your area, either build the course ahead of time or have the materials ready and complete it when the couple are walking their equine. Identify the start and end zone for the course.

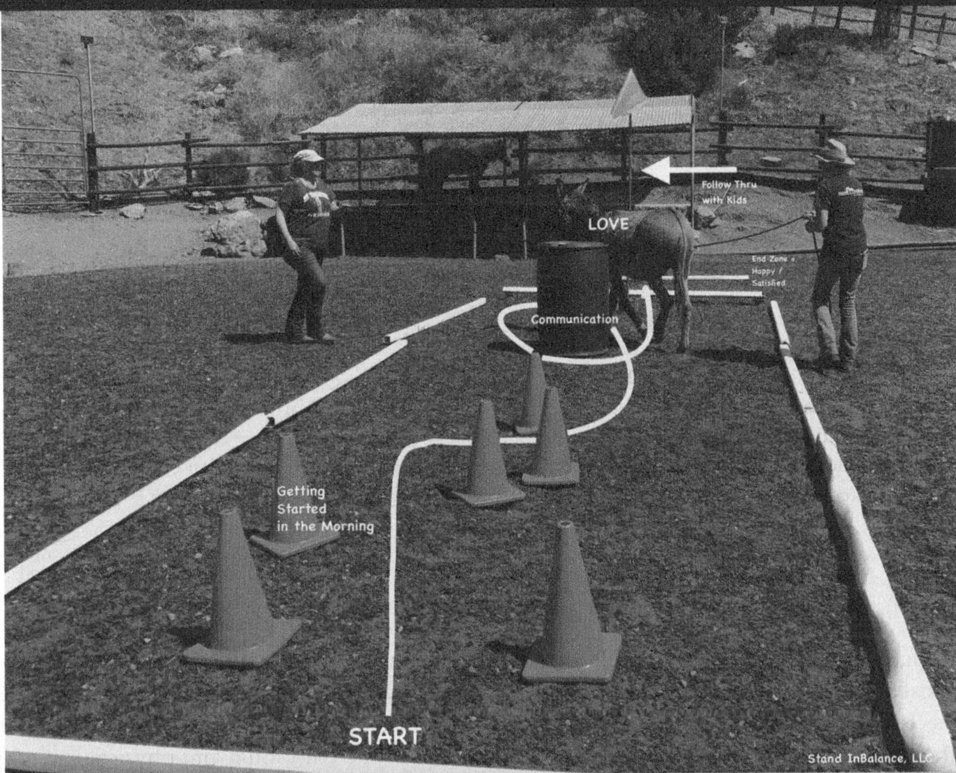

FIG. 23.1. Navigating a Day with PTSD Obstacle Course for Couples.

Directions

1. Ask the couple to go into the arena and choose one equine they would like to work with for the session. Leave the rest of the equines in the arena. Option: Take out the remaining equines.
2. Connect up with your equine so you can walk together. You can have them halter the equine or already have halters on.
3. Take a walk with your equine and identify:
   - a goal the couple wants to work on
   - 3–4 challenges to achieving that goal.
4. Therapist writes the goal on tape and places it in the "end zone" of the course.
5. Write each challenge on duct tape and then ask the partners to place them on 3–4 different obstacles in the obstacle course.
6. Have them name a strength they need to stay connected with to work through their challenges. Write this on a 3 × 5 index card and clip it to the halter, or write it on tape and place on the horse/donkey.
7. Explain the obstacle course and demonstrate how the couple must move their equine through the course and stop in the end zone. Demonstrate how the partners must each stand outside the course while the equine stays inside the rails. Use the labels they have chosen for the goal, strength, and obstacles as you describe the course.
   - You must start here and your "strength" must go through this obstacle—two cones.
   - You then must weave this obstacle—cones.
   - Your "strength" must then make a complete circle around this—barrel.
   - You must get over this "challenge"—pole.
   - You must get over this "challenge"—raised rail.
   - You must end your day calmly in your "goal"—end zone.
8. Determine a consequence in case they get pulled in or the horse goes out; for example, start over or pause, recenter, and continue. Ask them "What do you think should happen if you get pulled into your obstacles or your 'strength' [whatever they have labeled the horse/donkey] goes out?" Option: The therapist determines the consequence.

9. Go and attach the shorter lead line so they each have a lead rope.
10. Ask them to take their horse to the start line.
11. Before they start the course, ask them to state the goal and the challenges.
12. Ask them to go ahead and move their horse through their "day." Option: No talking to each other as they go through.

Discussion

Topics for discussion include:

- What did they notice about how their day went?
- How did they connect with each other and their "strength"?
- How did they communicate with each other?
- How did they handle having different resources? (One long rope and one short rope.)
- How did they handle it when their day got thrown off course—they step in or their equine steps out?
- Were there any other unexpected distractions, challenges that came into their day (other equines, etc.)?
- What did they learn that they can take home and implement to improve their day?

Guidelines

Prior to conducting EAP, clinicians need to be properly trained and certified. In addition to following general ethical guidelines, working with equines requires awareness of safety considerations and animal welfare. The Equine-Assisted Growth & Learning Associations (Eagala, 2015) Code of Ethics is a good reference that provides standards for practitioners that address the emotional and physical safety of clients as well as equines. When following the Eagala model, clinicians conduct sessions alongside an equine specialist. At Stand InBalance (Coleman's Equine Interactive Program in the Santa Monica mountains in California), most sessions include both a clinician and an equine specialist. However, when providing a depth psychology approach with an individual or couple, an advanced clinician with equine expertise may work independently to deepen the treatment process. Whenever providing treatment for special populations, such as different ethnic groups or veterans, clinicians should obtain specialized training and obtain consultation as needed.

CASE EXAMPLE

Jason and Carla (pseudonyms) were referred for equine-assisted couples therapy by Jason's individual therapist. Jason, a 44-year-old Caucasian male, is a retired sergeant who had been deployed three times to Afghanistan. After being wounded in combat, Jason underwent four surgeries and was diagnosed with PTSD and mild traumatic brain injury (mTBI). He and his wife Carla, a 41-year-old Caucasian female, have been married for 19 years and have three children. Since Jason's injury four years ago, Carla takes primary responsibility for the household, the children, and Jason's needs. She also works as a physician's assistant and has become increasingly resentful regarding Jason's lack of follow-through with daily routines and care of the children. He is often unmotivated, irritable, and frequently spends his time watching TV or playing video games. This has been increasingly draining and frustrating for Carla as indicated by her statement, "I know he has problems but this is like having four children instead of three!" Jason reports lack of motivation and difficulty "feeling much of anything." He rarely leaves the house and their social support system is extremely limited due to Jason's anxiety about crowds and interacting with others.

An exploration of marital history and their own individual family of origin history revealed that even before his injury, Jason's multiple deployments and his difficulty expressing his thoughts and feelings had been problematic for them. Jason grew up as the fourth of five children in an alcoholic family where he learned that the best way to protect himself was to "stay in his room and do his own thing" as much as possible. Jason's avoidant attachment style has been further exacerbated by his PTSD. Carla was the eldest of two girls in a family where her father was rarely home due to his work and her mother struggled with depression and anxiety. Carla coped with her own anxiety by managing her mother and her sister. Carla stated that she has always struggled with feeling inadequate and unsure about her own value. As we explored these challenges it became clear that Carla would frequently micro-manage Jason and criticize him in a passive-aggressive attempt to feel heard and valued. Thus, Jason and Carla were stuck in a vicious cycle of emotional disconnect and heated, angry attempts to connect.

Over the past few years, Jason had undergone various forms of treatment with minimal results. At the time of referral, Jason was receiving cognitive processing therapy (CPT) and was making some progress. Carla was skeptical that things would really change and stated that she did not trust him to follow through on daily tasks and commitments. In the initial EAP assessment, they both expressed a desire to rebalance their relationship. Jason reported a lost sense of identity and stated that he would like to be more motivated and independent. They both voiced a desire for improved communication, connection, and a stronger family unit.

The first few sessions focused on gathering family history, the impact of Jason's PTSD on them as a couple, and exploration of their attachment dynamics. In addition, psycho-education regarding PTSD, mTBI, and depression helped create a joint understanding of the ways in which Jason's "invisible" injuries were impacting their relationship.

EAP was used to assess their current dynamics as well as provide an opportunity for them to practice teamwork, affect regulation, communication, and mindfulness skills. Early exercises, such as choosing an equine to walk together, revealed how little Jason communicated his thoughts, feelings, and ideas to his wife, and how difficult it was for Carla to let Jason take the lead. The challenge for their sixth session was "Navigating the Day."

They labeled the aspects of the course as follows:

- Obstacles: Cones = Getting started in the morning
- Barrel = Communication
- Raised Pole = Follow-through with the kids
- Strength you are taking through the course = Love
- End Zone = Happy and satisfied.

The following transcript analysis are about pseudonym clients.

Table 23.1
Transcript Analysis of Case Example at the Beginning of the Intervention

Transcript	*Analysis*
Counselor: Go choose your "love" to go through the course with you.	Staying with the metaphor of their strength, which they designated as love.
Counselor: How did you guys decided on this donkey as "love"?	Asking them to articulate how they made their choice.
Counselor: We thought about going with the big bay horse but decided that since Jason really connected with this one last week we'd use him.	She has made an effort to join with Jason.
Counselor: So Jason, tell me about your connection with "love"	Emphasizing Jason has made a connection as well as keeping the experience of his attachment with "love," which is also analogous to Carla.
Counselor: Well last week he was really cooperative with us and it was great to hang out with him.	It had been empowering and pleasurable for Jason that they were able to come together with the donkey and be effective in walking and grooming him.

(Continued)

Transcript	Analysis
Counselor: Yes, last week there was a lot of love all the way around for the three of you.	Counselor is heightening the loving feelings and shifts in attachment that are developing between the couple.
Counselor: Yeah, that's true—it was really nice last week... which is pretty funny because that's the donkey that was most stubborn before.	She is acknowledging that there has been a shift and that last week's connection has helped her join with Jason in choosing "love" this week.
Counselor: Right... I actually recall you both saying he was a lot like "stubborn Jason" and what a difference it made to look underneath the stubbornness.	Consciously calling attention to how just like the donkey, Jason is often "stubborn," which is actually about avoidance of anxiety. When this is acknowledged and attended to, things can shift and there can be more loving connection.

After connecting with "love" (the donkey), the therapist attached the second, shorter lead rope or the halter (leaving it open for them to choose who had the longer lead rope) and asked them to take "love" to the start of their "day." After stating their challenges and the goal out loud, Carla and Jason began navigating the obstacle course. There were several challenges that showed up as they made their way through: First, "love" jumped out of the course as they were "getting started in the morning" (navigating cones); then after starting over, they had clearer verbal communication about how to navigate "love" (donkey) through the course but when it came to going around the barrel (communication), Carla got pulled into the course—she did not let go of her rope so they could effectively navigate by handing off ropes to each other as needed—and they had to start over again. On the third go-round, Jason let go of his rope and Carla could not keep "love" inside the course. During their fourth attempt, they got all the way around the barrel (communication) and then, with Jason's lead rope trailing on the ground, Carla quickly ran the donkey over the pole (follow-through with kids) and into the end zone (happy/satisfied)—even though Jason said "hey wait." Jason stood by the side for a few moments and then walked over to join her as the donkey succeeded in pulling/dragging them out of the end zone and over to his herd mates at the other end of the arena. At this point we circled up to process how their "day" went.

Table 23.2

Transcript Analysis of Case Example Continued

Transcript	Analysis
Counselor: So how did it go? And what have you guys noticed so far?	Open ended questions so they can share their experience.
Client, Carla: Well, we finally got through!	She is focused on their having "survived" the day versus the actual experience and its ramifications.
Counselor: So you survived the day—what was that like for you?	Asking her/them to deepen their process.
Client Jason: Well, we made it to the end.	Jason is also concretizing the experience and avoiding any emotions or possible conflict with Carla.
Counselor: Yes you did, that was a challenging day! So how did you do that?	Asking them to reflect on the experience and connect up with what worked before looking at the problematic patterns.
Client, Carla: It was hard to get in sync at first. **Client, Jason:** Yeah, once we figured out how to move through the cones it got easier.	They start to consider how they had to come together and communicate with each other to effectively start the day.
Counselor: Yes, there was a lot of navigating with "love" to get going. What worked?	Asking for more specifics.
Client, Carla: We had our game plan and talked it through. It really helped when Jason told me what he was thinking. **Client, Jason:** At first, the donkey didn't know what we were trying to do, but once we got a clear plan of how we were going to weave the cones it got easier.	They identify how important it was for them to create a plan and communicate with each other.

Transcript	*Analysis*
Counselor: What was going on for you guys with the lead ropes? **Client, Jason:** We had to change up the ropes... I wasn't sure we were allowed to do that... Client, Carla: Yeah, we did switch them around [toss them back and forth to each other]. I actually wasn't sure how well that would go, but it worked.	Calling their attention to the challenges around "give and take" regarding control and responsibilities. They are speaking to how hard it has been for Carla to let go of control and for Jason to take responsibility and control. Yet it is that give and take that actually works even though they aren't sure it is OK or that it will be successful.
Counselor: Yeah, so you had doubts, but handing off lead back and forth to each other actually worked! I'm curious—something happened there around "communication" and then once you got to the end of your day "love" really made a beeline to other end of the arena? What happened?	Counselor is reinforcing that sharing responsibility and control for things actually is effective for them even though they tend to doubt it. She then gently confronts how something shifted when Carla took control and didn't wait for Jason.
Client, Carla: Yeah, true. I guess I kind of rushed it at the end—I just wanted to get it done. I figured here is an opportunity—just do it. Geez, just like at home!	Focusing on the donkey helps lower defensiveness and Carla is able to speak to how the end experience mirrored what happens at home.
Counselor: There was pressure to finish up? I wonder how aware you were of "love" and what "love" needed or if that gets lost... feeling as though you have to "manage" everything and get it done? You get through the day, but then there isn't really any hanging out with "love" in "happiness and satisfaction." And, I'm wondering what happened for you Jason?	Counselor brings their attention back to where there was a rupture and asks them to examine the process and how the donkey was mirroring their shift back into old dynamics that undermine loving feelings and secure attachment. Although the counselor saw that Carla took control and did not let Jason reconnect so they could finish together, it is important for them to come to this rather than just being "told" about their dynamics. Counselor is also asking Jason to speak up about not being listened to during the end of the exercise.

As Carla and Jason processed their experience with the donkey, they were able to reflect on and discuss how they worked through difficulties regarding the morning and communication. They were then able to examine how much pressure Carla typically feels at home at the end of the day, which when combined with her difficulty letting Jason take responsibility and Jason's difficulty asserting himself often leads to disconnection, dissatisfaction, and resentment. As they each acknowledged and took responsibility for these dynamics "love" (the donkey) walked over to stand by them and nudged Jason for a head scratch. As Jason put his arms around both Carla and "love," Carla was able to lean into and "lean on" Jason in response.

I encouraged them to notice the positive shifts that were occurring and suggested that we come back to the exercise next week. As often happens after such a key session, Jason and Carla were able to reflect on and utilize improved communication and awareness throughout the week to help them increase their trust and sense of security in each other. While the following session of Navigating a Day with PTSD was not flawless, they were more connected and playful with each other, and they were able to complete the exercise and spend time hanging out with "love" in "happiness and satisfaction."

SUMMARY

As illustrated in case of Jason and Carla, EAP actively engages clients to create greater connection and trust in each other. In order to effectively work through challenges with the equines, clients have to learn to move from detachment and avoidance to engagement and cooperation. The affirmative experiences combined with deeper understanding gained through reflection with the therapist result in changes that strengthen the couples' attachment bond and mitigate the sequel of traumatic experiences. Equine-assisted couples therapy is a potent modality that can help partners learn to stay present in the moment, regulate their affect and communicate more effectively, which leads to a deeper, more satisfying connection with each other.

The following session note example is about pseudonym clients.

Stand InBalance
EMPOWERING YOUR AUTHENTIC SELF

Progress Note

Date: ____________

Client(s) / Organization: [Put clients full name]

Session Length: **50 min** **90 min** (circled) **120 min** **other** ____________

Therapist / Facilitator(s): Val Coleman, Ph.D. [add any co-counselors/ Equine Specialists]

Equine(s) involved in session (list any comments or concerns):

✓ **Condina** **Lucius** **Cosmo** ✓ **Cooper** **Millie** **May** ✓ **Bubba** ✓ **Bella-Rose**

Activities: Navigating the Day – Obstacle Course

Subjective: Both Jason and Carla stated that they'd had an "okay" week. Carla noted it had been a busy week with getting the kids back to school after the holidays.

Observations: Jason and Carla were cooperative and committed to working through the exercise even when it was challenging. They identified goal as: Happy & Satisfied. Challenges as: Getting started in the morning, communication, and follow through with the kids. They chose Love = Bubba as their strength for getting through the course.

Themes: Continued focus on Attachment issues and links to family of origin dynamics. Jason struggled to speak up and express his needs and feelings. Carla had difficulty letting go of control and recognizing Jason's contributions – end of obstacle course: taking over and managing everything at the end of the day at the expense of staying connected with Jason and having his help.

Plan: They will reflect on exercise during the week. Plan to do the course again next week to further re-alignment of roles, decrease disconnect, and reinforce increase in secure attachment bonds.

Signature: Sign full name, title

FIG. 23.2. Session Progress Notes.

Stand InBalance
EMPOWERING YOUR AUTHENTIC SELF

Progress Notes

Date:___________

Client(s) / Organization:____

Session Length: 50 min 90 min 120 min other __________

Therapist / Facilitator(s): ____

Equine(s) involved in session (list any comments or concerns):

❑ Condina ❑ Lucius ❑ Cosmo ❑ Cooper ❑ Millie ❑ May ❑ Bubba ❑ Bella-Rose

____

Activities:____

Subjective:

Observations:

Themes:

Plan:

Signature: ____

FIG. 23.3. Session Progress Notes—Blank.

REFERENCES

Bowlby, J. (1988). *A Secure Base.* New York: Basic Books.

Eagala (2015). *Fundamentals of the Eagala Model.* Santaquin: Equine Assisted Growth and Learning Association.

Fonagy, P. (2001). *Attachment Theory and Psychoanalysis.* New York: Other Press.

Gunter, J. (2007). *Teaching Horse: Rediscovering Leadership.* Bloomington, IN: AuthorHouse.

Johnson, S. M. (2003). A Therapist's guide to primary relationships and their renewal. In S. M. Johnson and V. E. Whiffen (Eds.), *Attachment Processes in Couple and Family Therapy* (pp. 3–17). New York: Guilford Press.

Khaylis, A., Polunsy, M. A., Erbes, C. R. Gewirtz, A. & Rath, M. (2011). Posttraumatic stress, family adjustment, and treatment preferences among National Guard soldiers deployed to OEF/OIF. *Military Medicine, 176*, 126–131. Retrieved from http://militarymedicine.amsus.org/doi/pdf/10.7205/MILMED-D-10-00094.

Mikulincer, M. & Shaver, P. R. (2007). *Attachment in Adulthood: Structure, Dynamics, and Change.* New York: Guilford Press.

National Center for PTSD (2016). *How Common is PTSD?* Retrieved from www.ptsd.va.gov/public/PTSD-overview/basics/how-common-is-ptsd.asp.

Pietrzak, R. H., Goldstein, M. B., Malley, J. C., Rivers, A. J., & Southwick, S. M. (2010). Structure of posttraumatic stress disorder symptoms and psychosocial functioning in Veterans of Operations Enduring Freedom and Iraqi Freedom. *Psychiatry Research, 178*(2), 323–329.

Price, J. L. & Stevens, S. P. (2017). *Partners of Veterans with PTSD: Research Findings.* Retrieved from www.ptsd.va.gov/professional/treatment/family/partners_of_vets_research_findings.asp.

Rheem, K. D., Woolley, S. R., & Weissman, N. (2011). Using emotionally focused couples therapy with military couples. In B. A. Moore (Ed.), *The Handbook of Counseling Military Couples* (pp. 89–112). New York: Routledge.

Rodrigues, C. S. (2014). *Dyadic Examination of Posttraumatic Stress Symptoms, Relationship Satisfaction, and Potential Mediators in Military Couples.* Doctoral dissertation. Retrieved from http://search.proquest.com/openview/e81b93ab0f7baf42f45a5e7ed9e7ef10/1?pq-origsite=gscholar&cbl=18750&diss=y.

Taft, C. T., Monosn, C. M., Schumm, J. A., Watkins, L. E., Panuzio, J. & Resick, P. A. (2009). Posttraumatic stress disorder symptoms, relationship adjustment, and relationship aggression in a sample of female flood victims. *Journal of Family Violence, 24*, 389–396.

Weissman, N., Batten, S., Rheem, D., Wiebe, S., Pasillas, R., Potts, W., Barone, M., Brown, C. & Dixon, L. (2017). The effectiveness of emotionally focused couples therapy with veterans with PTSD: A pilot study. *Journal of Couple & Relationship Therapy.* Retrieved from http://dx.doi.org/10.1080/15332691.2017.1285261.

24

The Four Agreements in Equine-Assisted Therapy for Relationships

Corey L. DeMala-Moran

INTRODUCTION

The Four Agreements (Ruiz, 1997) is a small book with a big impact. This is true not only for individuals, but for couples and families, as well. Written by Don Miguel Ruiz, this book utilizes four agreements that can not only change lives, but also change relationships. And in a day and age where, according to the American Psychological Association (2017), 40–50% of marriages end in divorce, we could certainly use some help.

I share *The Four Agreements* with all of my clients, and have found it extremely helpful when introduced to couples in conjunction with equine therapy. As you will see, not only are these "agreements" key for building and maintaining healthy, happy relationships, but also they fit ideally with our work with horses. Together, *The Four Agreements* and equine therapy can help heal broken relationships and build a solid foundation for new ones.

THE FOUR AGREEMENTS

1. **Be impeccable with your word:** Speak with integrity. Say only what you mean. Avoid using the word to speak against yourself or to gossip about others. Use the power of your word in the direction of truth and love.
2. **Don't take anything personally:** Nothing others do is because of you. What others say and do is a projection of their own reality, their own dream. When you are immune to the opinions and actions of others, you won't be the victim of needless suffering.
3. **Don't make assumptions:** Find the courage to ask questions and to express what you really want. Communicate with others as clearly as you can to avoid misunderstandings, sadness, and drama. With just this one agreement, you can completely transform your life.
4. **Always do your best:** Your best is going to change from moment to moment, it will be different when you are healthy as opposed to sick. Under any circumstance, simply do your best, and you will avoid self-judgment, self-abuse, and regret.

As you can see, these are simple and yet incredibly challenging rules to live by. Yet, if you did follow them, even in small ways, life and relationships would change for the better.

In this work, I use *The Four Agreements* themselves, as well as the rest of the book as the foundation. I also include mindfulness practices, as well as internal family systems (IFS) (Schwartz, 2008) that can help to identify and work through any blocks or resistance that may come up.

In my experience, adding horses to this work truly takes it to the next level. Horses, by nature, are masters of living by *The Four Agreements*. Horses are impeccable with their words. They are honest and non-judgmental which allows us a powerful template from which to learn and grow. As prey animals, horses are extremely in tune to the congruence of those beings around them. A predator does not express its intent on the outside (at least if it wants to eat). A successful predator is the wolf in sheep's clothing, not the wolf dressed as the wolf. Therefore, the horse's survival depends on its ability to pick up on this. And they pick it up in us as well. I often hear clients say, "I can't be anxious, angry, nervous, etc., around horses." Not so. Clients just have to be able to recognize how their feeling and then let the horse know. If you don't know how you are feeling, don't worry. The horse will tell you if you are ready to listen. When clients can learn to do this, relationships of all kinds start to improve. In building relationships with horses, clients begin to understand how what they say, as well as how they say it, matters, not only towards others, but also towards themselves. As they learn to be impeccable with their words, internally and externally, the horses will respond differently. The quality of their work with the horses will improve, illuminating the powerful effects of the first of *The Four Agreements*.

Horses are also wonderful teachers in regards to not taking things personally. They respond to the present moment and then go "back to grazing." There is no value in taking things personally for horses. Their survival depends on getting back to grazing as quickly as possible. There is no value for us in this either, other than increased levels physical, emotional and psychological suffering.

When we can learn not to take things personally in our relationships, we can actually listen and hear what the other is expressing and needing, as well as hearing and speaking for our own needs and feelings. When we are stuck taking things personally, we are often sunk before we even try and communicate. A great example of this is standing with a client and a horse in the summer time. While grooming the horse, the client notices the horse stomping her feet. When I ask the client what he thinks about that, he says, "Well, this horse doesn't like me. Just like my wife. Always mad at me about something." When we remind the client about the second of *The Four Agreements*, and he doesn't make the stomping about him, he is open to explore what is really going on. It's summer in New York and flies are plentiful. "Oh, I get it. The flies are the problem." Now we can find a solution. When we take things personally, we get stuck in the shame spiral and connection is lost.

Much like the second of *The Four Agreements*, the third helps us to stay open and find the courage to communicate openly and honestly. Our brains are wired to make assumptions. We fill in the gaps with whatever we have experienced in the past. This is wonderful for survival, but thriving, not so much. Not only is the third Agreement about becoming aware of the stories we tell ourselves, it also is about communication. As with the other Agreements, self-awareness is key. We must develop the courage to seek clarity of our own feelings and needs, and of the needs and feelings of others. So often I see couples that have relationships built on false assumptions from their pasts. Not only do they have no idea what their partner needs, they don't know what they need either. In working with horses, clarity and communication are key to success. If you don't know what you want the horse to do and how to communicate it to them, good luck. And if you are stuck in your assumptions, it is hard to even get started.

Fourth of the *The Four Agreements*, always do your best, is really the key to the whole process. In exploring this agreement with couples and families, I often see a huge increase in compassion, connection, and courage. In working with the horses, clients are able to try something new, explore what their best is in that moment, and find compassion for themselves. When they are able to watch their partners and family members do the same, compassion grows for each other as well.

As always, safety is the number one priority. It is important to know your horses and your clients and find experiences that fit for both. Another thing to always keep in mind is "trauma" and "dissociation." I encourage clients to have an understanding of both. Working with couples where one or both partners have suffered trauma can make things more difficult and caution must be taken. This work is incredibly healing for trauma; we just have to go slow and let the clients be our guide.

The goal of using *The Four Agreements* with couples and families is to help clients gain more self-awareness, increase self-regulation, and build connection and compassion for themselves and each other. I look to improve communication and listening skills as well as the ability to read their partner's non-verbal body language and recognize what he or she needs in moments of both crisis and calm.

The materials needed for this work can be as simple as a horse and a space. You can weave *The Four Agreements* into whatever methodology you use. The most important thing is to educate your clients about *The Four Agreements* and get them thinking about it in their lives and relationships. I find it helpful to go over this one at a time and then discuss how they all work together.

I have used this work in many different ways from weekly individual and couples sessions, monthly group work, and in the form of both day and weekend retreats. I have even done several daylong couples intensives. If I am beginning with a new couple, either in weekly sessions or in a retreat/workshop format, I will start by going over *The Four Agreements* and having a discussion about how they are currently living or not living by them. I then talk about how doing so would change their relationship and work with them to get them to agree to work on living by them both in session and at home. I also talk about any areas they have fears or concerns about working together around these Agreements. If at all possible, I talk about these areas out with the horses, either outside a paddock, arena, or the barn. This allows for the horses to be a part of the process, because the horses will always contribute to the processing. Having an equine specialist present at this time is helpful, as he or she can watch the horses and look for anything that might be helpful to direct the clients' attention to during this initial process.

Next, I will have the clients watch the herd, or meet the horse, if you only have one. Ideally, a herd is best as it allows the clients to watch how horses interact and do relationship. Then I will have each partner choose a horse they want to work with. Once they have each chosen their horse, I will allow them to get to know the horse by grooming or just simply being with the horse either in the stall or an arena/round pen. I will do this one at a time first, allowing them to get to know their horse and then together, allowing them time to get to know each other's horse. I will remind them of *The Four Agreements* and we will discuss the experience in reference to them. This could take one session or several depending on the clients. The key is to construct your sessions around building the relationship between clients and their horses, and then using what transpires there to bring clarity, compassion, and connection to the relationship between the clients and the individuals with whom they are looking to strengthen a relationship. The specific activities can be whatever you want, so long as it is safe and helping the clients learn to move toward a healthy relationship. The important thing here is to continuously apply *The Four Agreements*, allowing clients to become more aware of how they are or are not working in their relationships and how things could change if they did.

In relation to multicultural issues, just be sure to have a clear understanding of the culture of the couple, both past and present. This will help you to formulate activities and interventions that are respectful and productive.

CASE EXAMPLE

The clients for this case example are Joe and Stacy (pseudonyms). Joe is a 35-year-old, Caucasian, male electrician and Stacy is a 34-year-old, Caucasian, female high school teacher. They have been married for five years and together for seven years. The couple came to treatment because of constant fighting and lack of communication. Stacy stated she is "at her wits' end" with Joe and Joe reported he is tired of taking the brunt of her anger. Both Stacy and Joe have had some horse experience trail riding and Stacy rode periodically as a child.

The following is a part of their fourth session. In the first three sessions, I got a history from both, went over *The Four Agreements*, discussed safety, they then observed the herd and, lastly, chose a horse for each to work with. In the last session, each person spent time grooming their own horse, first separately and then together. Joe worked through the "fly" issue, gaining insight into how he takes things personally, both in relation to his horse stomping her feet, as well as in relation to his wife. This session, a 90-minute couple session, each client will be asked to move their horse around the round pen, a few times in each direction at whatever speed feels comfortable to them. There is a lunge whip in the center of the pen if needed and I discuss the use of this tool at the beginning of the session.

The following transcript analysis are about a pseudonym clients.

Table 24.1

Transcript Analysis of Case Example

Transcript	*Analysis*
Counselor: I would like you to take the Applause [horse] into the round pen and move him around in each direction a few times. You can do this at whatever speed is comfortable for you and Applause.	At this time, I will also check in to see that the client is inside their window of tolerance and if not, we will do some breathing or other grounding exercises to lower arousal level.
Counselor: How are you feeling about this?	Checking in to see if client is present and inside their window of tolerance. If needed, you can also check in with the client's body as well as your own.
Client, Stacy: I am OK. Let's see if I can get this horse to do what I want. I certainly can't get him to.	Client is already struggling with the first, second, and third Agreements.
Counselor: Remember the agreements and try to focus your intention, Applause and the relationship you have with him. *The client is now facing the horse with the lunge whip pointing at the horse. Applause is relaxed but won't move.*	Keeping the Four Agreements at the center and helping client to be able to focus on her intention and the relationship.
Counselor: How is it going?	I can see the client is stuck and after about ten minutes of this interaction, I check in.
Client, Stacy: Not well. He doesn't listen either. No one respects me, not even this stupid horse.	Not only is the client taking it personally, they are making assumptions and not being impeccable with their word. Imagine how using *The Four Agreements* could change this whole scenario.
Counselor: What is your intention? What do you want from Applause right now?	Clarity is key and I want the client to recognize how their body language.
Client, Stacy: *Starting to cry.* I just want him to come to me, no matter how I am feeling.	This is great insight and exactly what the client wants from their spouse.
Counselor: What is your body language saying, you want?	This helps the client to recognize their non-verbal "words" and the power they carry.
Client, Stacy: Oh, my gosh, I didn't even realize I am actually pushing him away. I do that with you my spouse, don't I?	Client is recognizing what a pattern.
Client, Joe: Yes, it's not that I don't love and respect you. I'm trying to come towards you, but it's like you have that whip pointed at me at the same time.	Having the partners watch each other with the horses is so powerful and can help each individual find compassion for the other, and for his or herself.
Counselor: How could *The Four Agreements* help here?	Bringing it back to *The Four Agreements* helps to keep us on track.
Client, Stacy: I could put the whip down, both here and with my words towards my spouse. I know they are awfully harsh sometimes. And I could be clear with what I want rather than getting caught in the assumptions I make up in my head. I also need to realize I am doing my best, and so is he. I'm sorry.	Although sometimes it takes many sessions for this kind of insight, the horses help us to realize our patterns much faster. They always know what needs to happen. Trust the process.
Client, Joe: I love you. I know I have to do my best, especially around not taking things so personally. You have a lot going on with work and your dad and just need me to be here for you.	Including the partner in the discussion is an important part of the process and allows for positive experiences in communication and conflict resolution.
Counselor: What do you guys notice about Applause?	Always bring it back to the horses.
Client, Stacy: I put the whip down and he is right here with me. And my spouse is too.	Applause literally put his nose right on her heart. They know the way!

REFLECTION

The clients came into the session in their usual space of conflict. Stacy was angry and frustrated and Joe was resigned and distant. As Stacy worked with a horse named Applause in the round pen, it became clear to her that she was sending mixed messages to both the horse and her husband. Stacy began by trying to chase Applause around the pen, and when that didn't work, she picked up the lunge whip "tool" and pointed it at him. He turned to her and she stood there facing him and him facing her. When I asked her what she wanted, she said that she "just wants him to come to her no matter what." We then discussed her body language and she was able to realize that she was both wanting him to come to her and pushing him away at the same time. This brought about an insightful discussion around this same pattern in their relationship. We concluded by talking about how living *The Four Agreements* could help them to break free from this pattern and find more compassion and connection for themselves and each other.

Next session, we will revisit this session and then Joe will take time in the round pen with his horse.

REFERENCES

American Psychological Association (2017). *Marriage and Divorce*. Retrieved from www.apa.org/topics/divorce.

Ruiz, D. M. (1997). *The Four Agreements*. San Rafael, CA: Amber-Allen Publishing, Inc.

Schwartz, R. C. (2008). You Are the One You've Been Waiting For: Bringing Courageous Love to Intimate Relationships. Oak Park, IL: Trailhead.

25

Equine-Assisted Psychotherapy with Couples and Families

A Relational Approach

Shelley Green, Michael Rolleston, and Monica Schroeder

INTRODUCTION

Expanding on the extensive use of equine-assisted psychotherapy (EAP) with at-risk adolescents (Burgon, 2011; Ewing, MacDonald, Taylor, & Bowers, 2007), clients struggling with addictions (Dell, Chalmers, Dell, Sauve, & MacKinnon, 2008) eating disorders (Sharpe, 2014) and trauma (Adams, Coady, & Yorke, 2008; Coleman, 2012; DePrekel, 2012), equine models have increasingly been utilized with couples, families, and groups to improve relationships, highlight strengths, normalize concerns, and enhance the overall therapeutic process (Green, 2013, 2014, 2017; Masini, 2010; Trotter, 2012). This chapter describes a relational, strength-based approach to EAP when working specifically with couples and families. As Lipchik (2002, p. 127) observes, "The importance of relational ties is a powerful resource for therapy." Incorporating a strength-based, relational stance that honors client solutions offers unique opportunities for the enhancement of couple and family relationships through EAP.

DESCRIPTION OF THE PROBLEM

Couples and families experiencing high conflict or crisis present challenging dynamics that can at times exhaust the resources of even the most resilient therapist. Traditional talk therapy may not always be the most effective or powerful tool, and may even exacerbate troubling patterns of interaction and communication. EAP, with its experiential focus, can be used as a means of disrupting repetitive patterns of interaction and offering clients an opportunity to notice and experience these interactions in a different context. Through their interactions with the horses, clients can attempt new behaviors in the moment, and effective processing of client interactions with the horses can allow translation of these new behaviors into their everyday lives.

RATIONALE FOR EQUINE-ASSISTED PSYCHOTHERAPY

EAP sessions offer the opportunity to assess and gather information about clients' patterns of interaction while simultaneously strengthening relationships. Integrating horses into clinical work with couples and families allows clients to experience the development of stronger relationship connections, greater trust, and enhanced ways of communicating (Hayes, 2015). Hayes highlights EAP's fit with relational work when he notes:

> The success, contentment, and well-being of every human are all directly tied to the quality of their relationships with themselves and others. To have successful relationships, humans, just like horses, must learn and have modeled for them qualities that will create and establish mutual love, trust, and respect.
>
> (Hayes, 2015, p. 93)

Equine-assisted interventions can highlight themes such as love, support, connection, trust, and respect. When clients find ways to partner with a horse during a session, they create a relationship with the horse, and may learn about their own capacity for relationship-building, connection, and trust. This relationship can mirror many of the qualities that characterize a familial or couple relationship, making their time with the horse relevant to the clients' lives outside of the session.

THEORETICAL APPROACH

Therapeutic approaches to working with couples and families that are informed by a relational focus view the couple or family exclusively in terms of their relationships to one another, allowing the therapist to pay attention to the patterns of human interaction, rather than to specific deficits or inadequacies of the individuals (Green, 2011). This focus allows the therapist to attend to mutual, reciprocal interactions in relationships occurring in a recursive process (Fisch, Weakland, & Segal, 1982), minimizing attention to blame and individual notions of deficiency, and allowing clients' unique solutions to become apparent. From a solution-focused approach to therapy, it is believed that a small change in the behavior of an individual can have far-reaching effects on the behaviors of others involved (de Shazer, 1985). By honoring clients' solutions, EAP with couples and families focuses on exploring exceptions to the problem, highlighting strengths in the relationships, and building on what is already working.

RELATIONAL ETHICS

EAP requires careful attention to ethical concerns, relevant with our clients and also in our relationships with the horses, who are our partners in this endeavor. A relational ethics perspective (Pollard, 2015) prioritizes respect, engagement, embodied knowledge, and responsibility for the other. Within this framework, all actions must consider our interconnectedness and, thus, the impact of our actions on each other. The clinical work described here is informed by this relational understanding of ethical decision-making.[1] As Pollard (2015, p. 366) observes, "Engagement requires an understanding of the complexity of each situation, each person's perspective, and each person's vulnerabilities." This framework informs all of our decision-making and interactions with clients, with horses, and with each other.

CASE EXAMPLE—COUPLE

Our work with couples is informed by the brief, systemic, relational principles described above. We offer a non-pathologizing, strength-based approach that highlights our clients' unique resources while acknowledging their struggles. In the case example that follows, we illustrate a single-session intervention that we conducted as a component of an intensive couples therapy program; the ongoing intensive work was conducted by our colleagues at Couples on the Brink (couplesonthebrink.com). As the session began, we learned that Meredith and Greg (pseudonyms),[2] both in their late 30s, had been married for ten years and shared a passionate, creative, synergistic relationship inspired by their common ground as artists. When they met, each had been committed to never marrying, but they fell in love deeply and quickly, and married each other three weeks later. They described many years of intimacy, connection, and passion, but were both devastated by the recent conflicts that seemed to threaten the stability and future of their relationship. As they said, "How could we be so in love and so miserable?"

We discussed content very briefly, and then began the equine session, inviting the couple to simply meet and greet the two horses they would be working with, noting what they observed about each. Almost immediately, the couple were entranced by the horses, in tune with their behavior and responses, and eager to connect, although Meredith was a bit more reserved. At one point, early in the session, the mare that they had chosen to call Do-Little became very interested in Greg, attempting rather forcefully to engage him by rubbing her head up and down his side and crotch. Meredith observed carefully, and when asked what she was noticing, commented that Do-Little was "trying to get Greg's attention the way I do—by demanding it—and he hates that." The other horse, Sanchez, she noted, was standing close by, quietly concentrating her gaze on Greg. Meredith commented that this is the style Greg would prefer, and would be open to receiving.

As the couple became increasingly comfortable and engaged with the horses, we asked them to find a way to catch a horse and take it for a walk; we provided no direction regarding how they were to do so, what tools they should use, whether they should work together or independently. As the session progressed, we observed Greg and Meredith's very different styles of engaging with the horses (Meredith animated, directive, and frustrated, and Greg patient, quiet, and careful). They worked independently, although Meredith frequently asked for Greg to come and help her, which he chose not to do. When asked about this, Meredith described similar interactions in their relationship, in which she repeatedly requests Greg's help and he refuses. Greg did not disagree, and stated that he often felt afraid that if he were to give in to her requests, he would be overwhelmed by her needs and not be able to remain productive as an artist. He also noted that Meredith frequently asked him for help with practical issues, but rarely for "matters of the heart," which would be much more important for him.

At this point in a typical two-hour session, we might have asked the couple to construct an obstacle course or a safe space to help us further make sense of their struggles and their responses. However, Greg and Meredith's interactions with the horses had been so intuitive, and their observations so metaphoric and thoughtful, that we chose instead to use the following intervention, described and analyzed below.

The following transcript analysis are about a pseudonym clients.

Table 25.1

Transcript Analysis of Case Example—Couple

Transcript	*Analysis*
Therapist: Greg and Meredith, what we would like for you to do now is take the halters off the horses, and to and array the horses, and yourselves, in a way that represents how you would like for your relationship to look right now.	Our team's rationale and intent: This request was intentionally vague. We made no suggestions as to whether they should work together, discuss a plan first, or simply proceed. Consistent with our focus on client strengths, we wanted to respect this couple as artists—creative, synergistic individuals who had a history of collaborating to develop beautiful works of art. We also wanted to find a way to engage their passion for each other, for freedom, and for connection.
Greg and Meredith did not respond verbally to our request, nor did they speak to each other at all. Instead, within 15–20 seconds, they had arranged the two horses nose-to-tail, with themselves in the middle, arms outstretched, fingertips lightly touching the sides of each horse. Initially, they were in a "spooning" position (see photo below), with Meredith's back to Greg. However, she quickly turned to face him, and they gazed silently into each other's eyes, tears streaming down their cheeks. The horses stood quietly in the position the couple had created with them.	Our team's observations: We watched this interaction with awe, as this couple had struggled for over half the session to decide how to catch a horse and take it for a walk, utilizing halters, lead ropes, balls, and hula hoops. The horses had been very clear in their disinterest and reluctance to cooperate. However, within an incredibly brief amount of time, Greg and Meredith managed to silently convey their wishes and create the synergy they needed to orchestrate this beautiful tableau. The horses responded quietly and immediately, and stood in the desired position until the couple broke their intense gaze and embraced, crying. At that point, the horses moved out of the position but remained close by, with their noses within our circle as we processed what had just occurred.

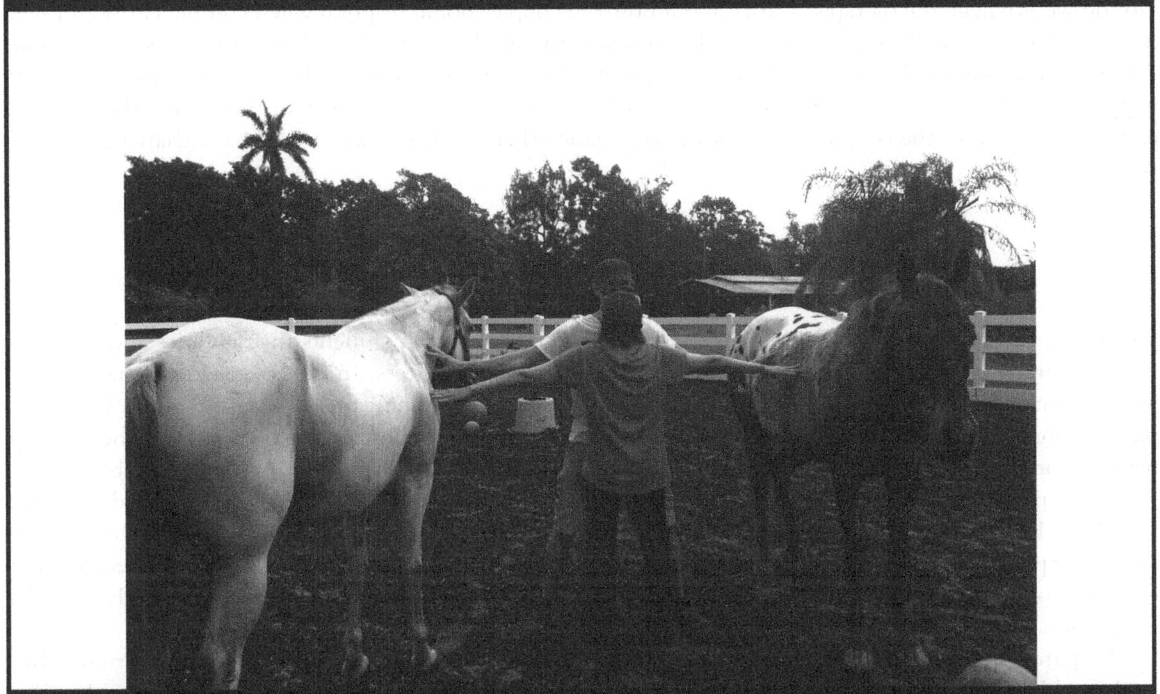

FIG. 25.1.

Table 25.2
Transcript Analysis of Case Example—Couple Continued

Transcript	*Analysis*
Therapist: We are just wondering if you can tell us what is happening for you both right now?	**Our team's rationale and intent:** We did not exclaim over what happened nor attribute any meaning or value judgment; instead we left the palette clean for the couple to bring to life in the way that was meaningful for them, thus honoring their solutions and their understandings of the encounter.
Greg: In just this moment with the horses, we connected in a way that filled me up, instead of draining me. I have thought in the last few months that if I let Meredith in, her constant demands would deplete me and I wouldn't be able to do my work. But just now, I felt filled up, instead of needing to fill her up. I didn't think that could happen in a such a brief, powerful moment. **Meredith:** I felt so connected to you, and so fulfilled, and so strong. And the horses stayed by our sides the whole time. They were in this with us.	**Our team's observations:** We too were surprised that this couple could have created such a powerful and connected experience that could transform how they thought about need, desire, demands, and connection. We were also deeply moved personally, and wanted to acknowledge the power of the moment while maintaining our focus on what had just occurred rather than on our own responses.
Therapist: If you could give a name to what you two have created here with the horses, what would it be? **Meredith:** I would call it our "cradle," as I felt cradled by these horses and by our connection. I hope that we can return to our cradle when we need to in the future. I hope we will always have it.	**Our team's response:** The therapist had taken a picture of the couple in their "cradle" with the horses, as it had seemed so powerful and intense. The therapist showed them the picture during this conversation and they asked for it, so she texted it to them as a reminder of their ability to connect even when struggling.
Therapist: How do you believe you will each find ways to return to this beautiful place you have created together, when you experience difficulties in the future? **Meredith:** We are going to frame this picture and display it in our home, as a reminder of how we learned to embrace our "heart connection." Of all of our life and therapy experiences, this time with the horses has been the most powerful. We will never forget it.	**Our team's rationale:** Consistent with our model, we wanted to simply honor this couple's unique solution to their conflict and distress, and to invite them to consider how this brief but powerful moment could enhance their responses in the future, when they felt challenged and disconnected.

We don't see any session or event, regardless of how powerful or compelling, as a "fix" to the problem. Nor do we privilege the therapist's story about how the couple should respond when conflicts arise. Rather, we see that couples will always have struggles to deal with, but that they can find ways to access their unique strengths and connections so that those struggles don't overpower them. We believe the experiences that happen with the horses are "embodied" ones, and that the image and memory of these embodied experiences can remain in the couples' repertoire and enhance their resilience when they have challenges in the future.

CASE EXAMPLE—FAMILY

We engage the families we work with in a strength-based manner that highlights their abilities and taps into their resources, placing the family at the center of the therapeutic process. In the case example that follows, we will discuss an intervention that was utilized during a five-session family intensive case at Stable Place (stableplace.org). Prior to the first session, we learned that Zachary (a pseudonym), 16 years old, had been living with his former foster parents, Betty and Robert (pseudonyms), for the past two years. This move back to his foster parents was prompted by unfit living conditions at his adoptive parent's home. They described the move as difficult but necessary for Zachary, who expressed his at-home struggles during a weekend visit with his former foster parents. At our first interaction, they described themselves as a loving family who cares deeply about their relationships with one another, and are hopeful to move forward with officially adopting Zachary in the near future.

The parents, Betty and Robert, arrived at the first session with Zachary eager to get started. They explained how their hope was to use these sessions as an opportunity to bring their family together in a way that focused on improving their trust, communication, and relationships. As their first equine session began, we invited the family to meet and greet the two horses they would be working with, paying close attention to what they observed about each horse. With both horses, Zachary was the first to approach and pet each. Betty was close behind, while Robert stood at a distance until the rest of the family invited him to come closer. Once the family was comfortable with the horses and acclimated to the barn, we invited them to choose one horse to work with in today's session. We asked the family to halter this horse as a team without communicating with one another verbally. After the halter was comfortably adjusted on the horse by the family, we asked the clients how they were able to get the halter on without talking to each other. Betty mentioned they needed to trust in the process a bit more than they usually would, and Zachary explained how he was noticing the family communicating with their eyes in order to let each other know what they needed. Since these interactions seemed to be exceptions to what usually happens with the family, we were curious how today they were able to so quickly and confidently try something they were not accustomed to when it involved trusting the process and communicating with each other in a different way that works.

We used this opportunity as a comfortable segue into our ensuing activity that highlights themes of trust and communication. In this single-session activity, called Lines of Communication, we invited the family to affix two lead ropes onto the halter they already adjusted on their horse of choice. Once the lead ropes were connected to the halter, we asked the family to lead the horse with both lead ropes wherever they would like without verbally communicating with one another. Outside of asking the clients to take the horse for a walk while refraining from verbal communication, we provided no indication of how they were to complete the activity, where they could lead the horse, and whether they should work individually or as a family. How this intervention transpired is described and analyzed below.

The following transcript analysis are about a pseudonym clients.

Table 25.3

Transcript Analysis of Case Example—Family

Transcript	*Analysis*
Therapist: Now that the horse is ready to go, we would like for you all to figure out a way to walk with the horse using both lead ropes and no verbal communication.	**Our team's rationale and intent:** This request was intentionally vague. We made no suggestions as to how they should work together, where they should lead the horse, or if they should explore other means of communication. Consistent with being client-centered, we wanted the family to work through these uncertainties together in a way that fits for them. We also wanted to find a way to engage the family by highlighting their communication skills and methods of working together (i.e., who takes the lead, who tries to communicate differently, who, if any, disregard the guidelines, etc.).
Betty and Zachary were the first to attempt the activity. Zachary took one lead rope and immediately started walking forward while Betty stayed beside the horse with the other lead rope. After a few steps forward, the horse planted its hooves and remained stationed in one spot. After a bit of tugging from Zachary while Betty stood quietly beside the horse, he eventually turned around and signaled something with his head and eyes. This signal seemed to mean, "let's go," as the three of them began moving as one. Once they began moving, the three of them walked as a group with Zachary leading the way until they decided they had gone far enough.	**Our team's observations:** We noticed Zachary and Betty were quick to go first while Robert observed. As each of them grabbed a lead rope, it seemed as though Zachary was ready to create movement immediately. However, it did not take long for Zachary to shift his immediacy and turn around toward Betty and the horse to communicate something. Once this moment of connecting back with one another occurred, the horse and Betty's demeanor seemed to shift in a way that indicated they were ready to walk. This quick shift in their approach and communication was something we noted and were interested in asking about.
Therapist: We are wondering how you guys created movement and how you decided where to go once you got that movement?	**Our team's rationale and intent:** We did not explain what occurred from our perspective nor attribute any meaning to what happened; instead, we encouraged the family to explain what happened from their perspective and explore their own meaning they attributed to their approach and style in this activity.
Betty: It seemed like once Zachary turned around and checked in with me and the horse, we were able to begin moving. It felt like we all got on the same page in this moment. Once we got on the same page, there was literally and figuratively no looking back. **Zachary:** When we weren't moving I decided to turn around and communicate with my eyes to Betty and the horse. I wanted them to start walking forward with me but knew I couldn't say anything. I think we just went with it once we started moving and didn't worry about where we were going. I just wanted us to keep moving forward. **Robert:** I noticed Zachary being very quick to get started and get moving. I think once he slowed down and checked in with who was behind him, they all were able to get ready to move together.	**Our team's observations:** We also noticed how movement seemed to occur as soon as all three members of the group, Zachary, Betty, and the horse, were able to get connected in some way, and, in turn, become comfortable with moving ahead together. It appeared all the connection that was needed transpired from a shift in Zachary's approach where he slowed down, turned back to the others in his group, communicated to them in a different way how he was ready to proceed, and began walking as soon as he noticed the other two were ready to go together.
Therapist: Zachary, would you like to attempt this again, and this time with Robert? **Zachary:** Sure. Should we use the same horse and hold the same ropes? **Therapist:** I'll leave that up to you two.	**Our team's rationale and intent:** Michael offered Zachary and Robert an opportunity to work through this activity together. We purposefully left the specifics up to the clients as a way for them to problem-solve and manage through these decisions in a way that challenges them to work together. As a new group attempts the activity together, we pay close attention to any similarities or differences in the approach or completion of the activity that may be worth inquiring about.

(Continued)

Transcript	*Analysis*
Zachary and Robert were able to create movement quite quickly. Again, Zachary appeared to take the lead as Robert and the horse followed closely behind. They walked along the outside fence of a large paddock until they made it all the way to the other side before stopping.	**Our team's observations:** In our work, we pay close attention to any similarities or differences within, or across, activities that might be worthwhile to point out. In this case, we noticed how Zachary quickly decided to take the lead on each occasion without first checking in with the others. We wondered how this might relate to the way the family communicates, or attempts to communicate, outside of the barn and how this works for them.
Therapist: Zachary, I noticed you took the lead and began moving forward without checking in with anyone again. Does this relate at all to how you work with your family in your everyday life? **Zachary:** Yes, I tend to just go for it and see what happens. **Robert:** Yes, Zachary does tend to take the lead and run with it at home without checking in with us. We are hopeful that he will check in with us more often prior to forging ahead without much plan or perspective on how we feel about it. We are always here looking out for his best interest, but I'm not sure Zachary always notices that or thinks we are there to help him. Instead, it seems like he thinks we are trying to hold him back from what he wants.	**Our team's rationale and intent:** At different points in a session, we do our best to help the client make sense of what is going on for them in the moment and how this might relate back to their everyday life outside of the barn. Our hope is these connections might help a client make better sense of their situation and/or give them the opportunity to explore different ways of approaching what hasn't been working for them.
Therapist: Now, I'd like to invite all three of you to work together this time to create movement.	**Our team's rationale and intent:** We hoped this invitation would allow the clients an opportunity to work together as a family. We also were interested in the dynamic that might transpire with three participants and only two lead ropes.
Zachary, Betty, and Robert placed themselves in a way that had Zachary on one side of the horse and Betty and Robert on the other side. Zachary was holding one lead role while Betty and Robert were both holding the other lead rope. It appeared as if they all took a moment to look at each other, check that they were ready to go, and proceeded with Zachary taking the first step. The family walked two full times around the paddock before stopping with Zachary a step ahead at all times, Betty close to the horse without much slack, and Robert at the end of the rope Betty was holding.	**Our team's observations:** It appeared as if the family intentionally was letting Zachary take the lead in this activity. We wondered what sort of meaning this had for the family and what their hope was by letting Zachary make the first move and stay one step ahead throughout.
Therapist: We noticed you all were able to create movement with some ease. How were you able to figure out who was doing what and where you were going? **Betty:** Well, I think Robert and I let Zachary take the lead in this activity, as we have been trying to do more of this at home recently as he gets older. We hope Zachary can continue to show us that we can trust when he takes the lead, and he won't just move ahead without checking in with us or considering how we feel about it. **Robert:** We waited for the indication from Zachary that he was ready to go, and followed close behind him. Betty and I decided to go on the same side of the horse and hold the same rope in order to let Zachary have full control over the other rope. For us this represents us giving Zachary more freedom and control as he gets older, yet staying close beside to encourage him heading in the right direction or getting him back on track when he is headed in the wrong direction.	**Our team's rationale and intent:** We hoped by inquiring about the way they worked together and how they decided to do so, we could approach their collaboration in a more indirect way that does not place our judgment or value on the process they used.

Transcript	*Analysis*
Therapist: How did you know what direction to head when you were all together? **Betty:** I'm not sure we knew exactly where we were going but we did stay along the outside fence in order to use it as a guideline to keep us on track. Getting us on the right track can be difficult at times, but it is even more difficult for us to stay on track once we get something that's working.	**Our team's rationale and intent:** We hoped to end our first session with the family in a way that left them thinking about the direction they were heading when they were all together. For us, this is synonymous with moving ahead together into the future and how they would like to do so. We hoped this would set a strong foundation for the sessions, themes, and conversations to come.

At the conclusion of the activity we invited the family to reflect on what they noticed in their communication and their work with one another that indicates individual and familial strengths they would like to carry with them into the future. We also asked the clients to think about what this outside fence, or track, might represent for the family when it comes to guiding their communication, trust, and work together. We encouraged the family to take note of any moments prior to our next session where they notice their strengths, and what might be different in these situations that allow them to communicate and work together in a way that fits for them. We invited the family to four more sessions, which we utilized as an opportunity to highlight strengths and weave themes together surrounding communication, trust, and coming together as a family.

The following session note example is about pseudonym clients.

STABLE PLACE, INC.
Initial Session Case Note

Client Name/Client #: Betty Smith/2017-000 (Family)	
Date, Time, and Duration: 07/01/2017 9:00 am 1.5 Hours	**Session Participants:** Michael (Therapist), Valerie (Equine Specialist), Betty, Robert, and Zachary (clients)
Problem Definition: Betty described a unique family situation that has put her and Robert, Zachary's former foster parents from when he was an infant, as the guardians for him now as a teenager. She mentioned he has been back with them for the past two years and they have been struggling with trust, honesty, and bonding as a family. Betty mentioned currently Zachary strongly opposes being adopted by them, as he expressed interest in being with a younger family, but they are hopeful his perspective will shift as they begin to improve as a unit.	
Desired Solutions: Betty discussed initiating therapy for her family with the hopes of improving their trust and communication while strengthening their familial relationships. She mentioned a desire to focus on bonding as a family and being honest with each other about what they are hopeful for when it comes to getting more settled as a family. They also hoped to use these sessions as a means of bonding and exploring what each person needs from the others.	
Equine Activities: For our first session, we started with a simple meet and greet with two of the horses we would be working with throughout the week. After the clients became comfortable with the horses, we proceeded into our first structured activity called Lines of Communication.This activity has a theme revolving around communication and working together where two lead ropes are affixed to one haltered horse with the objective of taking the horse for a walk together without using verbal communication. Our hope was to elicit some therapeutic conversation pertaining to the family's communication style, as well as highlight what they do well when it comes to working together and negotiating where they would go and how they would get there.	
Therapist Notes/Observations: The therapist noticed a number of occasions during the session where the family was able to communicate their needs to one another in ways that allowed everyone to get on the same page. When the family seemed to be on the same page, they appeared to work well together. They established roles, created movement, and identified their path by communicating in new ways and trusting in each other's process during the activity.	
Date of next session: 07/02/17	
Amount Paid: N/A	**Balance Due:** N/A
Therapist Signature and Date:	Michael Rolleston, MS Oct 12, 2017
Supervisor Signature and Date:	Shelley Green, PhD, LMFT Oct 12, 2017

FIG. 25.2. Session Case Example Notes.

[Your Logo/Organization Here]

Initial Session Case Note

Client Name/Client #:	
Date, Time, and Duration:	**Session Participants:**
Problem Definition:	
Desired Solutions:	
Equine Activities:	
Therapist Notes/Observations:	
Date of next session:	
Amount Paid:	**Balance Due:**
Therapist Signature and Date:	
Supervisor Signature and Date:	

FIG. 25.3. Session Case Notes—Blank.

NOTES

1 Pseudonyms are used in both case examples to protect client confidentiality. For an in-depth theoretical discussion of this specific case, see Green (2014).

2 Ibid.

REFERENCES

Adams, C., Coady, N., & Yorke, J. (2008). Therapeutic value of equine-human bonding in recovery from trauma. *Anthrozoos, 21*(1), 17–30.

Burgon, H.L. (2011) "Queen of the world": Experiences of "at-risk" young people participating in equine-assisted learning/therapy. *Journal of Social Work Practice: Psychotherapeutic Approaches in Health, Welfare and the Community, 25*(2), 165–183.

Coleman, V. (2012). Reclaiming boundaries through equine assisted counseling. In K. S. Trotter (Ed.), *Harnessing the Power of Equine Assisted Counseling: Adding Animal Assisted Therapy to Your Practice* (pp. 27–40). New York: Routledge.

Dell, C. A., Chalmers, D., Dell, D., Sauve, E., & MacKinnon, T. (2008). Horse as healer: An examination of equine assisted learning in the healing of First Nations youth from solvent abuse. *Pimatisiwin: A Journal of Aboriginal and Indigenous Community Health, 6*(1) 81–106.

DePrekel, M. (2012). Equine facilitated psychotherapy for the treatment of trauma. In K. S. Trotter (Ed.), *Harnessing the Power of Equine Assisted Counseling: Adding Animal Assisted Therapy to Your Practice* (pp. 59–71). New York: Routledge.

de Shazer, S. (1985). *Keys to Solution and Brief Therapy.* New York: Norton.

Ewing, C., MacDonald, P., Taylor, M., & Bowers, M. (2007). Equine-facilitated learning for youths with severe emotional disorders: A quantitative and qualitative study. *Child and Youth Care Forum, 36*(1), 59–72.

Fisch, R., Weakland, J. H., & Segal, L. (1982). *The Tactics of Change: Doing Therapy Briefly.* San Francisco: Jossey-Bass.

Green, S. (2011). Power or pattern? A brief, relational approach. *Family Therapy Magazine, 10*(6), 9–11.

Green, S. (2013). Horses and families. In A. Rambo, C. West, A. Schooley, & T. V. Boyd (Eds.), *Family Therapy Review: Contrasting Contemporary Models* (pp. 256–258). New York: Routledge

Green, S. (2014). Horse sense: Equine assisted single session consultations. In M. Hoyt and M. Talmon (Eds.) *Capture the Moment: Single Session Therapy and Walk-In Service.* Williston, VT: Crown House Publishing.

Green, S. (2017). Equine assisted psychotherapy. In J. Carlson & S. Dermer (Eds.), *The Sage Encyclopedia of Marriage, Family, and Couples Counseling.* Thousand Oaks, CA: Sage.

Hayes, T. (2015). *Riding Home: The Power of Horses to Heal.* New York: St. Martin's Press.

Lipchik, E. (2002). *Beyond Technique in Solution-Focused Therapy.* New York: Guilford Press.

Masini, A. (2010). Equine-assisted psychotherapy in clinical practice. *Journal of Psychosocial Nursing and Mental Health Services, 48*(10), 30–34.

Pollard, C. (2015). What is the right thing to do? Use of relational ethic framework to guide clinical decision-making. *International Journal of Caring Sciences, 8*(2), 362–368.

Sharpe, H. (2014). Equine-facilitated counselling and women with eating disorders: Articulating bodily experience. *Canadian Journal of Counselling and Psychotherapy, 48*(2), 127–152.

Trotter, K. S. (2012). Harnessing the Power of Equine Assisted Counseling: Adding Animal Assisted Therapy to Your Practice. New York: Routledge.

Section 13

PROFESSIONAL DEVELOPMENT

26

Partnering with Horses to Train Mental Health Professionals

Shelley Green[1]

INTRODUCTION: STATEMENT OF THE PROBLEM

Students enrolled in university-based mental health training programs typically spend 2–3 years immersed in didactic coursework focused on developing their understanding of a range of clinical theories and models, building competence in applying techniques specific to those models, and insuring that they understand the legal and ethical codes that guide the profession. While clearly this is the foundation for training informed, thoughtful, and ethical practitioners, a missing link in many training programs is attention to the self-of-the-therapist. A therapist's awareness of self—socially, emotionally, interpersonally—and of what he or she brings to each therapeutic encounter is critical to the process of sound ethical practice. As Timm and Blow (1999) observe, each of us is informed, often outside our own awareness, by significant events and life experiences that have contributed to our development as individuals. These experiences may inform our responses—in more and less positive ways—when our clients describe similar moments in their lives. Timm and Blow (1999) advocate for doing self-of-the-therapist work that explores both the restraints and resources that arise out of a therapist's life experiences. Additionally, Simon (2006) has proposed that family therapy training, specifically, be guided by a four-stage process that begins with an exploration of the trainees' personal worldview and ends with the therapists' developing nuanced skill in a model that most closely aligns with their personal understanding of the human condition. Within the first stage, trainees would be asked to explore their own life decisions, with the goal of understanding the worldview that informed those decisions and life structures (including political, social, spiritual, and personal beliefs).

Given that clinical training programs are typically rigorous and based on highly structured curricula developed to cover as many models, theories, and practices as possible, self-of-the-therapist work has at times become marginalized and is non-existent in many training programs. Discussing where (or whether) to include this work, including relevant literature and assignments designed to promote self-refection and awareness, does not always lead to consensus among faculty and administrators. Additionally, developing the means to invite students into such reflective discussion can be challenging when students themselves may be more focused on gaining clinical competence and remembering details of models to pass comprehensive and licensure exams.

THEORETICAL FOUNDATIONS OF OUR EQUINE-ASSISTED TRAINING APPROACH

An innovative response to this training dilemma has been developed in the Family Therapy program at Nova Southeastern University (NSU), by incorporating an equine-assisted training model into the self-of-the-therapist explorations of the students. All family therapy coursework at NSU is informed by a brief, systemic, relational approach to therapy (Cade & O'Hanlon, 1993; Flemons, 2002; Flemons & Green, 2007, in press; Green, 2012, 2014; Watzlawick, Weakland & Fisch, 1974) that privileges the clients' worldview and honors their solutions (deShazer, 1985). Therapy models are informed by a strength-based, non-pathologizing stance that seeks to make sense of all behaviors in context, rather than to diagnose or pinpoint dysfunction. Students in the NSU programs have the opportunity to take two electives in Equine-Assisted Family Therapy. In these courses, students learn about both the fundamentals of equine-assisted therapies and the components of their own personal experiences that may inform their relationships with clients. Informed by our commitment to a non-normative, non-pathologizing approach, we invite the students to explore connections between their interactions with the horses and the ways they have experienced, and responded to, similar situations in their personal and professional lives. As past struggles and challenges become relevant, our focus is on the resources students have acquired through meeting those challenges, and on how they may experience something new with the horses that has relevance for responding to challenges in the therapy room.

The courses are taught through our NSU Family Therapy collaboration with Stable Place, a local non-profit equine-assisted therapy program. Stable Place provides the setting, horses, and PATH Intl. certified equine specialists and is an integral component of the course delivery. All staff (therapists and equine specialists) at Stable Place are trained directly through the NSU courses, and the method for facilitating and processing activities is consistently informed by the relational, strength-based model described above.

The first course (Introduction to Equine-Assisted Family Therapy) addresses the world of animal and equine-assisted therapies, and includes attention to therapeutic riding, hippotherapy, and equine-assisted learning models. Students become acquainted with the literature in the field, including research on the effectiveness of equine-assisted models, and they are introduced to various national organizations that train and certify equine professionals, such as Eagala and PATH Intl. The course is taught in a hybrid approach, with half of the class sessions taking place at the Stable Place facility, offering students hands-on experience with the horses and allowing them to learn first-hand about equine assisted sessions. A central component of this introductory course involves exploring how the students' experiences with and reactions to the horses mirror their responses in the clinical setting. Activities are intentionally designed and processed in a way that metaphorically attends to the students' understanding of their strengths and growth areas as therapists, whether in terms of building trust and rapport, establishing connections, promoting change, or dealing with fear and anxiety in the room. The horses provide a rich and potentially transformative partnership for exploring and understanding how to bring their "best selves" into the room with clients. As one student observed:

> Since the horses are attuned and connected to each participant in equine-assisted therapy (EAT), they also pick up on what therapists bring into session. This course really highlighted that, by allowing training therapists to be participants, and by allowing them to experience the powerful sessions for themselves. The activities allowed for each clinician to be self-reflective, mindful, and intentional each time they worked with the horses during class. Each course activity made a way for the clinicians to explore their therapeutic orientation, their style of working and their personal values in an experiential way.

The advanced course—also a hybrid, with alternate weeks taking place at the barn—invites students further into a process of self-reflection regarding the particular strengths, areas of growth, values, beliefs, and worldviews that accompany them each time they enter the therapy room. The course is grounded in a mindfulness approach, and students are encouraged each week (in the classroom and at the barn) to attend to engaging in the experience in a mindful, fully present manner. This contributes to building a context of self-reflection, awareness, and introspection, which then translates well to our work with the horses. Course readings encompass the triad of equine-assisted therapy approaches, mindfulness and meditation, and self-of-the therapist literature. These readings guide class discussions and inform equine-based activities as well. Barn days are structured specifically to maximize students' awareness of their ways of approaching clients, building trust, developing rapport, dealing with fear and anxiety, and embracing challenge and change.

Activities are often simple (e.g., finding the horse's heartbeat and listening to gut sounds, hoof cleaning, taking the horse for a walk) and always require a significant level of self-awareness. For example, in one activity, students are blindfolded (if they are comfortable—or willing to be uncomfortable), and asked to simply touch and connect with one of the horses for several moments. Then as they are able, they are asked to find a way to partner with the horse that allows them to move the horse and to move along with it in a direction that is mutually desired. An equine specialist maintains connection with the lead rope and manages the proximity and pacing of the horse at all times, but the student is in charge of direction and movement. Students often report experiencing a trance-like phenomenon, in which they become aware only of themselves and the horse, moving in sync. Processing of this activity is powerful, focusing on the student's self-awareness, as well as his or her ability to connect and join with the horse, to manage the anxiety of the unknown, and to understand what creates change and movement. The relevance to therapeutic encounters is clear, and metaphors abound in our conversations. As one student described her response to this activity:

> During our very first day at the barn [Advanced Class], I had a trance-like connection with the horse I was working with. I was blindfolded and completely attuned to the way the horse moved, and the direction the horse took me on, trusting my equine specialist with my life. That experience taught me about the joining that occurs with clients in a way that does not necessarily require spoken language, but a humanness that begs for collaboration.

Weekly journal assignments and online postings offer students the opportunity to process their reactions to barn day experiences; these descriptions often become the basis for extended conversations in the classroom. Following is a student's journal description of her response to hearing the horse's heartbeat:

> The heartbeat exercise was so profoundly beautiful for me. I decided to use a firm but soft approach with my left hand on Paris [one of our horses], while joining with her. I had the intention of sending her loving kindness. I mapped my hand path in short firm strokes before making my way down to her chest area. She allowed me to find her heartbeat with ease. After listening to the soft and slow "ba-beat" a few times, I realized that my eyes were closed and I was smiling from ear-to-ear. It felt like such a gift that she was trusting me enough to hear this very private part of her body. Later, I realized that clients are trusting us to listen to their very private stories and this is also a gift, as well as a responsibility.

DESCRIPTION OF TECHNIQUE—MOVING THE HIPS

The activity I have chosen to address in more depth here involves an equine training exercise that our Stable Place team learned in a clinic led by horse trainer Richie Wingfield (www.richiewingfield.com). This exercise, although originally developed to assist riders with gaining trust and leadership with their horses on the ground, also has strong resonance for our students in terms of exploring how they have previously responded to fear, anxiety, and challenge. Students have the opportunity to try something new and to experience a transformative moment in terms of their relationship with that fear or anxiety through participation in this simple exercise.

This activity typically takes place late in the semester, after students have had many opportunities to interact with the horses and develop greater confidence and comfort with them. Students are asked to first consider a fear or challenge they have faced or are facing in their development as a therapist and/or as a person. They then write this challenge/fear on a small index card and we tape it to the hindquarters of the horse of their choosing. The student then holds the lead rope and walks toward the horse's hindquarters, utilizing their intentionality, energy, and focus to ask the horse to step under with the inside hind foot, thus disengaging the hindquarters. The equine specialist is, as always, in close proximity, monitoring the horse's movements and response to the student therapist's efforts to produce the desired movement.

Fundamentally, our equine-assisted training of students is not based on developing their horsemanship skills, and it is also not a venue in which the facilitators become therapists to the students. Both of these ethical and professional considerations are discussed at length with the students at the beginning of the term. This activity, as well, is not intended to help the students learn ground work or become adept at showing leadership to the horse. Rather, it is designed and intended to allow the students to alter their relationship with fear or anxiety (Flemons, 2002; Flemons & Green, 2007, in press) through an experiential moment that requires them to *move toward*, rather than away from, their fear. The horse's hindquarters, as the engine (and kicking end) of the horse, represent metaphorically the power and source of the fear, and by entering into a relationship with that fear rather than seeking to avoid it, students have a completely non-verbal, often emotional, and consistently powerful experience.

CASE EXAMPLE

Elena is a 53-year-old Family Therapy doctoral student with a rich professional background that preceded her interest in becoming a therapist. She is a confident, outgoing person and therapist, but she also struggles with the lasting effects of an injury from an accident that occurred two years prior. Her fears around pain and re-injury at times prevent her from fully participating in experiences that matter to her. Throughout the semester, she had been cautious and aware of avoiding any equine-assisted activities that might have been risky for her physically, and she had experienced some frustration at those limitations (as she had in her personal and professional life). Following is an excerpt from her session with Casper, another of our horses, along with my brief descriptions and explanations.

Table 26.1

Transcript Analysis of Case Example

Transcript	*Analysis*
Therapist: You are welcome to share the fear you have identified with your classmates, or you may certainly keep it private if you choose.	As this is a class, rather than a therapy group, it is critical to attend to privacy and self-disclosure choices, and to ensure that the facilitator does not act as a therapist to the student.
Student: OK, I'm just going to think about it myself as I go through this activity with Casper.	Student seemed to be experiencing some anxiety and chose to keep the content of her fear private at the beginning. This was honored.
Therapist: So I'll help you tape the fear onto the horse's hindquarters. *Does so.* And now I'm going to ask you to focus completely on that card as you walk towards the horse's back end and ask him to move his hips over. Does that make sense?"	The facilitator explains the activity briefly, with little extraneous detail, and with an emphasis on the focus (the card representing the fear).
After an initial struggle with inertia and the horse simply followed client in a circle, the client observes as our equine specialist does a brief (silent) demonstration that allows the client to consider what she needs to change in terms of her intentionality. She then begins to dance with the horse as he gracefully moves and circles. **Therapist:** Beautiful; watch that fear, notice how it's changing.	As mentioned previously, our goal is not to teach horsemanship skills. However, an equine specialist may offer to demonstrate a skill that simply seems impossible until viewed. No verbal instructions are given, and there is no emphasis on doing it the "right way." Students are asked simply to observe what works and to find their own path. Consistently, those paths vary widely. In this instance, following the demonstration, the client was able to find her own method of creating a beautiful dance with the horse.
Student: *Continues to dance with the horse, down a hill, in perfect rhythm; she is visibly crying, and yet seems simultaneously joyous.* I'm doing it! I'm letting it go! I'm letting it go!	There is very little verbal discussion during the student's experience; we prefer to allow each student to "have their moment," and any processing that is desired can come later, in the form of simple observations, connections to strengths, relevance to clinical work, and positive transformation.

REFLECTIONS

The student later described this session in her journal, continuing to process and make sense of her experience with Casper the horse in relation to her life experiences and what she brings to each session as a therapist. Following is an excerpt:

> Today I focused on my injury as I placed my obstacle card on his hip. At first, I was channeling my intention but I did not realize that it was up to me to *initiate* the movement. How freaking obvious! I can't believe I was just "willing" Casper to move with me, as if he could read my mind, without the follow through of my body. It was a profound experience for me in that I truly felt myself letting go for the first time with any of the horses. I know my injury was previously blocking me in a tentative stance with them, despite the fact that I love them all and want to be close with them. I have just been holding back for fear of re-injury. Since my obstacle was my injury, some part of me was able to just release the "hold back" and truly let go. I felt tears just gushing out of me and true joy filling my body as we spun around and around. I felt like I was in a flow state, or trance. I remember realizing that we were starting to go down a hill, but we both just kept going. It was the strangest most beautiful thing. We both seemed to trust the other one that everything would be okay.

The icing on the cake was when Casper stomped on my injury card as it flung off his hip. How appropriate! It was as if we both knew exactly what to do, once I made my mind up and invited him to join me, through my intention and my follow through. As I reflect back on my dance with Casper, I realize how visceral and immediate the impacts of equine work can be. I struggled with my injury for two years and, in one session with Casper, I was able to recognize the unintentional role I was playing in remaining stuck in my fear. Casper helped me see that and, in the process, he expanded my insight as a human being, and my vision as a therapist. In this sense, the experience was truly transformative and, ultimately, healing.

The type of learning that this student experienced is the norm, rather than the exception, in the equine classes. We strive to offer each student many opportunities to engage with the horses in ways that allow for personal and professional transformations. The horses offer something that is simply not available or possible in classroom-based, didactic contexts. The student's final words reflect our strong belief in the power of this partnership with horses to create change and to enhance the training of our therapy students:

> The learnings are visceral, as opposed to intellectual. For someone like me, who is always "in my head," this is a great way to engage my whole body/mind/spirit in the learning process. It is hard to forget this kind of learning.

NOTE

1 With special thanks to the staff of Stable Place Equine Assisted Therapies in Fort Lauderdale for their ongoing collaboration and enthusiasm for this work; to Richie Wingfield for his wonderful, warm spirit and exceptional horse training skills; and to the students of the NSU Equine Assisted Family Therapy courses for their unflagging passion and commitment to this way of learning.

REFERENCES

Cade, B. & O'Hanlon, W. (1993). *A Brief Guide to Brief Therapy*. New York: W. W. Norton.

deShazer, S. (1985). *Keys to Solution in Brief Therapy*. New York: W. W. Norton.

Flemons, D. (2002). Of One Mind: The Logic of Hypnosis, the Practice of Therapy. New York: W. W. Norton.

Flemons, D. & Green, S. (2007). Just between us: A relational approach to sex therapy. In S. Green & D. Flemons (Eds.), *Quickies: The Handbook of Brief Sex Therapy* (revised edition, pp. 126–170). New York: W. W. Norton.

Flemons, D. & Green, S. (in press). Therapeutic quickies: Brief relational therapy for sexual issues. In S. Green & D. Flemons (Eds.), *Quickies: The Handbook of Brief Sex Therapy* (3rd edition). New York: W. W. Norton.

Green, S. (2012). Horses and families: Bringing equine assisted approaches to family therapy. In A. Rambo, T. Boyd, A. Schooley & C. West (Eds.). *Family Therapy Review: Contrasting Contemporary Models*. New York: Taylor & Francis.

Green, S. (2014). Horse sense: Equine assisted single session consultations. In M. Hoyt & M. Talmon (Eds.), *Capture the Moment: Single Session Therapy and Walk-In Service*. Williston, VT: Crown House Publishing.

Simon, G. M. (2006). The heart of the matter: A proposal for placing the self of the therapist at the center of family therapy research in training. *Family Process, 45*(3), 331–344.

Timm, T. M. & Blow, A. J. (1999). Self-of-the-therapist work: A balance between removing restraints and identifying resources. *Contemporary Family Therapy, 21*(3), 331–351.

Watzlawick, P., Weakland, J. & Fisch, R. (1974). *Change: Principles of Problem Formation and Problem Resolution*. New York: Norton.

INDEX

For Product Safety Concerns and Information please contact our EU representative GPSR@taylorandfrancis.com Taylor & Francis Verlag GmbH, Kaufingerstraße 24, 80331 München, Germany

Batch number: 10733532

Printed by Printforce, the Netherlands